The U.S. Health System
Origins and Functions
Sixth Edition

Camille K. Barsukiewicz, PhD

School of Urban Affairs and Public Policy

University of Memphis

Memphis, Tennessee

Marshall W. Raffel, PhD

Professor Emeritus of Health Policy and Administration

The Pennsylvania State University

University Park, Pennsylvania

Norma K. Raffel, PhD

Health Service Research

State College, Pennsylvania

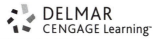

DELMAR
CENGAGE Learning™

Australia • Brazil • Japan • Korea • Mexico • Singapore • Spain • United Kingdom • United States

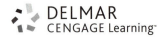

The U.S. Health System: Origins and Functions, Sixth Edition
Camille K. Barsukiewicz, Marshall W. Raffel, Norma K. Raffel

Vice President, Career and Professional
    Editorial: Dave Garza

Director of Learning
    Solutions: Matthew Kane

Managing Editor: Marah Bellegarde

Senior Acquisitions Editor: Tari Broderick

Product Manager: Natalie Pashoukos

Editorial Assistant: Ian Lewis

Vice President, Career and
    Professional Marketing: Jennifer Baker

Marketing Director: Wendy Mapstone

Marketing Manager: Michelle McTighe

Marketing Coordinator: Scott Chrysler

Production Director: Carolyn Miller

Production Manager: Andrew Crouth

Senior Content Project
    Manager: James Zayicek

Senior Art Director: Jack Pendleton

For product information and technology assistance, contact us at
Professional & Career Group Customer Support, 1-800-648-7450

For permission to use material from this text or product, submit all requests online at cengage.com/permissions. Further permissions questions can be e-mailed to **permissionrequest@cengage.com**

Library of Congress Control Number: 2009927154

ISBN-13: 978-1-4180-5298-0

ISBN-10: 1-4180-5298-1

Delmar
5 Maxwell Drive
Clifton Park, NY 12065-2919
USA

Cengage Learning products are represented in Canada by Nelson Education, Ltd.

For your lifelong learning solutions, visit **delmar.cengage.com**

Visit our corporate website at **cengage.com**

Notice to the Reader

Publisher does not warrant or guarantee any of the products described herein or perform any independent analysis in connection with any of the product information contained herein. Publisher does not assume, and expressly disclaims, any obligation to obtain and include information other than that provided to it by the manufacturer. The reader is expressly warned to consider and adopt all safety precautions that might be indicated by the activities described herein and to avoid all potential hazards. By following the instructions contained herein, the reader willingly assumes all risks in connection with such instructions. The publisher makes no representations or warranties of any kind, including but not limited to, the warranties of fitness for particular purpose or merchantability, nor are any such representations implied with respect to the material set forth herein, and the publisher takes no responsibility with respect to such material. The publisher shall not be liable for any special, consequential, or exemplary damages resulting, in whole or part, from the readers' use of, or reliance upon, this material.

Printed in United States of America
1 2 3 4 5 XXX 13 12 11 10 09

CONTENTS

PART THREE
The Changing Health Care Environment / 213

PREFACE

Whether you are considering a career in health administration, direct patient care, health policy and planning, or health care finance, an understanding of the varied and interconnected aspects of the U.S. healthcare delivery system is essential. Understanding is complicated by the rapid rate of change occurring in our healthcare system. Managed care, market forces, regulation, and technology development contribute to the rapid change.

Since the failure of comprehensive health care reform efforts of the mid-1990s, changes brought about by market forces, greater emphasis on data collection for outcomes measurement, increased cost constraints, integrated organizations, and incremental approaches to regulation have made understanding the healthcare system imperative not only in our professional lives, but in our role as health care consumers. Where once we were provided with a health insurance plan by our employer, we are now asked to choose among plans with varied benefits and varied costs to us. We may even be faced with the fact that our employer will no longer provide health insurance as one of our employment benefits. Where once we relied on our physicians' advice, we are now asked to evaluate, compare, and monitor alternatives to care.

Previous editions of this text have been rich in a historical approach to understanding health care delivery and applying that historical knowledge to current trends. The primary purpose for the sixth edition remains as a text for introductory courses in health care delivery systems. It retains some of its historical approach, while bringing broader attention to health care delivery and the unique challenges it faces in the United States today.

ORGANIZATION

The text has been divided into three major sections, each important to the delivery of health care services. Part I focuses on the external health care environment. Chapter I provides an introduction to the dynamic health care system in the United States. Chapter 2 discusses the cost of health care, trends in spending, some reasons for increasing costs, and attempts at containing costs.

Chapter 3 provides a background for how we pay for health care, including both historical and current trends in private health insurance and government programs. It discusses Medicare, Medicaid, managed care, and the phenomenon of the uninsured population in a system largely defined as an employment-based insurance system. Chapter 4 is a new chapter that discusses health status and health care utilization. Chapter 5 is an overview of physician training, licensing, and credentialing.

Part 2 focuses on the internal health care environment—the organizations and persons who deliver health care. Chapter 6 introduces other personnel that are key to the delivery of medical services, including personnel in areas that might be referred to as "alternative medicine."

The emphasis in Chapter 7 changes somewhat to health care organizations, beginning with ambulatory care, or outpatient services. Chapter 8 discusses acute inpatient care, primarily hospital care, and the dramatic market changes facing this segment of health care delivery.

Chapter 9 discusses mental health services and systems. Chapter 10 addresses the many facets of long-term care and the challenges brought about by an aging population. Chapter 11 is a new chapter that provides an overview of the public health system and its transition from public health to community health.

Part 3 addresses changes in the health care environment. Chapter 12 discusses the importance of information management systems and the application of technology, especially the electronic medical record, to improve the quality of care.

Chapter 13 brings the text to a conclusion with a look toward innovative approaches that organizations can take to address issues of quality of care and outcomes of measurement, a look at what remains to be done, and the challenges we continue to face.

NEW TO THIS EDITION

Brand new chapters on the topics of public health, technology development and information management systems, and health status and health care utilization have been added to the sixth edition. Exhibits in every chapter stimulate discussion on the various chapter topics. Activity-based Learning Questions and Question of Ethics sections have been updated for this edition. Updated references with related Web resources provide additional research opportunities as well.

INSTRUCTOR RESOURCES

Additionally, an online companion including the instructor's manual, PowerPoint presentations, and test banks, was created to accompany this text. The instructor's manual provides a sample course syllabus, suggested answers to the Exhibit discussion questions, talking points for the end-of-chapter ethics questions, as well as suggested individual and group activities and assignments.

ACKNOWLEDGEMENTS

While we have made an effort to include a comprehensive view of U.S. health care delivery, there is much room for further study. The text is not meant to be a study of health care policy; therefore, the "why" of many changes faced in health care delivery may require further inquiry. The health of the nation is not totally a result of medicine and health care delivery. Economics, culture, education, values, and many other factors determine the health of a nation. We hope that this overview stimulates further interest in the study of health care delivery in our nation and across the globe.

I would like to especially acknowledge Marshall and Norma Raffel and Delmar Cengage Learning for giving me the opportunity to write the sixth edition of this book. Additionally I would like to thank Alice Johnson for her assistance on many aspects of this project.

REVIEWERS

James R. Ciesla, PhD

Professor, Public Health and Health Education Programs
Northern Illinois University
Dekalb, IL

Cheryl G. Davis, D.H.A., CLS (NCA)

Associate Dean for Administration and Resource
    Development
Tuskegee University
Tuskegee, AL

Heather Dean

Health Services Administration Course Developer and
    Coordinator
Keiser University
Ft. Lauderdale, FL

Stephen DeRosa, MA

Adjunct Faculty
Merrimack College
North Andover, MA
    and
Chief Information Officer
Gateway Healthcare, Inc.
Pawtucket, RI

Robert M. Dyer, PhD

Assistant Professor, School of Government
Regent University
Virginia Beach, VA

Maria Kronenburg, MBA, PhD

Adjunct Instructor
Troy University
Norfolk, VA

George B. Moseley III, MBA, JD

Lecturer in Health Law and Management
Harvard School of Public Health
Boston, MA

Susan M. Radius, PhD, CHES

Professor and Program Director
Coordinator, Undergraduate Internship in Community
    Health Education
Towson University
Baltimore, MD

Marilyn V. Whitman, PhD

Internship Coordinator and Adjunct Instructor
University of Alabama
Tuscaloosa, AL

Chapter 1

Introduction

Health care in the United States is dynamic, constantly changing in its delivery mode, treatment methods, applications of technology, and payment mechanisms. In the early 1900s, physicians treated patients in the home, and patients paid physicians directly for their services. As discoveries in anesthesia and germ control emerged, physicians changed the location of care to hospitals. Previously, hospitals were considered the places where patients went to die. With advances in medical treatment, hospitals became the preferred choices for care. These hospitals also became the focus of physician training.

HEALTH CARE PROVIDERS

The simple days of referring to health care systems as physicians and hospitals soon changed. A *health care provider* is now the accepted term to include not only physicians and hospitals but also home health care agencies, nursing homes, dentists, rehabilitation organizations and therapists, chiropractors, and more.

Reduced payments forced health care providers to seek new patients and new sources of revenue while also increasing efficiency, resulting in a competitive market. The competitive market brought about what is referred to as system integration. System integration moved in two major directions. Horizontal integration, in its most basic form, is an attempt to deliver similar services to a broader area, as in hospital mergers. Vertical integration, on the other hand, is an attempt to combine providers of a wider range of services, as in a health care organization delivering physician services, hospital services, home care, and nursing home care under one business entity. These integrated entities have come to be known as "health systems," and we now look at individual hospitals, physicians, nursing homes, and so on, to see if they are part of a larger "system."

HEALTH CARE PAYERS

As medical care advanced, the costs of care increased. Prepaid care (insurance) emerged in the 1930s and throughout World War II until employment-based health insurance became the norm in the United States. However, employment-based health insurance did not protect all who needed health services. In 1965, after years of debate about universal health coverage, public payment systems (Medicare and Medicaid) brought health care within reach of many more Americans (the elderly and the very poor). The side effects of those public programs were greater utilization of services, the emergence of new hospitals, growth of existing hospitals, and increased costs. Many attempts were made to reform the payments systems to control costs. In the 1980s, Medicare hospital payment system was reformed from retrospective payment to prospective payment. The fixed payment system forced hospitals to run more efficiently.

Even though health care costs continue to rise, the focus of health care delivery continues to be on cure and on "sick care" rather than on prevention and wellness. At about the same time period as the major changes to Medicare payment systems, managed care began to grow and included prevention incentives.

The concept of managed care—case management for comprehensive care in the most efficient and effective way—is a sensible approach. Each person, whether healthy or sick, works with a primary care physician who establishes a long-term relationship with the patient. The primary care physician helps patients determine the appropriate provider of care and the appropriate setting for care when needed, and helps people prevent illness through lifestyle changes. Unfortunately, managed care has become controversial as a health care delivery system, often seen as cost containment through treatment denial. However, managed care has been successful in moving the trends toward wellness, instrumental in the move toward integrated systems of care, and has resulted in many new innovative approaches to health insurance. The purest form of managed care, the health maintenance organization, currently has only 20 percent of the insurance market, although modified managed care forms have grown dramatically.

Employer-based health benefits plans are another approach to providing health care coverage. Rather than purchase health insurance for their employees, employers may set aside their own funds to pay for employee health care expenses. Employees submit charges to their employer, and the charges are paid from the set-aside funds. This type of plan is more complicated than it sounds here, but a more specific description is provided later in the text. Other innovative systems are also discussed.

PATIENTS

The term *health care consumer* often replaces the term *patient* in modern discussions of health care. "Consumers" are expected to make more informed decisions when choosing health insurance coverage, choosing providers of care, and making lifestyle changes. Under this scenario, informed consumer decisions are expected to translate into lower health care costs through a more competitive health care market. Providers of care, whether hospitals, physicians, clinics, or others, will disclose their outcomes of care to compete for consumers and insurance contracts. Consumers will use this information to choose providers of care when they become patients (consumers of care).

CHANGE AS A CONSTANT

In today's health care environment, change is happening at all levels. Change will continue to occur as new technology is developed, costs continue to be a concern, and organizations of all types struggle to adapt to their environment.

Health care delivery changes occur through health policy, organizational approaches, and consumers' commitment to healthier lifestyles. Although the term *health care system* is not quite the oxymoron that it was in the twentieth century, it remains short of true system behavior.

True systems thinking involves looking at health care delivery with a broader, more encompassing view. It requires consideration of how each sector influences the operation of other sectors. It involves viewing the patient as a whole patient rather than as body parts that are treated by each specialty of medical care. More than that, it involves looking at health care as a part of societal needs taking into account education, income, occupation, lifestyle, living conditions, and so on. Providing medical interventions is only a small part of every person's journey to health.

It remains to be seen if prevention can take precedence over the belief that every disease can be cured, and whether integrated systems of health care delivery can provide more comprehensive and consistent care to all Americans. Although managed care has helped bring some attention to prevention and healthy lifestyles, it has not been the answer to eliminating health disparities among different segments of the population. New and broader approaches may be needed.

POPULATION HEALTH

Not all health care is comprised of individuals seeking care from individual health care organizations. The public health sector provides a large portion of health care. The focus of public health is on the health of the community rather than the health of individuals. The public health sector's responsibility is largely based on issues not under the control of individuals, such as water quality, air quality, immunization of the population, and so on.

Although communicable disease was once the major challenge of public health, current priorities are based on chronic care issues. Healthy People 2010, launched by Health and Human Services Secretary Donna Shalala and Surgeon General David Satcher in January 2000, has the following two overarching goals:

1. To help individuals of all ages increase life expectancy and improve their quality of life

2. To eliminate health disparities among different segments of the population

As a result of these goals, more attention is being paid to lifestyle issues with a focus on the population as a whole. Smoking, sedentary lifestyles, and unhealthy food choices are just some of the health education areas being stressed. Obesity rates are on the increase in all ages, races, and economic levels. Chronic illnesses are a larger problem than acute illnesses. All require the attention of individuals, health care providers, and government policy makers.

Health disparities are a major concern. Studies have shown that certain minorities receive less care and lower quality care compared to similar people from nonminority groups. Even controlling for age, income, health insurance, and education, the disparities remain, indicating the possibility of a degree of bias in health care delivery. Studies continue to flush out the reasons for the disparities and address them head on.

SUMMARY

This text, designed as an overview of the U.S. health care system, provides both a historical and a current view of the delivery of health care in the United States. We begin with a view of the cost of care, the evolution of payment mechanisms for health care services, and an introduction to the health status of the U.S. population and determinants of health care service utilization.

We continue with a discussion of the health care system through historic and current information regarding various providers of care: physicians, hospitals, ambulatory services, mental health services, public health services, and long-term care services.

The remaining text focuses on some of the newer trends in the continually changing health care environment. Although other "industries" across the economy have developed widespread use of computers and information management, health care is far behind in technology development for information management. Technology is highly incorporated in medical interventions, yet scarce in information gathering that can foster improved quality of care and error prevention. We consider why this phenomenon is true. We also look at some of the current issues of importance to health care reform and how our system may look in the future.

Each chapter asks the reader to consider difficult questions that do not always have one right answer. We call them "Questions of Ethics," but they are questions that pose difficult policy directions—for organizations, consumers, and the nation. Somewhat more "hands-on" exercises are included in the "Activity-Based Learning" section of the chapters. Exhibits are provided in each chapter that are also meant to stimulate discussion of the chapter topic.

PART ONE

The External Environment of Health Care Delivery

Chapter 2

Health Care Costs

CHAPTER OBJECTIVES

After completing this chapter, readers should have an understanding of the following:

- Trends in the cost of health care
- Reasons for the rising cost of health care
- Effects of the rising cost of health care
- Efforts to stem the rising cost of health care

INTRODUCTION

Health care cost containment has been a buzz phrase for over a decade in the United States. To understand why there is such a focus on cost containment, it is important to understand the costs associated with health care delivery. This chapter provides a background on the trends in health care costs, the causes of increases in costs, and the efforts to reduce those costs.

Technological advances spawned the increased demand for medical care. The increased use of medical care, in turn, increased the cost of medical care. The technology and costs both caused major changes in the health care delivery system in the United States. Neither is the sole cause of change; together they are not the causes of change, yet neither can be ignored. The large elderly population is soon to be exacerbated by the number of baby boomers who will become eligible for Medicare when they turn 65 beginning in 2011. It is widely known that the older people get, the more health care services they will require. Although Americans are living longer lives, the latter portion of their lives often brings chronic illness.

TRENDS IN HEALTH CARE COSTS

If we placed a current dollar value on all goods and services a country produces during any one year, the resulting sum would constitute what is known as the **gross national product (GNP)** or **gross domestic product (GDP)**. Economists have been able to use such figures as a rough index of a nation's economy. These figures indicate the increasing or decreasing wealth in a society from one year to the next as a comparative measure of the economic vitality and productive capacity of one country against another. The United States has historically used the GNP figure, but began using the GDP in late 1991. In the transition from GNP to GDP, both figures were used at different times for a number of years.

EXHIBIT 2–1

June 29, 2007

Time Has Come to Address Soaring Health Care Costs

BYLINE: Michael Kinsman

Talk to any business owner—from one at the tiniest company to one at a giant corporation—and you'll find out that health care benefits is the one workplace issue that gives everyone the frights.

They would be foolish not to worry about the rising costs of providing health care.

Health care is often the most expensive employee benefit and it only makes sense that trying to control its cost is a practical business tool.

Recently, the Society for Human Resource Management reported that health care costs are expected to rise 11.2 percent next year, down slightly from the past year.

This is part of a long-running pattern at which the cost of health care greatly supersedes the inflation rate or other increases in the cost of doing business.

How could you ignore this?

The implications of health care cost containment are not pretty. Every worker should be aware of them and thinking about them.

Let's look at the issue of the large employers. These companies usually offer the best benefits packages.

To be competitive and attract the best employees, they typically have a solid benefit package that includes health care coverage and some type of pension provision, whether it is a traditional defined-benefit plan or making contributions into 401(k) accounts.

But now the biggest companies are feeling global pressure. Foreign operators can pay lower salaries and fewer benefits than in the United States and jobs that can be relocated often are.

That ratchets up the pressure on U.S. companies to cut their payrolls by eliminating jobs and reducing health care benefits for those who remain.

Now, let's look at small employers.

The National Federation of Independent Businesses reports that cost and availability of health care is the most crucial issue facing small businesses. And, because an estimated 99.7 percent of all U.S. business have 500 or fewer employees, this is a big headache.

The result of this is that fewer small businesses will likely be able to offer health care coverage in the future, and workers who enjoy those benefits today might find they are paying a higher share of the cost of health care or see their benefits eliminated.

This is not a new issue. It has been building for two decades. But the need for health care coverage has never been greater in our society. Today a moderately serious illness is enough to drive any middle-class household toward insolvency.

Government policies long have established work as the vehicle for most people to obtain medical benefits. Job tenures have gotten shorter and less secure and, at the same time, health care costs have spiraled upward.

This double whammy is putting the squeeze on everyone. But workers who have taken health care benefits for granted can no longer do that.

Isn't it time to figure out a way to give adequate and affordable health care coverage to everyone, instead of relying on the good intentions of employers to provide it?

Copyright 2007 Copley News Service

Visit Copley News Service at www.copleynews.com.

Discussion Questions

This news article illustrates the frustrations many sectors feel over the cost of health care and spiraling insurance costs.

1. What are the main issues the author of the article identifies?

2. Have you observed the same issues the author discusses?

3. Do you agree with him?

The health sector has long accounted for one of the largest shares of the GDP in the United States, as measured by the percentage of the GDP credited to it (for example, the costs for physicians, nurses, optometrists, dentists, therapists, and other health workers; and the hospitals, nursing homes, health insurance companies, community health agencies, public health departments, and support for medical research). Over the years, the health sector has captured a growing share of the GDP. In 1960, for example, national health expenditures constituted only 5.2 percent of the GDP. Since that time, they have risen steadily to 16.0 percent of the GDP in 2005 (National Center for Health Statistics 2007). All indicators point to a continued rise (see Table 2–1).

Also important, the public (government) sector has paid for an increasing share of all national health costs over the years. In 1929, for example, only 13.6 percent of the total health expenditures were from tax sources (Raffel and Raffel 1994). The 13.6 percent was for the following:

- The health services provided by the armed services, the Veterans Administration, and other federal government hospitals

- Health services provided by state and local health departments

- Care in state and local government general hospitals for psychiatric care and mental retardation

- Limited monies provided by the federal government for medical research (mainly through grants)

Since that time, government expenditures have risen to the point that, in 2005, government at all levels was responsible for 45.4 percent of all health expenditures. This percentage has been relatively constant since 2000 (see Table 2–1).

The increase in the government's share of the GDP for health care prior to the 1970s can be attributed to activities such as medical research; the **Hill-Burton Act**, which for many years provided construction grant monies for hospitals and other health facilities; and programs such as disabled children's services, mental health services, and other programs that, in their own way, added to the total public share. By 1970, there was a sharp rise in federal government expenditures. This was due largely to the

TABLE 2–1 Gross Domestic Product and National Health Expenditures: United States, Selected Years 1960–2005

	1960	1970	1980	1990	2000	2003	2004	2005
Gross domestic product (in billions)	$526	$1,039	$2,790	$5,803	$9,817	$10,961	$11,713	$12,456
Percentage								
National health expenditures as percent of GDP	5.2	7.2	9.1	12.3	13.8	15.8	15.9	16.0
Distribution Percentage								
National health expenditures	100.0	100.0	100.0	100.0	100.0	100.0	100.0	100.0
Private	75.3	62.4	58.1	59.8	55.9	55.1	54.9	54.6
Public	24.7	37.6	41.9	40.2	44.1	44.9	45.1	45.4

SOURCE: Centers for Medicare and Medicaid Services. 2005. Office of the Actuary, National Health Statistics Group, Nation Health Expenditure Accounts, National health expenditures. Retrieved from www.cms.hhs.gov/statistics/NationalHealthExpendituresData.

implementation of **Medicare** and **Medicaid**. The growth in the public sector in subsequent years can be attributed to growth in the expenditures for these two programs for the most part.

By 2005, 83.6 percent of all monies spent for health was for personal health care, which consists of the cost for hospital care, physician services, dental and other professional services, drugs, eyeglasses, nursing home care, and related items (National Center for Health Statistics 2007). Public health activities, research and construction of medical facilities, program administration, and the net cost of private health insurance (the difference between the premiums collected and the benefits paid) account for the remaining 16.4 percent (see Table 2–2).

TABLE 2–2 National Health Expenditures Distribution Percentage, Per Type of Expenditure: United States, Selected Years 1960–2005

Type of National Health Expenditure	1960	1970	1980	1990	2000	2003	2004	2005
Distribution Percentage								
National health expenditures	100.0	100.0	100.0	100.0	100.0	100.0	100.0	100.0
Health services and supplies	90.6	89.6	92.1	93.4	93.4	93.6	93.5	93.6
Personal health care	84.7	84.0	84.8	85.1	84.2	83.4	83.5	83.6
Hospital care	33.3	36.8	39.8	35.2	30.8	30.3	30.5	30.8
Professional services	30.2	27.6	26.5	30.4	31.5	31.3	31.3	31.3
Physician and clinical service	19.4	18.7	18.5	22.1	21.3	21.2	21.2	21.2
Other professional service	1.4	1.0	1.4	2.5	2.9	2.8	2.8	2.9
Dental services	7.1	6.2	5.2	4.4	4.6	4.4	4.4	4.4
Other personal care	2.2	1.7	1.3	1.3	2.7	2.9	2.9	2.9
Nursing home and home health	3.2	5.7	8.4	9.1	9.3	8.6	8.5	8.5
Home health care[1]	0.2	0.3	.9	1.8	2.3	2.2	2.3	2.4
Nursing home care[2]	2.9	5.4	7.5	7.4	7.0	6.4	6.2	6.1
Retail outlet sales of medical products	18.0	14.0	10.1	10.4	12.6	13.2	13.2	13.0
Prescription drugs	9.7	7.3	4.7	5.6	8.9	10.1	10.2	10.1
Other medical products	8.2	6.6	5.4	4.7	3.7	3.2	3.0	2.9

(continues)

TABLE 2–2 (Continued)

Type of National Health Expenditure	1960	1970	1980	1990	2000	2003	2004	2005
Government administration and net cost of private health insurance	4.4	3.7	4.8	5.5	6.0	7.1	7.3	7.2
Government public health activities	1.5	1.9	2.5	2.8	3.2	3.0	2.8	2.8
Investment	9.4	10.4	7.9	6.6	6.6	6.4	6.5	6.4
Research[3]	2.5	2.6	2.1	1.8	1.9	2.1	2.1	2.0
Construction	6.9	7.8	5.7	4.9	4.7	4.4	4.4	4.4

[1] Freestanding facilities only. Additional services of this type are provided in hospital-based facilities and are counted as hospital care.

[2] Includes personal care services delivered by government public health agencies.

[3] Research and development expenditures of drug companies and other manufacturers and providers of medical equipment and supplies are excluded from "research expenditures," but are included in the expenditures class in which the product falls in that they are covered by the payment received for that product.

SOURCE: Centers for Medicare and Medicaid Services. 2005. Office of Actuary, National Health Statistics Group, National Health Expenditures Account, National health accounts, National health expenditures. Retrieved from www.cms.hhs.gov/NationalHealthExpendData.

MULTIPLE CAUSES OF INCREASED HEALTH CARE COSTS

Inflation

Factors accounting for the health sector's increasing share of the nation's GDP can best be seen in personal health care expenditures, for this is where the big growth occurs. One factor in the rise of the health sector's share of the GNP is **inflation**—inflation that affects all sectors of the economy, as well as inflation that is specific to the health sector. Economy-wide inflation during the 1980s accounted for nearly half of the rise in personal health care costs. The cost of everything—food, electricity, telephones, gasoline, automobiles, and labor—rose. However, the cost of health care rose at a greater rate than other areas of the economy (see Table 2–3). Health sector inflation stems from the introduction of new technology and the costs associated with its operation, the costs of equipment and drugs, and the rising cost of highly skilled professional personnel. However, total costs also grew from increased consumption of services.

As a labor-intensive sector and as a traditionally heavy employer of unskilled labor (as well as skilled labor), the health care sector is acutely sensitive to congressionally mandated raises in Social Security rates, to raises in the minimum wage, and to state or federal legislation mandating new employee benefits. However, employment in the health care services is projected to increase some 22 percent from 2006 through 2016. Growth will be slowest in hospitals, with much larger increases in long-term care, home health, and ambulatory care (Bureau of Labor Statistics 2008). Health services continue to be one of the largest areas of employment in the United States (see Table 2–4).

TABLE 2–3 Annual Change Per Capita in Health Care Spending (Per Type) and Gross Domestic Product (GDP), 1994–2004

Year	All Services	Hospital Inpatient	Hospital Outpatient	Physician	Rx Drugs	Other	GDP
1994	3.5%	−2.3%	8.0%	2.1%	5.1%	12.3%	4.9%
1995	4.2	−3.7	7.0	2.6	10.7	8.6	3.4
1996	4.2	−4.6	7.0	2.2	10.8	12.0	4.4
1997	5.6	−5.4	8.9	4.1	11.4	11.8	5.0
1998	7.1	0.0	7.7	5.6	13.6	7.6	4.1
1999	9.9	2.6	11.6	6.7	18.1	5.5	4.8
2000	9.3	4.0	9.8	7.7	14.2	4.4	4.8
2001	11.3	8.6	14.5	7.8	13.5	9.1	2.1
2002	10.7	8.2	13.0	7.9	13.1	6.2	2.5
2003	8.4	6.1	11.1	6.4	8.9	5.8	3.9
2004	8.2	6.2	11.3	6.4	7.2	6.0	5.6

NOTE: GDP is in nominal dollars. Estimates differ from past reports due to data revisions by Milliman and the Bureau of Economic Analysis.

SOURCE: Center for Health System Change. 2005. *Tracking health care costs: Spending growth stabilizes at high rate in 2004, Data Bulletin No. 29, June 2005*. Health care spendiwng data are the Milliman Health Cost Index ($0 deductible). Gross domestic product is from the U.S. Department of Commerce, Bureau of Economic Analysis.

TABLE 2–4 Employees in Health Services sites, United States 2000–2005 (in thousands)

Site	2000	2001	2002	2003	2004	2005
All Health Services Sites	12,211	12,558	13,069	13,615	13,817	14,052
Offices and clinics of physicians	1,387	1,499	1,533	1,673	1,727	1,801
Offices and clinics of other health practitioners	1,030	1,054	1,128	1,255	1,303	1,328
Nursing and professional care facilities	2,245	2,236	2,404	2,478	2,476	2,463
Hospitals	5,202	5,256	5,330	5,652	5,700	5,719
Home health care services	548	582	636	741	750	795
Other	1,799	1,931	2,038	1,816	1,861	1,946

SOURCE: U.S. Department of Labor, Bureau of Labor Statistics. 2006, January. Current Population Survey: Employment and Earnings, Table 18, and unpublished data. Retrieved from www.bls.gov/cps/home.htm#annual.

Prior to major revisions in hospital payment systems in the mid-1980s, critics of the health field focused on inefficiencies that drive up costs unnecessarily—hospitals made more money if patients stayed longer. The economic pressures of **prospective payment systems** (**PPS**—discussed in more detail in Chapter 3), reduced fee schedules, and **capitation** payments, as well as regulatory devices such as **certificate of need (CON)** programs, self-referral restrictions, and **fraud** and **abuse** legislation have driven out some of the inefficiencies that existed. These efforts tend to suppress demand and decrease services. However, some may limit access for many who need care, thereby contributing to a lesser quality of care and higher costs in the long run.

The Aging Population

Population increases contribute to a rise in the use and intensity of services. U.S. population has continually increased, owing to a greater number of births than deaths and to more immigration than emigration. These increased numbers of people raise the basic demands on the health care system. The aging of the U.S. population accounts for a significant share of increased health care costs. People are living longer lives, but not necessarily healthy later years. Along with greater longevity comes a variety of acute and chronic debilitating diseases, the diagnosis and treatments for which are very costly.

Technology

As we look at the health sector and its rising costs, we note immediately that technological advances have been enormous: new drugs permit more effective treatment of disease; organs can be transplanted; new anesthetics are safer and often more effective; new instrumentation permits the electronic monitoring of patients who require intensive care and high-risk surgery; a variety of sophisticated diagnostic and therapeutic radiological devices have been implemented (for example, computed tomography [CT] scanners, magnetic resonance imaging [MRI], and cobalt therapy units); autoanalyzers and an array of other laboratory equipment allow faster, more accurate, and more sophisticated analyses; new metals and materials are less toxic to the body; laser therapy and surgery techniques are more advanced; and so on.

The developmental costs of new pieces of equipment are typically high, and many require highly trained (and more costly) technicians to operate them. The very development of this new technology increases utilization and accompanying expenditures. New drugs and new anesthetics likewise frequently lead to expanded services and increased utilization and costs.

Hospitals and physicians often employ technology and use a greater number of diagnostic tests because of concern over an increase in malpractice claims. Referred to as practicing defensive medicine, the substitution of tests for professional judgment may or may not always improve the overall quality of care, but it certainly increases costs.

Medical care is more than just treatment and medications, and both society and the medical community have begun to realize the therapeutic benefit of a pleasant and caring environment. A homelike room, pleasant surroundings, and accommodation for family involvement are new advances in care delivery, although they may not be technology driven. Although medical necessity has been the definition that health care payers use, the comfort and caring that lead to healing are now a component of patient-centered care.

Health Care Utilization

Along with technological advances have come a number of other changes in the organization and utilization of health care services that have affected the overall cost picture. The increase in obesity in adults as well as children also increases the risk of chronic diseases such as diabetes and heart failure (Anderson et al. 2007). The number of patient visits to physician offices has decreased since the turn of the century (National Center for Health Statistics 2007). Although the number of hospital admissions had decreased dramatically since 1980, they began rising in 2000, and the average length of stay steadily decreased but has stabilized since 2000 (see Table 2–5).

TRENDS IN HEALTH CARE COSTS

Costs for the Aging Population

The impact of an aging population has been particularly significant on the overall cost picture. In 1995, approximately 33.5 million people in the United States were age 65 and over—about 12.8 percent of the population. After 2010, when the **baby boomers** start to enter this age group, this share of the population will begin to increase dramatically. The 2005 U.S. Census Bureau report on the 65 and over population has a particularly striking illustration of the effect of the baby boom population on the total population (see Figure 2–1). By 2050, 20 percent of the

TABLE 2–5 Hospital Admissions and Average Length of Stay, Per Type of Hospital Ownership: United States, Selected Years 1975–2005

Type of Ownership and Size of Hospital	1975	1980	1990	2000	2003	2004	2005
Admissions	**Number**						
All hospitals	36,157	38,892	33,774	34,891	36,611	36,942	37,006
Federal	1,913	2,044	1,759	1,034	973	1,000	952
Nonfederal*	34,243	36,848	32,015	33,946	35,637	35,842	36,054
Average length of stay	**Number of days**						
All hospitals	11.4	9.9	9.1	6.8	6.6	6.5	6.5
Federal	20.3	16.8	14.9	12.8	11.5	11.6	11.6
Nonfederal*	10.9	9.6	8.8	6.6	6.4	6.4	6.3

NOTE: Data are based on reporting by a census of hospitals.

*The category of nonfederal hospitals comprises psychiatric, tuberculosis and other respiratory diseases hospitals, and long-term and short-term general and other special hospitals.

SOURCE: American Hospital Association Annual Survey of Hospitals. Hospital Statistics, 1976, 1981, 1991–2007 editions. Chicago, IL. In National Center for Health Statistics. 2007. *Health, United States, 2007 with chartbook on trends in the health of Americans*. Hyattsville, Maryland.

population is expected to be in the 65 and over age group. Major causes of higher numbers of elderly are large increases in the oldest of the elderly population because of longer life expectancy and the large number of people approaching the oldest ages. The population aged 85 and over was 4.2 million people in 2000, and is projected to increase to almost 10 million by 2030. The population aged 100 years and over was 37,000 in 1990, and grew to 50,000 in the 2000 census (He et al. 2005).

More than other age groups, the elderly are afflicted with a number of debilitating and degenerative conditions, such as heart disease and cancer, which make a heavy demand on health resources. Their conditions are more life threatening and complicated, and are often multiple. The results are longer hospital stays, use of more specialized hospital services, and attention of more personnel. In 2005, for example, although 4.8 days was the average length of short stays in hospitals for all patients, those 65 to 74 spent an average of 5.3 days and those 75 years and over spent an average of 5.7 days (see Table 2–6).

Because of advances in knowledge, surgical and anesthetic techniques, and monitoring devices, more elderly people can be successfully treated surgically than in years past. Consider the days of hospitalization for an aging population in 2005:

- 554.2 days per 1,000 people for the total population
- 1,398.5 days per 1,000 people for those 65 to 74 years of age
- 2,593.9 days per 1,000 people for those 75 years and over (National Center for Health Statistics 2007)

Continuing concern for the solvency of the Medicare health insurance trust fund stems from longer-than-average lengths of stay, higher number of days of care, and costs per hospital stay for the aging population (see Table 2–7). These statistics also raise the more fundamental policy question of whether we will be able to afford the continued allocation of resources to health care at current growth rates.

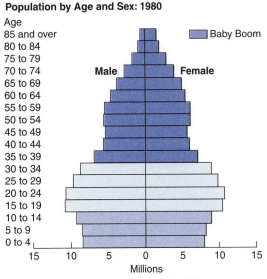

Population by Age and Sex: 1980

Note: The reference population for these data is the resident population.

Source: U.S. Bureau of the Census, 1983, Table 44. For full citation, see references at end of chapter.

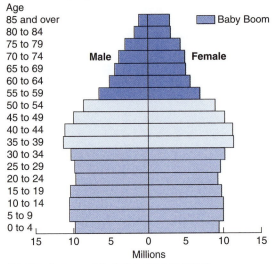

Population by Age and Sex: 2000

Note: The reference population for these data is the resident population.

Source: U.S. Census Bureau, 2001, Table PCT12. For full citation, see references at end of chapter.

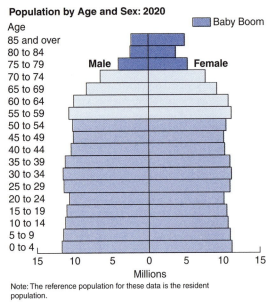

Population by Age and Sex: 2020

Note: The reference population for these data is the resident population.

Source: U.S. Census Bureau, 2004. For full citation, see references at end of chapter.

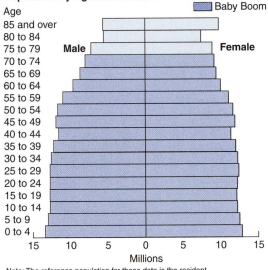

Population by Age and Sex: 2040

Note: The reference population for these data is the resident population.

Source: U.S. Census Bureau, 2004. For full citation, see references at end of chapter.

Figure 2–1 Estimated Growth of the Baby Boom Population

SOURCE: He, W., M. Sengupta, V. Velkoff, and K. DeBarros. 2005. *U.S. Census Bureau, current population reports*, P23-209, 65+ in the United States: 2005. Washington, DC: U.S. Government Printing Office. Retrieved from www.census.gov/prod/2006pubs/p23-209.pdf.

TABLE 2-6 Days of Care and Average Length of Stay in Nonfederal Short-Stay Hospitals, According to Age: United States, Selected Years 1980–2005

Characteristics	1980	1990	2000	2002	2003	2004	2005
	Average length of stay in days						
Total	7.5	6.5	4.9	4.9	4.8	4.8	4.8
AGE							
Under 18 years	4.5	4.9	4.4	4.5	4.5	4.5	4.7
18–44 years	5.3	4.6	3.6	3.7	3.7	3.7	3.7
45–54 years	7.5	6. 2	4.8	4.8	4.8	4.9	4.9
55–64 years	8.8	7.2	5.2	5.1	5.1	5.1	5.1
65+ years	10.7	8.7	6.0	5.8	5.7	5.6	5.5
65–74 years	10.0	8.0	5.7	5.6	5.4	5.4	5.3
75+ years	11.4	9. 2	6.2	6.0	5.8	5.8	5.7
	Days of care per 1,000 population						
Total	1,297.0	818.9	557.7	570.9	574.6	568.7	554.2
Age							
Under 18 years	341.4	226.3	179.0	195.2	195.5	193.2	191.8
18–44 years	818.6	467.7	309.4	322.7	333.9	339.7	334.9
45–54 years	1,314.9	699.7	437.4	456.7	477.2	491.1	471.1
55–64 years	1,889.4	1,172.3	729.1	752.2	735.9	735.2	712.4
65+ years	4,098.3	2,895.6	2,111.9	2,085.1	2,088.3	2,048.6	1,988.3
65–74 years	3,147.0	2,087.8	1,439.0	1,411.9	1,428.9	1,405.2	1,398.5
75+ years	5,578.8	4,009.1	2,851.9	2,795.0	2,776.1	2,714.9	2,593.9

NOTE: Data are based on a sample of hospital records.

SOURCE: National Center for Health Statistics. 2007. *Health, United States, 2007 with chartbook on trends in the health of Americans*, Table 99. Hyattsville, Maryland.

Personal Health Care Expenditures

Table 2–8 provides a detailed breakdown of the nation's health expenditures for 2005. The $1,661.4 billion for personal health care represents 83.6 percent of all monies spent that year on health (National Center for Health Statistics 2007). Personal health care is the treatment and caring function of the health sector; it excludes public health activities, research, and construction of health facilities. Although planners are seeking to slow construction and to cut costs in other areas, the principal focus for cost containment is the personal care sector.

TABLE 2-7 Expenses for Health Care and Prescribed Medicine According to Age: United States, Selected Years 1997–2004

	Population in Millions			Total Expenses					
				Percentage of People with Expenses			Mean Annual Expense Per Person		
Characteristic	1997	2000	2004	1997	2000	2004	1997	2000	2004
Under 65 years	237.1	243.6	256.5	82.5	81.8	82.9	$2,163	$2,333	$3,028
65+ years	34.2	34.8	37.0	95.2	95.5	97.1	$6,999	$6,735	$8,906

SOURCE: National Center for Health Statistics. 2007. *Health, United States, 2007 with chartbook on trends in the health of Americans*, Table 128. Hyattsville, Maryland.

Hospital care accounts for $611.6 billion, or 30.8 percent, of all personal health care expenditures. Physician services come next, accounting for $421.2 billion, or 21.2 percent. Prescription drugs account for $200.7 billion, or 10.1 percent. These three components account for 62.1 percent of all personal health care expenditures, and the government seeks most urgently to address these three elements (see Table 2–8). The other components of personal health care do not make as heavy a demand on government resources; however, the government has made attempts to limit these costs also. Drug and medical sundries consist of over-the-counter purchases; drugs that are provided in hospitals, nursing homes, and directly by physicians are charged to these categories. Prescription drugs are currently the focus of great concern. As new prescription drugs are developed for many conditions previously having no drug therapy, costs to consumers increase. Congress has added a drug benefit to Medicare because of the overwhelming costs to many seniors, and this adds new considerations to controlling overall health care costs.

Health care costs involve a number of entities paying for those costs. The first column of figures in Table 2–9 shows the total amount spent in a number of health categories. The table shows who pays for each category (the public or private sector) and how (consumer payments, health insurance, federal government, state/local government, or other groups). Note that, of the $611.6 billion spent on hospital care in 2005, about 3.3 percent or $20 billion was paid out of pocket (directly by patients) because the patients had no health insurance, their benefits had been used up, they had **co-pays** or **deductibles**, or because their insurance

did not cover all of the expenses. For the remaining costs (96.7 percent of the expenditures for hospital care), **third-party payers** (principally the insurance companies and government) made the payments.

Medicare accounted for 29.5 percent or $180.4 billion of all hospital expenditures; Medicaid accounted for 17.3 percent or $105.8 billion. Private health insurance was responsible for 35.5 percent or $217.1 billion. These figures represent expenditures for hospital care, not hospital costs or hospital charges. Hospitals as well as other health care providers may well charge much higher prices for their services. However, payments from insurance companies and government programs are adjusted down to a fee schedule that has been previously agreed upon when a provider agrees to participate in a particular insurance plan. Just as a person determines what type of insurance policy to purchase, health care organizations determine what programs they will participate in as providers of care (this will be explained in greater depth in Chapter 3).

Turning to physician services figures in Table 2–9, patients paid $42 billion or 10.1 percent of the total $421.2 billion spent in that category. This figure might suggest how inadequate health insurance is in this area. However, the percentage of the total physician costs paid by patients has been decreasing steadily, particularly since the 1990s (National Center for Health Statistics 2007). The amount patients paid includes co-payments, **coinsurance** payments, and deductibles for care in physicians' offices, a type of care not usually covered by fee-for-service insurance plans. The theory of "**moral hazard**" would argue that such first-dollar coverage (that is, insurance

TABLE 2-8 National Health Expenditures According to Type of Expenditure: United States, Selected Years 1960–2005

Type of National Health Expenditure	1960	1970	1980	1990	2000	2004	2005
Amount in billions of dollars							
National health expenditures	$27.5	74.9	253.9	714.0	1,353.3	1,858.9	1,987.7
Health services and supplies	$24.9	67.1	234.0	666.7	1,264.4	1,738.9	1,860.9
Personal health care	$23.3	62.9	215.3	607.5	1,139.9	1,551.3	1,661.4
Hospital care	$9.2	27.6	101.0	251.6	417.0	566.9	611.6
Professional services	$8.3	20.6	67.3	216.8	426.7	581.1	621.7
Physician and clinical service	$5.4	14.0	47.1	157.5	288.6	393.7	421.2
Other professional service	$.4	.7	3.6	18.2	39.1	52.6	56.7
Dental services	$2.0	4.7	13.3	31.5	62.0	81.5	86.6
Other personal care	$.6	1.2	3.3	9.6	37.1	53.3	57.2
Nursing home and home health	$.9	4.3	21.4	65.2	125.8	157.7	169.3
Home health care[1]	$.1	.2	2.4	12.6	30.5	42.7	47.5
Nursing home care[2]	$.8	4.0	19.0	52.6	95.3	115.0	121.9
Retail outlet sales of medical products	$4.9	10.5	25.7	74.0	170.3	245.5	258.8
Prescription drugs	$2.7	5.5	12.0	40.3	120.8	189.7	200.7
Other medical products	$2.3	5.0	13.6	33.7	49.5	55.9	58.1
Government administration and net cost of private health insurance	$1.2	2.8	12.2	39.2	81.2	135.2	143.0
Government public health activities	$.4	1.4	6.4	20.0	43.4	52.5	56.6
Investment	$2.6	7.8	19.9	47.3	88.8	119.9	126.8
Research[3]	$.7	2.0	5.4	12.7	25.6	38.3	40.0
Structure and equipment	$1.9	5.8	14.5	34.7	63.2	81.7	86.8

[1] Freestanding facilities only. Additional services of this type are provided in hospital-based facilities and are counted as hospital care.
[2] Includes personal care services delivered by government public health agencies.
[3] Research and development expenditures of drug companies and other manufacturers and providers of medical equipment and supplies are excluded from "research expenditures," but are included in the expenditures class in which the product falls in that they are covered by the payment received for that product.

SOURCE: National Center for Health Statistics. 2007. *Health, United States, 2007 with chartbook on trends in the health of Americans*, Table 124. Hyattsville, Maryland .

TABLE 2–9 Personal Health Care Expenditures for Hospital and Physician Services and Source of Funds: United States, Selected Years 1960–2005

	1960	1970	1980	1990	2000	2004	2005
Expenditure type	**Amount in billions**						
All personal health care expenditures[1]	$23.3	62.9	215.3	607.5	1,139.9	1,551.3	1,661.4
Hospital care expenditures[2]	$9.2	27.6	101.0	251.6	417.0	566.9	611.6
	Distribution Percentage						
All sources of funds	100.0	100.0	100.0	100.0	100.0	100.0	100.0
Out-of-pocket payments	20.7	9.0	5.4	4.5	3.3	3.3	3.3
Private health insurance	35.8	32.5	36.6	38.9	34.6	35.6	35.5
Other private funds	1.2	3.2	5.0	4.1	5.2	4.5	4.5
Government[3]	42.2	55.2	53.0	52.5	56.9	56.7	56.8
Medicaid[4]		9.6	9.1	10.6	17.0	17.1	17.3
Medicare		19.4	26.1	27.0	29.9	29.4	29.5
	Amount in billions						
Physician services expenditures	$5.4	14.0	47.1	157.5	288.6	393.7	421.2
	Distribution Percentage						
All sources of funds	100.0	100.0	100.0	100.0	100.0	100.0	100.0
Out-of-pocket payments	61.7	46.2	30.4	19.2	11.2	10.1	10.1
Private health insurance	29.8	30.1	35.5	42.7	47.4	48.3	48.3
Other private funds	1.4	1.6	3.9	7.2	7.7	6.7	6.4
Government[3]	7.2	22.1	30.1	30.9	33.8	34.9	35.3
Medicaid[4]		4.6	5.2	4.5	6.6	7.1	7.1
Medicare		11.8	17.0	18.6	20.2	20.7	21.2

[1] Includes all expenditures for specified health services and supplies other than expenses for program administration, net cost of private health insurance, and government public health activities.
[2] Includes expenditures for hospital-based nursing home care and home health agency care.
[3] Includes other government expenditures for these health care services, for example Medicaid State Children's Health Insurance Program (SCHIP) expansion, care funded by the Department of Veterans Affairs, and state and locally financed subsidies to hospitals.
[4] Excludes Medicaid SCHIP expansion and SCHIP.

SOURCE: National Center for Health Statistics. 2007. Health, United States, 2007 with chartbook on trends in the health of Americans, Table 125. Hyattsville, Maryland. Data are compiled from various sources by the Centers for Medicare and Medicaid Services.

coverage for the total costs of physician office visits) should not be part of any insurance package because it encourages frivolous visits to the physician. Under fee-for-service plans, first-dollar coverage encourages billing for extra visits by the physician. Under **managed care** plans, however, visits to a primary care physician are encouraged, both for prevention of disease and early treatment, which helps avoid costly hospital care. Again, some of the out-of-pocket expenses represent payments toward co-payments or noncovered services (a more detailed explanation of insurance, Medicare, Medicaid, and managed care is provided in Chapter 3).

Under Medicare, a physician who accepts assignment agrees to accept 80 percent of what Medicare determines to be a reasonable fee from Medicare after the deductible has been met, and the physician agrees to bill the patient only for the balance—that is, only 20 percent of the fee set by Medicare. In a growing number of states, state laws require physicians to accept assignment in all cases as a condition for retention of their license to practice medicine in that state. Federal legislation regulates the amount that physicians may charge in nonassigned cases (115 percent of the approved amount). Nearly half of the population eligible for Medicare has taken out additional health insurance, which pays the deductible and the coinsurance (the 20 percent) portion of the allowed charges. These supplementary insurance policies (known as **Medigap** insurance) also cover the deductible and coinsurance charges under the hospital portion of Medicare. All of these contribute to the reduction in the percentage of total costs a patient pays directly.

Another significant component of the sum paid directly by patients to physicians represents monies paid by patients not enrolled in Medicare for surgical and in-hospital medical care to cover charges over and above what the insurance company pays. Also in this category are payments by people who do not have health insurance.

Looking at nursing home care in Table 2–10, patients paid some 26.5 percent or $34.9 billion of the total $121.9 billion spent in that category in 2005. Though the cost per day in a nursing home is substantially less than in a hospital, the length of stay is typically much longer, and the population in nursing homes is well over 65 years of age by a large majority (average age of a nursing home resident is over 80). Medicare pays for skilled nursing care up to only 100 days, provided that the patient had first spent three days as an inpatient in a hospital (Medicare 2007). After the twentieth day, patients have to pay a significant part of the cost ($124.00 per day in 2007). Many elderly people do not meet the initial hospitalization requirement. Other Medicare patients do not need skilled nursing care, but instead need custodial care (help with dressing, bathing, eating, and so on), for which Medicare does not pay.

Though federal expenditures for nursing home care under Medicare have been slight (15.7 percent or $20.7 billion), they are substantial under Medicaid; the federal and state governments under the Medicaid program paid 43.9 percent or $57.9 billion of all nursing home expenditures in 2005. Medicaid pays for intermediate and custodial care, but only after nursing home residents "spend down"—that is, use any personal funds

TABLE 2–10 Personal Health Care Expenditures for Nursing Home Care, Prescription Drugs, and Other Personal Health Care and Source of Funds: United States, Selected Years 1960–2005

	1960	1970	1980	1990	2000	2004	2005
Expenditure type	**Amount in billions**						
All personal health care expenditures	$23.3	62.9	215.3	607.5	1,139.9	1,551.3	1,661.4
Nursing home care	$0.8	4.0	19.0	52.6	95.3	115.0	121.9
	Distribution Percentage						
All sources of funds	100.0	100.0	100.0	100.0	100.0	100.0	100.0

(continues)

TABLE 2-10 (Continued)

	1960	1970	1980	1990	2000	2004	2005
Out-of-pocket payments	77.3	52.0	37.2	36.1	30.1	26.6	26.5
Private health insurance	0.0	0.2	1.2	5.6	8.3	7.5	7.5
Other private funds	6.3	4.8	4.2	7.2	4.8	3.7	3.7
Government	16.4	43.0	57.5	51.1	56.9	62.2	62.3
Medicaid		23.3	53.8	45.8	44.1	44.8	43.9
Medicare		3.5	1.6	3.2	10.6	14.9	15.7
Amount in billions							
Prescription drugs	$2.7	5.5	12.0	40.3	120.8	189.7	200.7
Distribution Percentage							
All sources of funds	100.0	100.0	100.0	100.0	100.0	100.0	100.0
Out-of-pocket payments	96.0	82.4	70.3	55.5	27.7	25.2	25.4
Private health insurance	1.3	8.8	14.8	26.4	49.4	47.4	47.4
Other private funds	0.0	0.0	0.0	0.0	0.0	0.0	0.0
Government	2.7	8.8	14.9	18.1	22.9	27.3	27.2
Medicaid		7.6	11.7	12.6	16.7	19.1	18.6
Medicare		0.0	0.0	0.5	1.7	1.8	2.0
Amount in billions							
Other personal health care	$5.3	11.8	36.2	105.5	218.1	285.9	306.1
Distribution Percentage							
All sources of funds	100.0	100.0	100.0	100.0	100.0	100.0	100.0
Out-of-pocket payments	84.5	78.9	64.6	50.4	39.0	34.6	33.9
Private health insurance	1.6	3.3	15.3	24.6	25.1	23.6	23.5
Other private funds	4.2	3.6	4.3	4.7	3.8	3.2	3.2
Government	9.8	14.2	15.8	20.2	32.2	38.6	39.5
Medicaid		3.3	3.9	6.5	15.9	20.1	20.6
		1.1	3.8	7.1	9.7	12.1	12.6

SOURCE: National Center for Health Statistics. 2007. *Health, United States, 2007 with chartbook on trends in the health of Americans*, Table 125. Hyattsville, Maryland.

and assets available until they are poor enough to qualify for Medicaid funds.

Despite the fact that hospital, physician, and nursing home services make up almost 70 percent of health care expenditures, other areas deserve attention. The rising cost of prescription drugs has gained much attention of late, particularly for senior citizens who are often on fixed incomes and require continuing drug therapy for chronic ailments, and who are covered under Medicare, which did not cover prescription drugs until 2006 (see Table 2–10). Drug coverage became available through Medicare with the Medicare Prescription Drug, Improvement, and Modernization Act of 2003. Although the legislation was passed in 2003, the benefit did not become available until 2006. Expenditures by the government for this benefit are not yet available. Estimates, however, range from $395 billion to $534 billion over ten years (Welch 2004).

Another area to watch is the cost of "other professional services." As alternative medicine gains a foothold, many patients are seeking alternative treatments, and many third-party payers are willing to pay the cost of such treatment, which is often lower than the cost of traditional medical care. Included in these areas might be such services as chiropractic, massage therapy, herbal medicine, and acupuncture.

RESOURCES FOR HEALTH: ARE THERE ANY LIMITS?

The increase in health costs and the likelihood of continued increases raise the question of how much of the nation's resources should be allocated to the health sector. In 2005, 16 percent of the nation's GDP was spent in the health sector, a growing portion over the years. The increased spending has brought high-quality health care services to the population, contributing to its health and quality of life. However, the increase in funds for health care services means less money available for other purposes.

To the extent that consumers pay out of pocket for health care, the money cannot be spent for travel, clothes, food, transportation, entertainment, education, or a number of other things. Fortunately, consumers have to pay for only about 16 percent of this cost directly by out-of-pocket payments. For the remainder, all citizens pay indirectly through taxes and in the prices paid for purchases, which usually include a component to cover the employers' contributions for employee health insurance (Moskowitz 1999). As the costs of health care go up, and as the health care sector commands a growing percentage of the GDP, citizens pay one way or another. Although many Americans may feel that costs are getting out of hand, most people are reluctant to push for widespread health care reform that may mean less personal decision making regarding the type or quantity of health care they can seek. People are nonetheless displeased when they have to spend more for insurance or out of pocket, because other wants cannot then be met.

Attitudes Toward Change

There is a certain public ambivalence about the rising costs of health care. Although many Americans express concern over rising costs of care, most still believe that the government should do more to increase access to care, and still desire some form of universal health insurance, especially when confronted with the rising number of people who are uninsured for health care. Yet, the philosophical desire for universal coverage is often offset by a fear of a government-controlled health care system.

Those most concerned over rising health care costs are business and industrial leaders, health insurance companies, government, those who cannot afford health insurance, and those who must purchase health insurance individually rather than as part of a group. Historically, many large companies paid all of the health insurance premiums for their employees. Employers today see the rising cost of health insurance as a barrier to profits. The costs of health insurance are built into the price of the product or service or are hidden as a reduction in salaries paid to employees. Employers are concerned that, if costs continue to rise or if the insurance benefits they pay for are expanded and cost more, the passed-on costs could jeopardize their competitive positions in the marketplace.

Government and others who are concerned with public policy understand that, as the health sector commands a greater share of the GDP, less money will be available in the economy for development in other sectors—improvements in public education, research, and defense, to cite just a few examples. As suggested earlier, health care policy affects profitability and employment in all sectors of the economy, especially if consumers cannot afford new products because of expenditures they make in the health area. Thus, business and industrial executives are understandably among the leaders in the drive to contain health care costs. The rise in health care costs is threatening to them.

What Can Be Done about Rising Costs

In many cities and regions, businesses (for example, New York Business Group on Health, Colorado Business Group on Health, Dallas-Fort Worth Business Group on Health, Memphis Business Group on Health, Midwest Business Group on Health, and so on) are joining together to review and define their own health plan needs. In a cooperative effort, they seek "bids" from local physician-hospital organizations (PHOs—explained more fully in Chapter 3) or commercial insurance plans for health care coverage as a group. Together, they are able to purchase more affordable health insurance, and the PHO or commercial insurer receives a larger base of clients for a given period (perhaps one or two years). Business coalitions such as these allow employers to have a greater say in defining the health plan while having leverage to control costs. They also help employers to choose health plans that provide high-quality care based on a number of different criteria defined by the employers.

Commercial insurance companies are also unhappy about the rise in costs. As their payments rise, they must recover the costs through increased premiums from the insurance purchasers. When they raise their premiums, they run the risk of losing business to competitors, and they also get pressure from purchasers to do something about rising costs. The loss of business might entail not only health insurance but life and retirement policies as well. As nonprofit organizations, Blue Cross and Blue Shield face the additional problem of regulation by state insurance commissioners. They frequently have limits placed on the amounts they can pay in benefits and on how much they can charge for their policies; if the constraints make them less competitive, those they insure may shift to the competition.

Government's Response to Rising Costs of Health Care

Federal, state, and local government combined paid almost 45 percent—34.2 percent federal, 10.7 percent state/local—of all personal health care expenditures in 2005 (National Center for Health Statistics 2007). In recent years, these levels of government have sought to contain the rising costs in several ways: (1) through regulation (for example, certificate of need and rate control), (2) by reducing their efforts in some areas (for example, eliminating support for a variety of health education and health service programs), (3) by shifting costs

to the providers or to the consumers, (4) by paying hospitals and physicians less, and (5) by shifting the care of psychiatric patients from state psychiatric hospitals to noninstitutional and community services.

At the state level, the increases in Medicaid costs have outpaced increases in revenue in most states. Under these circumstances, the ability of a state to expand health services, improve education, or strengthen any of its other services is severely constrained. To trim costs, many states have moved people eligible for Medicaid into managed care programs rather than cutting back on Medicaid eligibility and services or cutting back in other areas. Alternatively, states can raise taxes, but run the risk of alienating voters. Often federal solutions are sought.

At the federal level, health care initiatives began when the economy was booming and the population was expanding. In recent years, however, the economy has had its ups and downs, and the population is aging. The resulting drain on the Medicare trust fund has already been noted. A conservative ideology in the Reagan-Bush years de-emphasized federal initiatives and actions in the health sector; the growing demands of other sectors precluded much action in the health area. The Clinton era, on the other hand, placed great emphasis on health care. A lengthy national debate resulted in a wide range of congressional proposals, from employer mandates to a single-payer universal health plan. A lack of consensus among competing interest groups, highly charged advertising to the public, and a very complicated (even unmanageable) proposal by the Clinton task force resulted in no action on the part of the government. Instead, market forces were allowed to take hold, resulting in a strong emphasis on managed care. The second Bush administration also looked primarily to market forces, except for action on a Medicare drug benefit (mentioned previously and described more fully in Chapter 3).

Political Choice or Moral Choice?

The health economist Uwe Reinhardt (2007a) believes that the perceived cost crisis in health care is actually a moral crisis. He points out that health care providers, both physicians and hospitals, provide uncompensated care to people who are poor and uninsured. At one time, **cost shifting** allowed providers to charge more to private insurance and government programs to help pay for the uncompensated care. However, these payers have decreased the amounts that they pay for care so that cost shifting is no longer possible. Reinhardt notes that federal and state programs for the poor "often, quite irresponsibly, pay less—sometimes much less—than the full cost of providing care to their beneficiaries. . . . Many U.S. hospitals already totter near the point of bankruptcy, mainly because of underpayment by government and the burden of their uninsured patients . . . private benevolence [providers who give uncompensated care to the poor] gives undue moral cover to politicians who shirk their duty" (p. 1020). Although it is true that the poor can receive medical care for acute illnesses, they often do not receive timely care or preventive care—once again inflating the cost of health care across the board (Reinhardt 2007a).

In determining the allocation of resources to health care, ideology plays a role, as does politics. The health sector has been expanding and commanding a greater share of the GDP, but policy makers have not determined if there is a right percentage. The health sector commands more than most other nations, but that may mean very little. The health sector is a major employer of both skilled and unskilled labor. Health workers pay taxes and spend money, thus fueling the nation's economy. As a heavy purchaser of supplies, drugs, and equipment, this sector generates employment in the firms that produce these goods, as well as in the construction industry because of the need for new buildings and for modernization of existing buildings. A new weapons system is sold with relative ease—a weapons system that may never be used—whereas the health system still has difficulty selling the need for new scanners, additional research dollars, more beds for long-term care, and the community health and social services that would demonstratively be used to improve health and the quality of life in general, as well as contribute to the nation's economy.

The health sector has inefficiencies and excesses. They are not to be condoned, but should be dealt with as they are identified and as effective solutions are devised. In the battle for resources, however, the health sector has seen a great shift in societal values. The health sector now uses the language of business and economics—customers (rather than patients), cost effectiveness, marketing of services, vendor payments, multi-institutional management, corporate structure, risk management, and the health industry—as though it were comparable to the automobile, banking, or airline industries. It uses businesslike language, speaking of health sector competition, antitrust, mergers and acquisitions, and leveraging capital. Health care has lost its beginnings as a social service, a societal need, and an altruistic undertaking.

Again from Reinhardt (2007b), we have this question, "'As a matter of national policy, and to the extent that a nation's health system can make it possible, should the child of a poor American family have the same chance of avoiding preventable illness or of being cured from a given disease as does the child of a rich American family?' That question has long been answered in the affirmative in most other industrialized nations. In the United State it evokes irritation" (p. 749).

Edwards et al. (1999) echoed these thoughts some eight years earlier in regard to the "I-Thou" and "I-It" attitude in the patient–physician relationship. The I-Thou attitude is one of true caring and valuing the other person. The I-It attitude regards the other person as a thing to be assessed, evaluated, or used. The authors describe the danger of a conversion of health care to business: "Unfortunately, a physician's I-Thou motivation to serve patients is susceptible to I-It conversion in response to strong and direct financial pressure from third-party payers. . . . Commercial concerns pressure doctors to see more patients, decreasing time available for each patient . . . severe time restriction is inefficient and dangerous as well as damaging to patient/physician rapport" (p. 22).

The health care sector certainly is not an island; it must coordinate with other sectors in society. In doing so, however, there is evidence to suggest that the health sector is failing to maintain and emphasize adequately the value component of its claim for resources, for the value element can assist society in making a more balanced choice in the allocation of resources.

Recent **Institute of Medicine** reports have focused on the quality of health services. The 2000 report, "To Err is Human," indicated that deaths caused by medical error could be from 44,000 to 98,000 each year. What's more, adverse events (errors causing injury) cause between $8.5 billion and $19.5 billion in health care costs. The 2001 report, "Crossing the Quality Chasm," calls for action to improve the health care system in all quality dimensions and specifically points to six goals: to make health care safe, effective, efficient, timely, equitable, and patient-centered.

"Cost containment," "industry integration," and "market-driven systems" have not been able to address issues of quality. A new view of health care costs is needed. Standards of care, patient outcomes, and computerized information systems are the current initiatives in improving the quality and reducing the costs of health care services and will be addressed in subsequent chapters.

SUMMARY

Health care costs are increasing both in real dollars and in percentage of the GDP. Economy-wide inflation, population increases, and technological advances all contribute to growth in health care spending. As additional monies are allocated to health care, other sectors of the economy do not have access to those same resources. The political dilemmas that flow from conflicting claims for use of the available monies are considerable. Though most consumers express concern over rising costs, they are insulated to a considerable extent because of their private health insurance, Medicare, Medicaid, or other third-party payment arrangements. The principal groups that are most concerned in the clash over access to resources are business and industrial leaders, insurers, government, and those who would like to buy health insurance but cannot afford it.

Various tactics to reduce the cost of health care have been attempted, all with limited success. Price controls, reduced-payment schemes, shifting of responsibilities between and among responsible parties, and regulation have all been part of the cost-containment efforts.

Most recently, competition in health care delivery has shifted the focus to outcomes analysis and standards of care to reduce variation in treatment. Outcomes analysis will allow health care providers to determine the highest quality of care at the lowest costs by comparing methods of treatment and eliminating ineffective, high-cost procedures and products. However, outcomes analysis requires financial investment in computer technology and research personnel. Some may view standards of care as intrusive and a violation of both physician and patient autonomy.

The business of health care delivery, although focused on containing costs, must also emphasize quality care. Changes in the financing of health care, discussed in Chapter 3, give us a better picture of the relationships among costs, quality, patient choice, and the debate over health care as a right or a privilege.

ACTIVITY-BASED LEARNING

Do you know the cost of a visit to a physician? If you have or a family member has recently visited the doctor, what was the cost of the visit? How much of it did you (or the family member) pay? How much did the insurance (if there was coverage) pay? Did this cover the entire bill, or was there a portion that seemed to disappear (through write-off)?

Is it possible to determine what the cost to the consumer and/or the insurance company would be for a specific surgical or diagnostic procedure? Call a local hospital to ask the cost of a typical surgical procedure such as an appendectomy or angioplasty.

A QUESTION OF ETHICS

- Is health care delivery a business venture? How is it the same as any other business? How does it differ?

- How much is enough? Should we, as a society, really be concerned with how great a portion of our economy is focused on health care?

REFERENCES

1. Anderson G., Grogner, B., & Reinhardt, U. (2007). Health spending in OECD countries in 2004: An update. *Health Affairs, 26*(5), 1481–1489.

2. Bureau of Labor Statistics, U.S. Department of Labor. 2008. *Career guide to industries, 2008–09 edition*. Health Care. Retrieved July 29, 2008, from http://www.bls.gov/oco/cg/cgs035.htm

3. Edwards, M., Garland, M., Bonazzola, M., & Crawshaw, R. (1999). "Care" that cares: Medicine's essential patient-centered ethic. *Pharos,* Fall, 20–23.

4. He, W., Sengupta, M., Velkoff, V., & DeBarros, K. (2005). *U.S. Census Bureau, current population reports*, P23-209, *65+ in the United States: 2005*. Washington, DC: U.S. Government Printing Office. Retrieved from www.census.gov/prod/2006pubs/p23-209.pdf

5. Institute of Medicine. (2001). *Crossing the quality chasm: A new health system for the 21st century*. Washington, DC: National Academy Press.

6. Institute of Medicine. (2000). *To err is human: Building a safer health system*. Washington, DC: National Academy Press.

7. Medicare. (2007). *Medicare premiums and coinsurance rates for 2007*. Retrieved from questions.medicare.gov/cgi-bin/medicare.cfg/php/enduser/std_adp.php?p_faqid=1847

8. Moskowitz, D. (1999). *Health care almanac and yearbook*. New York: Faulkner & Gray.

9. National Center for Health Statistics. (2007). Health, United States, 2007 with chartbook on trends in the health of Americans. Hyattsville, MD. Retrieved from www.cdc.gov/nchs/data/hus/hus07.pdf

10. Raffel, M., & Raffel, N. (1994). *The U.S. health system, origins and functions* (4ᵗʰ ed). Albany, NY: Delmar Publishers, p. 192.

11. Reinhardt, U. (2007a). U.S. health care stands Adam Smith on his head. *British Medical Journal*, *335*(7628), 1020.

12. Reinhardt, U. (2007b). The U.S. muddle over a child's right to health care. *British Medical Journal*, *335*(7623), 749.

13. Welch, W. (2004, March 18). Medicare cost estimates are no shock to some. *USA Today*. Retrieved from http://www.usatoday.com/news/washington/2004-03-18-medicare-costs_x.htm

Chapter 3

Paying for Health Care Services

CHAPTER OBJECTIVES

After completing this chapter, readers should have an understanding of the following:

- The origin and development of health insurance in the United States
- The variety of health insurance plans available
- The government programs of Medicare and Medicaid
- Alternative and emerging methods of paying for health care
- Problems inherent in each of the health care payment mechanisms

INTRODUCTION

Estimates vary concerning how many people in the United States are protected against the high costs of health care. Some estimate that insurance and government programs cover about 85 percent of the U.S. resident population. In 2007, U.S. Census Bureau figures indicated that nearly 46 million Americans were without any health insurance protection sometime during the year (DeNavas-Walt et al. 2008). Although the exact figures may change depending on the sources of data, the fact remains that many people are still unprotected from health care costs and must rely on whatever out-of-pocket funds they might have available to them or on charity to pay for care. For some people who are uninsured, securing access to care can be difficult. Even among those who are insured or who are enrolled in a government program, many are underinsured and do not have adequate protection against hospital, physician, nursing home, dental, and pharmacy charges. Both private insurance and government programs have shortcomings, and these are a cause for social concern.

THE INSURED POPULATION

The United States has what is primarily an employment-based health insurance system. The majority of people who have health insurance obtain it through their place of employment (group policies). However, some people, mainly the self-employed and others who are not eligible for group enrollment, have nongroup insurance (individual policies). The principal differences between group and individual coverage are that group insurance generally costs less and has a broader range of benefits. An estimated 67.5 percent of people with insurance have what is referred to as private insurance—policies with Blue Cross and Blue Shield or one of the large commercial insurance companies (Aetna, United HealthCare, CIGNA, and so on). Some 27.8 percent of those insured are protected against health care costs under government programs (DeNavas-Walt et al. 2008). Government programs include Medicare, an entitlement program principally for those age 65 and older, which also protects a small number of (approximately 3 million) younger people who fall into certain disability categories. More than 38 million people also received benefits in 2007 under Medicaid, a federal or state government program designed to pay for health care for certain categories of people who are very poor. Many of these people (some 5.5 million people in 2005) were Medicare enrollees who became **dual eligible**—also eligible for Medicaid because of their low income (DeNavas-Walt et al. 2008; CMS 2007a).

Protection against health care costs is also available through various other government programs for: (1) military personnel; (2) their dependents in the military system and through a program known as the Civilian Health and Medical Program of the Uniformed Services (CHAMPUS); (3) Native Americans and Alaskan natives through the Indian Health Service; and (4) veterans who are totally dependent through the U.S. Department of Veterans Affairs (see Table 3–1).

The figures cited about the number of people with insurance and otherwise protected are estimates, and the estimates vary depending on the rate of unemployment in the country, business conditions, and the changing eligibility standards for Medicaid and other government programs. Those not protected by health insurance or by government programs are not only individuals who are unemployed. These people may be employed part-time, between jobs, employed with incomes too high to qualify for Medicaid but not high enough to afford health insurance, working in some small businesses that do not offer health insurance, and who choose not to have health insurance (DeNavas-Walt et al. 2008). In fact, most of those without insurance in 2006 were in paid employment (see Table 3–2).

People who have the protection of health insurance often feel a sense of satisfaction, but inadequate coverage against the costs of medical care can be a cause for great social concern. Some health insurance policies exclude coverage for conditions that existed at the time of enrollment (preexisting conditions). Other policies insist that people with insurance must wait a certain period of time (typically one year) before the company will cover a preexisting condition. Most policies place a limit on how much is paid for hospital care, physician care, nursing home care, and the like through annual limits, lifetime limits, or fee schedules. In an effort to make people with insurance more aware of health care costs and therefore more responsible health care consumers, many policies require portions of the costs to be paid by the insured, including the following:

- Deductibles: money patients must pay (out of pocket) before an insurance policy provides benefits
- Coinsurance: a percentage of the costs of each service that people with insurance must pay along with the insurance payment (for example, a payment of 80 percent of the

TABLE 3–1 Coverage by Type of Health Insurance: 2004 and 2005

Insurance	% covered in 2004	% covered in 2005
Any private plan	68.2	67.7
Employment-based	59.8	59.5
Direct purchase	9.3	9.1
Any government plan	27.3	27.3
Medicare	13.6	13.7
Medicaid	13.0	13.0
Military	3.7	3.8
Uninsured	15.6	15.9

SOURCE: U.S. Census Bureau, Current Populations Survey, 2005 and 2006 Annual Social and Economic Supplements.

TABLE 3–2 **Work Characteristics of the Uninsured**

Characteristics	2005		2006	
	Number	Percentage	Number	Percentage
Total 18- to 64-year-olds	36,315	19.7	37,792	20.2
Worked during the year	26,293	18.0	27,627	18.7
Worked full-time	20,780	17.2	22,010	17.9
Worked part-time	5,513	22.1	5,618	22.9
Did not work	10,022	26.1	10,165	26.1

SOURCE: U.S. Census Bureau, Current Population Survey, 2006 and 2007 Annual Social and Economic Supplements.

cost by the insurance and 20 percent of the cost by the patient)

• Co-pay: a flat fee paid for each type of service (for example, a patient pays $20 for each physician visit or $5 for each prescription filled)

Why are there such a variety of policies with so many limitations that ultimately force a patient or patient's family to meet a significant portion of the costs of care? Why can't we have a comprehensive benefit structure for all people? What good is all the insurance if it does not protect?

The answers to these questions are rooted in at least two factors: social choice and historical developments that shaped the health insurance industry. In his 1974 book *Who Shall Live?* Victor Fuchs offered this explanation as it relates to social choice:

> The most basic level of choice is between health and other goals. While social reformers tell us that "health is a right," the realization of that "right" is always less than complete because some of the resources that could be used for health are allocated to other purposes. This is true in all countries regardless of economic system, regardless of the way medical care is organized, and regardless of the level of affluence. (p. 17)

Although most Americans express concern over the numbers of uninsured people, we have been unwilling to provide comprehensive coverage even for a limited population group—the elderly. As each year passes, benefits are cut and the elderly are forced to pay more. In theory, universal health care coverage is desirable. However, fear of increased taxes, government

control, and loss of some benefits by those with extensive health insurance, prevents us from moving toward implementing the theory. However, Menzel and Light (2006) remind us of an important factor:

> A common conservative argument against "government health insurance" is thus that people should take care of themselves. Paradoxically, however, this belief also forms an argument for universal health insurance: people need universal access to basic health care in order to maximize their ability to care for themselves. When people are ill, individual liberty and personal responsibility are quickly compromised. (p. 38)

A second answer to the questions posed earlier lies in the history of health insurance in the United States, and in the principles of health insurance rate structuring.

HISTORY OF HEALTH INSURANCE

The year 1929 is generally credited as marking the birth of modern health insurance. In that year, Justin Ford Kimball established a hospital insurance plan at the Baylor University Medical Center at Dallas for the schoolteachers of Dallas, Texas. As a one-time superintendent of the Dallas public schools, he was sensitive to the plight of schoolteachers, particularly so when he found many of them had unpaid bills at the hospital. Working from hospital records, he calculated that the schoolteachers as a group "incurred an average of 15 cents a month in hospital bills. To assure a safe margin, he established a rate of 50 cents a month" (Anderson 1975, 19). For those 50 cents per month, the schoolteachers were assured twenty-one days of hospitalization in a semiprivate room.

Kimball's success spread, and his approach became the national Blue Cross plan model: the concept of assuring the benefit not of cash but of service, the emphasis on semiprivate accommodations, and even the time frame of twenty-one days of benefits. Though 1929 is cited as the beginning, there were antecedents. Anderson (1975) notes the following, for example:

> Between 1916 and 1918, attempts were made by 16 state legislatures from New York to California to establish some form of compulsory health insurance, essentially a mechanism to help families pay for health services, which were already being felt as costly and unpredictable episodes. The necessary mass political support in the states was not present, however, and the solid opposition of the American Medical Association, insurance companies, and the pharmaceutical industry, not to mention business and industry opposed to unaccustomed payroll taxes, stopped the movement. (p. 17)

The Health Insurance Institute (1978) also cites antecedents:

> When health insurance began some 130 years ago, it met a far simpler need—coverage against rail and steamboat accidents. The nation's first health insurance company came into being in 1847. Three years later another company was organized specifically to write accident insurance. By 1864, coverage was available for virtually every type of accident. At the turn of the century, 47 companies were issuing accident insurance. . . .
>
> Both accident insurance companies and life insurance companies entered the health insurance field in the early 1900s. At the beginning, the insurance largely covered the policyholders' loss of earned income due to a limited number of diseases, among them typhus, typhoid, scarlet fever, smallpox, diphtheria, and diabetes.
>
> This was the birth of modern health insurance. The demand for the new product grew as the Depression of the 1930s deepened. Out of this emerged the Blue Cross service concept, which foreshadowed insurance company reimbursement policies for hospital and surgical care. Also during the 1930s, insurance companies began to emphasize the availability of cash benefit plans for hospital, surgical, and medical expenses. The first Blue Shield type of plan for surgical and medical expenses was formed in 1939. (p. 7)

In addition, the single hospital benefit plan was organized in 1912 at Rockford, Illinois; the Grinnell, Iowa hospital plan in 1921; and the Brattleboro, Vermont plan in 1927. Each offered payment for limited hospital services. However, the idea Kimball at Baylor developed was the model that spread. The American Hospital Association (AHA) asked Kimball to describe the Baylor plan at its annual meeting in 1931. Other hospital administrators also developed interest; by 1935, eleven states had fifteen hospital insurance plans, and six additional plans developed during 1936. "Concurrently, there was a move to create a coordinating agency of some sort to give the now rapidly growing movement a national focus and a broad base" (Anderson 1975, 36). This was done within the framework of the AHA, evolving over the years to a semiautonomous body and eventually to a completely independent Blue Cross Commission and, later, Blue Cross Association.

Anderson notes that the early leadership came not from hospitals but from early pioneers, farsighted individuals, some of whom were hospital accountants or **actuaries**. The hospitals, says Anderson, were "timid in their backing of prepayment." After all, it was a new idea, an experiment. "Originally, the plans covered only employees and not their dependents; the dependents were an unknown and feared quantity **actuarially**. But common sense and equity would shortly have it that dependents should be covered too, and so they were" (Anderson 1975, 43).

The Blue Cross movement surged ahead in the 1940s, with a nationwide enrollment of 6 million subscribers in 1940, spread through fifty-six independent Blue Cross plans. "By 1945, the enrollment was up to 19 million in eighty plans, and by the early 1950s, it was 40 million. By that time, private insurance companies were also coming up from behind after an early lack of interest in insuring against hospital costs" (Anderson 1975, 45).

The Health Insurance Institute (1978) states the following:

> During World War II, as a result of the freezing of wages, group health insurance became an important component of collective bargaining. Even greater impetus came in the postwar era when the U.S. Supreme Court ruled that employee benefits, including health insurance, were a legitimate part of the labor-management bargaining process. (p. 8)

As Blue Cross began to demonstrate the feasibility of covering hospital expenses through the insurance mechanism, pressures to do likewise for physician services also developed. The pressures accelerated following the 1932 report of the Committee on the Costs of Medical Care, with its challenge to organized medicine. In 1939, the California Medical Association established the California Physicians' Service, which was the first of what became known as the Blue Shield plans for payment of doctors' bills. Like Blue Cross, Blue Shield operated on a service benefits principle: The California plan provided complete physician services at a rate of $1.70 per month (Hawley 1949):

> Enrollment was limited to employed persons earning less than $3,000 per year. Physicians were reimbursed on a "unit" basis, the unit having a par value of $2.50 (the fee for an office visit), with other services being valued at multiples of this unit (unit value scale). (p. 36)

Two things are important to note in this historical development. First, California developed the unit-value scale. (A similar concept known as the relative-value scale was developed for Medicare in the 1990s and will be described later in this chapter, in the "Paying Physicians" section.) Most Blue Shield plans did not, however, use this method for establishing their schedules of payments. Second, the need to devalue the unit was acceptable to the medical profession because the plan was sponsored by medical society: The physicians were obligated to deliver the service regardless of what the plan could pay. The arrangement was acceptable to physicians because they had a say in the management of the plan. Throughout the Blue Shield movement, physicians had dominated the boards of directors not only because they underwrote the plan but also because the plans were truly their response to the challenge for national health insurance and because the plans met the American Medical Association's (AMA) principles of keeping medical matters in the hands of physicians.

A similar situation existed with Blue Cross. Participating hospitals agreed to accept the Blue Cross payment as full payment for care in a semiprivate room. If the Blue Cross plan could not pay the agreed-upon cost, then the hospital would accept whatever Blue Cross could pay and not bill the patient for any additional monies. Thus, Blue Cross offered its subscribers service benefits rather than lump-sum or **indemnity** benefits. In the early days of Blue Cross, quite a few plans had to pay hospitals less than 100 cents on the dollar, and hospitals tended to dominate Blue Cross boards. Both Blue Cross and Blue Shield have changed their board structures because the plan underwriting by the providers of service is now less a fact of life. Even when Blue Cross paid a hospital full cost, it was frequently discounted. Because the hospital was assured payment, the discounted amount was acceptable.

Both Blue Cross and Blue Shield were service-benefit plans, relying mainly on type of accommodation (semiprivate room) as the determinant of service-benefit eligibility. Blue Shield relied on income of the patient or patient's family. Blue Cross provided benefits for subscribers who used private rooms, and Blue Shield provided benefits for patients who were above income requirements, by having patients pay the additional charges, if any.

Blue Cross worked quite well. The Blue Shield service-benefit principle did not work well. The reasons for this failure were historical and developmental. When Blue Shield first began, physicians commonly charged patients on a sliding fee scale, charging wealthy people more to pay for care of the poor, and so on. The early Blue Shield payments for various services were designed for the going rate in the service-benefit income category. As the economy developed, and inflation along with it, the Blue Shield schedule of payments provided service-benefit payments for fewer subscribers because they were increasingly above the maximum income. Blue Shield made the same dollar payment for services rendered, but because the patient was above the service-benefit income level, the patient frequently had to pay an additional amount to the physician.

This situation led some Blue Shield plan executives to develop different types of contracts with different service-benefit income levels, allowance schedules geared to each level, and, of course, premiums geared to the allowances. However, still the Blue Shield service benefits, when geared to subscriber income, did not work well because of inflation and the difficulties in determining subscriber income. Patients were left to discuss their income level with their physicians, and both parties were reluctant to talk about money when patients were sick. Resulting misunderstandings were common. In time, many executives of Blue Shield plans (as well as commercial insurance and eventually Medicare) developed contracts with "usual, customary, and reasonable (UCR) allowances" (this will be described further in the "Paying Physicians" section later in this chapter).

Another problem Blue Shield faced with regard to service benefits developed as a result of the changing health system. Initially, radiology, pathology, and anesthesiology were hospital services that Blue Cross covered. During the 1950s and 1960s, many of the hospital-based physicians in these specialties moved out from under the hospital umbrella to do their own billing while still housed in the hospital, and many also established their own offices. Blue Cross generally was not allowed by law to pay for physician services as such, but only for hospital services. Blue

Shield rate structures were not geared to pay these professional services because they had never been calculated or anticipated in structuring the rates. For a while, subscribers were caught in a bind and had to pay the bills until Blue Shield was able to adjust its rates to incorporate these benefits. However, then Blue Shield had to encourage the groups, mainly the employers, to go along with the increased rates. Not all were willing to do so unless they had to, and those who worked with unions would not do so until the next round of collective-bargaining sessions began, when these new benefits could become a management concession.

Both Blue Cross and Blue Shield also faced similar situations in later years as new, often expensive, technology developed. If they paid for equipment under existing rates because payments were close to or at cost, hospitals would be encouraged to expand and pass the increased costs on to Blue Cross. The new equipment would be averaged with all other costs and be built into what all admissions would cost. If Blue Cross covered such items, a rate increase would eventually be necessary, and a rate increase would give competitors an advantage. The pressures on both Blue Cross and Blue Shield became even more acute as they acted as fiscal intermediaries (agencies handling the payments) for Medicare. The federal government sought to pressure the Blues (a term frequently used for the Blue Cross and Blue Shield movement) and others to stem rising costs. Pressure also came from state governments, which were affected by the rising costs of Medicaid. If the Blues held the line, the federal or state Medicaid program would benefit.

Generally, the Blue Cross plans provided great support and assistance to the developing Blue Shield plans. Typically, they used the same salaried sales forces, the same personnel systems, the same offices, and sometimes the same executive staffs. Although the governing boards were generally different and the corporations generally separate from a legal standpoint, in nearly all states, special enabling legislation for both plans made them legally different from ordinary insurance companies. In some states, there were bitter conflicts between the Blue Cross plan and local medical societies that sponsored Blue Shield. These conflicts even reached the national level in 1948, for example, when the AMA opposed a proposed merger of Blue Cross and Blue Shield at the national level for purposes of enrolling national accounts.

Why the conflict? The AMA's position was based on fear that it would be accused of restraint of trade. It also feared that Blue Cross, representing the hospitals, would dominate the national joint venture, and the views of medicine would not

be adequately represented (Anderson 1975). Like the conflicts within the states, this reflected an age-old fear on the part of physicians that nonmedical people would tell doctors how to practice medicine. Hospital executives, by the same token, were wary of physicians telling them how to run hospitals.

Though a mechanism for enrolling national accounts was eventually successful, the national Blue Shield and Blue Cross organizations did not successfully merge until 1978. Part of the reason for the successful merger was that, by 1978, under pressures from state insurance departments and the federal government, the Blue Cross and Blue Shield plans were less than surrogates for the providers; they were becoming true third-party payers.

HEALTH INSURANCE RATE STRUCTURING (PREMIUM CALCULATION)

Premium errors in the early days of Blue Cross came about because the plans did not have a reliable statistical base available for predicting what their utilization would be. No one else had the data either. A great deal of information had to be weighed into the equation for calculating what the premium should be. Not only did the amount paid to hospitals have to be calculated, but also an amount for overhead costs had to be included in the premium charged. Overhead costs included the salaries of those who worked for Blue Cross, office space, supplies, utilities, and so on.

Deciding on a rate to charge is complicated because Blue Cross worked with the **community rate** idea; in the beginning, it enrolled not communities but representative bodies or groups of the community—typically, groups of employees.

In a small group, perhaps less than twenty employees, Blue Cross would probably say that the small group is not typical for its rate and may respond by offering to write an individual contract or policy. However, it may not cover any preexisting conditions. Moreover, Blue Cross will charge more for a policy because of higher risks of determining the likelihood that subscribers may incur high health care expenses and higher administrative costs (contracting, billing, and so on, for four individual policies rather than one group). Thus, Blue Cross and Blue Shield typically offer nongroup enrollment for those who are not eligible for group enrollment.

Blue Cross is not the only health insurance available. In a competitive insurance market, insurers look for ways to entice employers to buy their plans. One way is through "**experience rating**" rather than community rating. Community rating was conducted through determining statistical probability of how many people in a group might experience a certain disease. Experience rating takes into account the probability of disease among a specific group based on age, occupational risk, lifestyles, and so on. A large insurance company could offer a health insurance policy with about the same benefits as Blue Cross at a lower cost if the group to be insured is low risk. It would base its rate on the group's experience (or performance). Alternatively, the insurance company could charge the same as Blue Cross but provide greater benefits. The commercial company does not need the unused premium money from the low-risk group to carry the losses incurred with a high-risk group, as does Blue Cross. If the commercial company enrolled a high-risk group, its rate would bear a relationship to its experience or anticipated claims performance.

With an experience-rated policy, the commercial insurance company is thus not likely to lose. At worst, it takes a loss for one year only and then adjusts its premiums accordingly the next year. If the competition takes away too many low-risk groups, Blue Cross is forced to seek a rate increase that, in turn, might make it noncompetitive.

Blue Cross has thus had to engage in experience rating also, simply to remain competitive and to keep a contingency fund. However, the process has undermined the concept of the community rate and has driven up health insurance costs. The result is higher premiums for those who are sicker.

In recent years, the underwriting by hospitals and physicians has been inconsequential because the economic pressures that exist today prevent any subsidization. Hospitals and doctors can no longer cost-shift (use higher payments from some patients to subsidize low, or no, payment from others). Instead, insurance rates rise, and health care providers are forced to operate more efficiently if payers begin to lower their payments to providers.

HEALTH INSURANCE TODAY

At one time, four basic groups provided protection against the costs of health care services: commercial insurance companies, the nonprofit Blue Cross and Blue Shield plans, health maintenance organizations (HMOs), and government plans. However, changes have occurred among third-party payers, just as they have occurred among health care delivery organizations. Many new forms and many hybrid forms of health plans are now available. The development of Blue Cross and Blue Shield has been discussed at length, but other forms of health plans existed earlier and continue to develop today.

Commercial Insurance

Most private health insurance companies (commercial insurance companies) restrict their business to group coverage, generally through places of employment; Aetna, Prudential, and CIGNA are examples of such companies. Other companies focus primarily on individual policies, and the benefits of these nongroup plans tend to be the most limited in terms of the amounts paid for care, the types of care covered, and who is covered.

The group commercial companies are able to be less restrictive, because they emphasize group enrollment. If a large group is enrolled, then all members of the group can be enrolled and no person will normally be excluded because of poor health. Some group commercial companies selectively exclude people with health problems from enrolling in small employee groups or charge higher rates for that person than for the rest of the small group members. This practice, known as selective medical underwriting, was designed to hold down the cost of the insurance for other employees, but undermines the very purpose of insurance as a way to spread the risk. Concern over selective underwriting has led many states to prohibit the practice.

The **Health Insurance Portability and Accountability Act of 1996 (HIPAA)** also made broad changes in health insurance availability, primarily by eliminating many of the practices of excluding people from coverage because of preexisting conditions. If a person had group coverage by one employer and moved to another employer, the second employer's insurance could exclude that person. This helped to reduce **job lock**—a term used to describe people who stay in jobs they don't really like or want, simply to maintain their health insurance. HIPAA also made individual health insurance coverage more available by mandating that companies providing group insurance must also provide an individual insurance product (U.S. Department of Labor 2007).

The benefits that group insurance companies provide tend to be more liberal than those that nongroup companies provide, but what is and is not covered vary depending on what the group wants and is willing to pay for. As with Blue Cross and

Blue Shield, the benefits may vary in terms of the number of days covered in hospital, the dollar amounts paid for surgical and medical care, whether office medical care is included, and whether nursing home care, home health services, dental, vision, and major medical expenses are covered.

Nearly all people enrolled in commercial insurance plans and the nonprofit Blue Cross and Blue Shield plans are covered for hospital and physician care; lesser numbers are covered for dental and vision care, though such coverage is growing. Major medical expense insurance, sometimes called catastrophic insurance, was first introduced in 1951, by the commercial companies and also became available through Blue Cross and Blue Shield plans. Typically, major medical insurance covers 80 percent of all residual medical expenses (that is, it covers 80 percent of all expenses that regular hospital, medical, and surgical policies do not cover) after the individual with insurance pays the deductible. The deductible may vary from $500 to $1,500 or more, depending on what the group wants and is willing to pay for. For catastrophic illness, the bills can mount, so these policies tend to pay 80 percent up to a maximum of perhaps $250,000 or more.

Both deductibles and coinsurance are mechanisms designed to limit costs and to give greater responsibility for the use of services to individuals with insurance. The assumption is that insured people will not likely incur unnecessary expenses by overusing medical care. High deductibles may reduce the potential to overuse care, however, for a person who really needs the added services, the costs can be significant and a deterrent to receiving needed care. In recognition of this problem, many policies now set a limit of $2,000 to $3,000, which the patient has to pay, after which the policies pay all costs. When an insurance company and a patient or two companies share the payment of costs, the policy is considered coinsurance.

Self-Insured Health Plans

Each state sets standards for fiduciary responsibilities, minimum coverage, reporting responsibilities, disclosure responsibilities to policyholders, and so on, for insurance companies. Within this framework, large interstate businesses have difficulty complying with multistate regulations when providing health insurance benefits to employees in diverse locations (for example, large companies like Ford, Federal Express, International Paper, or General Electric have manufacturing facilities and offices in many states). In 1974, Congress passed the Employee Retirement Income Security Act (ERISA). Although a major thrust of the legislation was to set standards for securing retirement plan funds,

the act also set regulations by which employers could establish self-insured health benefits plans. In other words, employers could set aside funds to pay for employees' medical expenses and pay them directly from the fund rather than purchasing a group plan from an insurance company. Self-insured plans were defined as employee health benefits plans and differentiated from health insurance. As such, health benefits plans were exempt from state regulations. Interstate employers could thus set up plans that were the same for all of their employees without regard to their geographic location.

ERISA also provided other benefits to employers who self-insured. Not only did the act remove state regulation from the benefits plans, but also the federal regulations covering these plans were very liberal. Federal regulations addressed the process rather than the content of employee benefits plans—reporting requirements, disclosure, and fiduciary conduct. Unlike state regulations, the federal regulations did little to set standards for minimum coverage, reduction, or termination of benefits. Employers had more latitude in deciding just what procedures or treatments that the benefits plans would cover.

Employer self-insured plans are often difficult to differentiate from health insurance for employees because employers often contract with well-known insurance companies to administer their plans. However, the difference is significant operationally. Although the issue is outside the scope of discussion in this text, ERISA has become problematic when states attempt to establish statewide universal health insurance for all residents because ERISA exempts employee benefits plans from any state regulations.

Government Plans

Government plans fall into another category of third-party payers for health care. In this category are a number of programs that have already been cited, such as those for military personnel and their dependents; for veterans with service-connected disabilities and disabilities not service-connected if they are unable to afford private care; and for Native Americans and Alaskan natives. The principal programs addressed here are Medicare and Medicaid. These programs were established when Congress amended the Social Security Act in 1965, adding to it Title XVIII (Medicare legislation) and Title XIX (Medicaid legislation).

Medicare

Medicare is a health insurance program for people age 65 and above, regardless of income or wealth. In 1972, provisions were added to cover people under 65 with long-term disabilities, and those who suffer from end-stage renal (kidney) disease (ESRD) that require a kidney transplant or dialysis treatment.

Medicare originally consisted of two parts: Part A primarily for inpatient care, and Part B for **ambulatory care**. **Medicare Part A** provides coverage for in-hospital care, skilled nursing care, hospice, and home health care. Part A benefits are financed by Social Security taxes and Medicare payroll taxes, require no premium payment by the beneficiary, and are automatic for those 65 and over. Although Medicare provides health care coverage without a premium cost to the beneficiary, it is not by any means free health care. Benefits require deductibles and coinsurance provisions that the enrollee pays.

Some of the benefits of Medicare Part A (for the year 2008) are as follows (Medicare 2008):

- Up to ninety days of inpatient care for each benefit period. A new benefit period begins after the patient has been out of the hospital or skilled nursing facility for sixty consecutive days. The inpatient hospital deductible is $1,024 for each benefit period. There is also a $256-a-day coinsurance for the sixty-first through ninetieth days, and a $512-a-day coinsurance for each "nonrenewable, lifetime reserve day (sixty extra days of hospitalization)."

- Up to 100 days in a skilled nursing facility, with Medicare paying the full cost for the first twenty days and the patient paying $128 a day for each day thereafter. To be eligible for this benefit, the patient must have been in the hospital for three consecutive days prior to being transferred to skilled nursing care.

- Unlimited home health visits by a participating home health agency for **intermittent care**, including skilled nursing, physical therapy, or speech therapy for patients confined to their home and needing care as certified by a physician. The deductible does not apply to home health visits.

- **Hospice** care in a home or homelike environment for the terminally ill. A wide range of medical and social services is available, including medical, nursing, and social work services, respite care, and short-term inpatient care, as well as homemaker services. All services are available without charge to the patient except for some sharing of the cost for outpatient drugs and inpatient respite care.

Many elderly have additional insurance to cover the Medicare deductibles and co-payments (referred to as Medigap, or Medicare supplemental insurance). A small number of people over 65 who are not automatically eligible for Medicare because of insufficient work experience for the necessary Social Security credits may receive Medicare coverage by paying a monthly premium ($423 in 2008).

Medicare beneficiaries must bear in mind one additional factor: Hospital care must be medically necessary and must be a type of care that only a hospital can provide. If the hospital's **utilization review** committee or another **peer review organization (PRO)** does not approve the hospital stay after the patient's admission (for example, the organization determines that inpatient care was not needed), then they may retroactively deny benefits, and the patient may have to pay all costs or the hospital may have to bear the loss.

Medicare Part B is supplementary medical insurance. It is optional, and Part A beneficiaries must pay for it if they agree to enroll; therefore, most people do subscribe to it (see Table 3–3). In fact, Part B enrollment is automatic unless recipients inform Social Security that they do not want coverage and to discontinue deductions for it from their Social Security checks. Part B provides the following important insurance benefits:

- Part B covers payment of reasonable physician charges after the patient pays the initial annual deductible ($135 for 2008).

- Part B covers hospital outpatient, ambulance, and emergency department services under the same $135 deductible.

TABLE 3–3 Medicare Enrollment—Aged Beneficiaries as of July 2006

	A and/or B	A only	B only	A and B
U.S. and outlying areas	36,255,198	2,125,510	362,356	33,767,332
U.S. only	35,224,339	1,645,432	350,330	33,228,577

SOURCE: Centers for Medicare and Medicaid Services. Retrieved from www.cms.hhs.gov/MedicareEnRpts/Downloads/06Aged.pdf.

Medicare pays 80 percent of the approved amount; the patient is responsible for the remaining 20 percent.

- Part B covers a number of other services and supplies, such as outpatient physical and speech therapy, diagnostic X-ray examinations, medical supplies, prosthetics, limited chiropractic services, and so on.

Medigap insurance may pay the deductibles and coinsurance of Medicare Part B, depending on the coverage the patient secures. For the year 2008, Part B cost Medicare beneficiaries $96.40 per month. Additional costs come out of federal general revenue. As health care costs go up, so do the premium charges, but the law requires that the premium increase to the recipient be limited to the percentage rise in Social Security income.

The Centers for Medicare and Medicaid Services (CMS), formerly the Health Care Financing Administration (HCFA), under the Department of Health and Human Services oversees the Medicare program. It handles some payments directly, but most payments for care are made by fiscal intermediaries for Part A and carriers for Part B, with whom CMS contracts. The contractors are mainly Blue Cross, Blue Shield, and commercial insurance companies. Contractors must rebid for the position approximately every three years.

Medicare clearly helps people who are aged and eligible to pay for needed health services. Many of the beneficiaries are on fixed incomes and may still have to pay considerable sums when hospitalization and skilled nursing facility care are necessary. Medigap, which helps with those expenses, is expensive in itself. Medicare Part A and B do not cover some expensive items, such as prescription drugs, hearing exams and hearing aids, and eyeglasses (Medicare 2007).

Although Medicare payments represent a sizable portion of most physicians' incomes, getting physicians to accept assignment in its early days was not easy. Some physicians would accept assignment in all cases, but many more accepted assignment on a selective or case-by-case basis, presumably basing the decision on whether they thought the patient could afford to pay more than the fee Medicare had established as being reasonable. Some physicians never accepted assignment. Massachusetts dealt with this issue by requiring that all physicians accept assignment in all cases if they wished to retain their license to practice there. A number of states have since adopted similar legislation.

Congress began to deal with this problem first by instituting a Medicare participating physician (MPP) program, whereby physicians who agreed to participate would accept all cases on assignment. Those who did not agree to accept all cases on assignment would have to bill all transactions to Medicare, but would not receive direct payments. Payment would go to the patients, and the physicians would have to bill the patients. They would not be able to make case-by-case decisions whether to accept assignment. Congress also directed that the names of all participating physicians be published so that Medicare patients could determine beforehand whether a physician was an MPP. Other incentives to participate include shorter turnaround time for payments, rollover of Medicare payment information to Medigap insurers to reduce paperwork for participants, and access to toll-free telephone numbers for support services. The number of physicians accepting assignment has thus increased significantly because of actions by various federal and state governments. Whether as a result of legislation or acceptance of Medicare, nearly 73 percent of physicians accepted new Medicare patients between 2004 and 2005 (Cunningham et al. 2006). Participation rates for physicians (MDs and ODs) in 2006 went up to 94.7 percent (see Table 3–4 in this text) (CMS 2006a).

As stated before, Medicare legislation that created Parts A and B was passed in 1965. More recent legislation and demonstration projects have brought about what are known as Medicare Parts C and D.

Medicare Part C is an option available to people eligible for Medicare. HMO or PPO plans provide care that Medicare approves. Although Part A and Part B allow choice of health care providers, Part C requires participants to choose doctors and other providers within their network. Participants must still pay the Part B premium and may actually be required to pay an additional fee based on the expanded services they may receive. Part C (also called Medicare Advantage) eliminates the need for supplemental Medigap insurance because deductibles and coinsurance costs are nonexistent. Small co-pays at the time of care may be required. Part C actually places participants in a managed care plan that makes Medicare somewhat invisible. Increased benefits to participants might be preventive services, vision care, and even prescription drugs. In administering Part C, CMS pays a flat fee per patient to the managed care plan. The managed care plan must "manage" the care of the members with appropriate preventive services and location-appropriate (inpatient versus outpatient) care. The managed care organization is at risk for paying costs greater than the amount Medicare pays to them (Medicare 2007).

TABLE 3-4 Participation Rates as Percentage of Physicians, by Specialty Selected Periods

Percent of Physicians Participating	2000	2001	2002	2003	2004	2005	2006
Physicians (MDs and DOs)	-	-	90.3	91.2	91.9	93.0	94.7
General practice	80.2	79.0	80.2	84.3	84.8	84.5	88.6
General surgery	93.3	92.5	92.8	95.6	95.5	95.2	96.2
Otology, laryngology, rhinology	91.8	91.3	91.7	93.9	94.5	94.1	95.1
Anesthesiology	93.7	92.3	92.3	95.5	95.4	95.1	96.8
Cardiovascular disease	95.8	94.4	94.3	96.4	96.1	96.1	97.1
Dermatology	90.8	90.1	90.1	92.4	92.9	92.6	93.8
Family practice	90.8	90.3	90.8	93.2	93.7	93.8	94.8
Internal medicine	90.7	88.7	88.8	92.2	92.9	92.9	94.8
Neurology	92.1	89.9	89.1	93.3	94.0	93.0	94.6
Obstetrics/gynecology	86.8	86.3	86.5	88.8	89.1	89.4	91.5
Ophthalmology	93.3	92.8	93.3	95.1	95.0	94.9	96.0
Orthopedic surgery	93.8	93.1	92.4	95.5	95.8	95.6	96.1
Pathology	93.6	92.2	92.0	95.4	95.3	94.4	96.4
Psychiatry	79.1	79.6	80.4	83.0	82.8	83.3	87.4
Radiology	95.3	91.9	91.6	95.7	95.6	95.4	97.4
Urology	94.6	93.8	93.6	96.0	96.2	96.1	96.9
Nephrology	95.1	93.6	93.6	95.5	95.6	95.4	96.7
Clinic/other group practice	91.6	92.7	93.5	93.4	92.1	91.7	82.7
Limited license practitioners (LLP):							
Chiropractor	59.4	63.0	64.4	65.2	70.4		
Podiatry—surgical chiropody	90.7	91.6	92.1	92.3	93.4		
Optometrist	78.4	80.0	80.6	82.4	83.1		

NOTE: Effective with the October 1, 1985 election period, carriers were instructed to count individuals only once.

SOURCE: CMS. 2006. Data Compendium, 2006 Edition, Providers and Suppliers, p. 59. Retrieved from www.cms.hhs.gov/datacompendium/18_2006_data_compendium.asp.

Although the direct costs of care that Medicare recipients bear are still considerable, the cost of benefits the government pays has been frighteningly high, far exceeding the early calculations when the legislation was being considered in the early 1960s. Expenditures by Medicare continue to rise, despite various cost-containment efforts, posing a political dilemma. If Medicare is to continue to meet its obligations, raising taxes to meet the rising demand and rising costs as we have in the past is not popular with wage earners and businesses. Some of the increased costs are being shifted to patients through higher deductibles and higher premiums for Part B. Denying access to some high-end services is an option for cost containment, but not one society has been willing to take.

Although Congress struggles with ways to deal with the cost of the Medicare problem, it also recognizes the shortcomings of the benefits. Congress recognizes that many seniors, although living longer active lives, are dependent on prescription drugs to help control chronic conditions such as heart disease, arthritis, diabetes, and the like. In a time of concern over cost containment, developing a plan to ease the cost of prescriptions for the elderly has not been easy. However, in 2003, former President George W. Bush signed into law the Medicare Prescription Drug Improvement and Modernization Act (*Medicare Part D*), providing a prescription drug benefit to seniors and other people eligible for Medicare. Participation is voluntary. Seniors who have Part A and Part B may elect to receive Part D drug benefits. Participants in Part C plans must obtain their drug coverage through the Part C plans (see Figure 3–1). Seniors may enroll during the period of November 15 and December 31 in one of many drug plans available. Plans may provide different drugs at different prices, with generic medications available in many drug categories. The standard Part D benefit features a $250 deductible, which, after meeting, enrollees pay 25 percent of the costs, up to $2,250. Enrollees then pay the full amount up to a limit of $3,600, at which time enrollees pay 5 percent of the cost and Medicare pays 95 percent of the cost. The gap in coverage between $2,250 and $3,600 is often referred to as the "doughnut hole."

Choosing a drug plan is confusing and difficult for many seniors. Bearing the costs of the first $250 and the gap referred to as the doughnut hole is also difficult for many seniors. It remains to be seen if Congress will again tackle drug coverage in the future to make it less complicated and less costly (see Table 3–5).

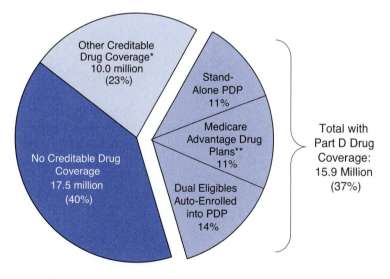

Figure 3–1 Prescription Drug Coverage Among Medicare Beneficiaries (as of February 13, 2006)

NOTE: * Includes employer/union, FEHBP, and TRICARE coverage.

** Approximately 560,000 dual eligibles are enrolled in Medicare Advantage drug plans and are reported in this category.

Numbers do not add to 100% due to rounding.

SOURCE: HHS, February 22, 2006. "Tracking Prescription Drug Coverage Under Medicare: Five Ways to Look at the New Enrollment Numbers," (#7466), The Henry J. Kaiser Family Foundation, February 2006.

TABLE 3-5 Basics of Medicare Coverage and Costs to Enrollees—2008

Program	Deductible	Other Provisions
Part A		
Inpatient hospital	$1,024 per admission	Daily coinsurance and limits $256/day coinsurance for 61–90 days
Skilled nursing facility care		$128 a day after first 20 days
Home health services		Intermittent care only
Hospice		
Part B		
Ambulatory care	$135 annually	80/20 coinsurance $96.40 premium per month
Part C		
Advantage	None, but may have co-payments for services	Handled as an HMO May be higher monthly premium
Part D		
Prescription drug coverage	$250	75/25 coinsurance up to $2,250
	$2,251 to $3,600	95/5 coinsurance

SOURCE: Your Medicare coverage. Retrieved from Medicare.gov.

Medicaid

Medicaid, authorized by Title XIX of the Social Security Act, is a federal and state-financed program to provide health insurance for low-income Americans: the categorically and medically needy. The principles of Medicaid were to (1) make medical services accessible to those who could not afford them; (2) provide medical services through "mainstream" American medicine; and (3) make payment directly to the provider of care for eligible patients.

Originally, the eligibility for benefits was determined through eligibility for cash assistance (welfare) through the Aid to Families with Dependent Children (AFDC) program (for single parents and children) and the Supplementary Security Income (SSI) program (for people who are aged, blind, or disabled). All states must cover these people as "categorically needy." States also covered the "medically needy"—people who have enough money to live on, but not enough to pay for significant specific medical costs they incur. The Personal Responsibility and Work Opportunity Reconciliation Act

of 1996 (welfare reform) drastically affected Medicaid programs. It replaced AFDC with the state-run Temporary Assistance for Needy Families (TANF) programs that separate eligibility for cash assistance from eligibility for Medicaid. The law made it easier for states to expand Medicaid to more working families and to offer families at least six months of Medicaid after they leave welfare for work. The federal government provided some $500 million in matching funds to support these changes. All states must still cover people who are "categorically needy" and "medically needy" (CMS 2000).

Medicare beneficiaries who have low income and limited resources may receive help paying for their out-of-pocket medical expenses from their state Medicaid program. Those who are eligible for both Medicare and Medicaid are referred to as dual eligible; in essence, Medicaid becomes their supplemental, or Medigap, insurance.

Each state must define income eligibility; determine the type, amount, duration, and scope of services; set the rate of payment for services; and administer its own Medicaid program (CMS 2005a). Medicaid standards for people with low incomes differ from state to state, most based on some percentage of the federal poverty level (see Table 3–6). These amounts are very low, excluding many people with what we would consider low incomes, but not low enough to qualify for Medicaid benefits.

Each state's Medicaid program must at least provide for inpatient and outpatient hospital services; physician services; medical and surgical dental services; nursing facility services; home health care; family planning services; rural health clinic services; laboratory and X-ray services; pediatric and family nurse practitioner services; federally qualified health center services; nurse or midwife services; and early periodic screening, diagnosis, and treatment (EPSDT) of children under 21. A state, at its option, may elect to pay for dental services, prescribed drugs, eyeglasses, intermediate-care facility services, and other services.

Medicaid is financed from general tax revenues. The federal government share currently ranges from 50 percent in the wealthiest states to 80 percent in those states with the lowest per capita personal income. Medicaid was originated as a fee-for-service, vendor payment program with payments made directly to the provider. Providers participating in Medicaid must accept the Medicaid payment as payment in full and cannot bill additional amounts to patients. Because those eligible for benefits have very low incomes, cost sharing through deductibles, coinsurance, or co-payments is not very logical.

Like Medicare costs, Medicaid costs have risen rapidly (see Table 3–7). In 2000, Medicaid covered 42.8 million people, and expenditures exceeded $168 billion; by 2005, more than 55 million people were covered, and expenditures were more than $ 257 billion (CMS 2007b). Costs have been of growing concern to both state and federal governments. In most states, increases in Medicaid expenditures are outpacing increases in state revenues. Because payments have not grown with inflation, more physicians are limiting the number of Medicaid patients they treat; some have withdrawn from the program totally. The refusal to participate is not just financially driven. Physicians experience difficulties with excessive paperwork, changing enrollment status of beneficiaries, long delays in payment, and other program deficiencies.

However, state governments are not sitting by idly. In the past, many were forced to reduce the number and scope of optional services and to be more restrictive about eligibility of the medically needy. Other options were to impose limits, such as those on the number of days for in-hospital care and on the amounts paid to physicians, hospitals, and nursing homes.

Rather than simply reduce the number of people eligible for Medicaid, state governments have tried many innovative

TABLE 3–6 2008 HHS Poverty Guidelines

People in Family or Household	48 Contiguous States and DC	Alaska	Hawaii
1	$10,400	$13,000	$11,960
2	14,000	17,500	16,100
3	17,600	22,000	20,240
4	21,200	26,500	24,380
5	24,800	31,000	28,520
6	28,400	35,500	32,660
7	32,000	40,000	36,800
8	35,600	44,500	40,940
For each additional person, add	3,600	4,500	4,140

SOURCE: *Federal Register*. 2008. Vol. 73, No. 15, January 23, pp. 3971–3972.

TABLE 3-7 **Medicaid Recipients and Payments for Selected Fiscal Years**

Year	Recipients (in millions)	Amount (in billions)	Average payment per recipient
1980	21.6	$23.3	$1,079
1990	25.3	$64.9	$2,568
2000	42.8	$168.3	$3,936
2003	52.0	$233.2	$4,487
2004	55.0	$257.7	$4,685

SOURCE: Centers for Medicare and Medicaid Services. Office of Information Services, Enterprise Databases Group, Division of Information Distribution, Medicaid Data System. Before 1999 Medicaid Statistical Report HCFA-2082. From 1999 onward, Medicaid Statistical Information System, MSIS. Retrieved from www.cms.hhs.gov/MedicaidDataSourcesGenInfo/Downloads/msistables2004.pdf.

approaches to stabilize their Medicaid programs. The state of Oregon extended Medicaid benefits to all residents who were below poverty level. This action added many more people to the Medicaid roles. To pay for the cost of care for these new Medicaid enrollees, the state mandated managed care for all Medicaid patients and developed a list of medical services in priority order based on the effectiveness of the services. The program does not pay for those procedures that have little or no beneficial effect, even though they were on the federal government's regular Medicaid list. The plan offers a basic benefit package that stresses prevention and covers most, but not all, of the usual Medicaid treatments. It goes beyond the customary Medicaid benefits by providing coverage for dental and hospice care, prescription drugs, routine physicals, and most transplants. A broadly representative commission of health professionals and community leaders developed the list of medical treatments and their prioritization. The federal government had to approve the plan but rejected it in mid-1992, because the prioritized list might have violated the federal Americans with Disabilities Act. According to Oregon's governor, the plan enjoyed the support of leading groups for people with disabilities in Oregon because they believed it would help more than harm those who had disabilities. The Oregon commission reorganized the list, deleted references to "quality of life," and extended coverage to some controversial treatments (Oregon Health Plan 1998). The Clinton administration approved the revised plan in March 1993, for a five-year demonstration period. The acceptance of the Oregon plan signaled that the Clinton administration recognized the need for drastic action and would give the states flexibility in dealing with the problems associated with health care reform.

By 2005, CMS approved waivers (called 1,115 waivers) for thirty-one states to expand Medicaid coverage to their populations (CMS 2005b). In many states, the waivers consisted of adopting managed care programs in an attempt to control costs and provide more comprehensive care to their enrollees. This approach shifts the risk from the state to the managed care providers. When the managed care plans have been given realistic budgets, they have been successful. However, in areas where payments to managed care programs are too low to provide care, the same problems have occurred as those found in fee-for-service Medicaid plans (see the next section for more about managed care).

Waivers are necessary for states to move toward implementing managed care Medicaid plans because of the original concept of the Medicaid program. The 1965 legislation emphasized that Medicaid recipients should receive care through "mainstream" American medicine. That meant care provided by private physicians in their offices, and choice of providers of care. Managed care, with its limited "panel" of providers and restrictions regarding in-network facilities, technically violates the original concept of the Medicaid structure—thus, the need to obtain a waiver from the federal government. With any innovative delivery plan, states must prove that recipients will receive benefits that are the same or better than those the federal government mandates. As of 2005, only two states, Alaska and Wyoming, did not include managed care in their Medicaid program (CMS 2005b).

In 1997, Congress also created the State Children's Health Insurance Program (SCHIP) to reach more children whose parents earn too much to qualify for Medicaid but too little to purchase health insurance. SCHIP gives the states three options for covering children: (1) design a new children's health insurance program, (2) expand current Medicaid programs, or (3) provide a combination of both. In 1998, 2 million children were enrolled in SCHIP plans in all fifty states. That number grew to over 6.6 million in 2006 (CMS 2007a). The program is funded by federal and state funds and is designed to cover children ages 18 and younger.

Managed Care

At one time, the terms *managed care* and *health maintenance organization* (HMO) were synonymous. However, managed care now describes a wider range of services and practices that have come to revolutionize the practice of medicine and the delivery of health care. In its broadest sense, managed care is a health care delivery system that, in some way, places providers in the position of managing the utilization of health care by consumers. Managed care has five very important characteristics:

1. A select panel of providers
2. Comprehensive health services
3. Quality tracking
4. Utilization review
5. Cost containment

There are various types of managed care, but the three broadest categories are perhaps HMOs, preferred provider organizations (PPOs), and point-of-services (POS) plans. These are described in the sections that follow, although with a reminder that they are not the only managed care plans available and that drawing distinctions among various managed care plans is very difficult in many instances (see Figure 3–2).

Health Maintenance Organizations

HMOs are perhaps the most restrictive of managed care plans. The term *HMO* may refer to a specific organization (such as Kaiser Permanente) or a health insurance plan (for example, Aetna, United HealthCare), which adds to the confusion and

makes descriptions even more difficult. The basic characteristics, however, are the same for the organization or the health plan.

The main characteristic is the gatekeeper concept. A **primary care physician (PCP)** or other health care professional is the case manager. All care for the patients is directed (in conjunction with the patient) through the PCP, including referrals to specialists, orders for diagnostic tests, and any surgical or other treatment procedures. As the case manager, the PCP receives payment on a capitated basis—a fixed payment per patient per month. By providing as much needed care as possible in-house, the PCP controls costs (for the HMO) often connected with specialty care. The PCP determines the appropriate setting for care by providing referrals when necessary. Other HMO network providers (contracted with the HMO for discounted fees) must provide services outside the realm of the PCP. If a patient chooses health services with a provider outside the network or seeks services without a referral from the PCP, the HMO will not pay for the service and the patient is responsible for any costs incurred; that is one way of shifting risk. However, the real shift of risk is to the PCP. The capitated fee is fixed. The PCP receives the same payment per month regardless of the number of times a patient is seen and regardless of the range of services the PCP provides. In some cases, the PCP may also be at risk for some of the costs associated with referring a patient for additional treatment—at risk either for admonishment by the HMO's administration (through utilization review) or through loss of income if a pool of money is withheld from the PCP to pay for specialty care.

Another very important feature of the HMO is the emphasis on preventive care. One very effective way of reducing overall health care costs is to keep the population healthy. Traditionally, health insurance has really been "sick care insurance," paying for services only when they are medically necessary. Therefore, traditional health insurances do not pay for routine exams or care that "rules out" illness. HMOs not only pay for routine exams, but they also encourage them and monitor that patients receive preventive care such as immunizations

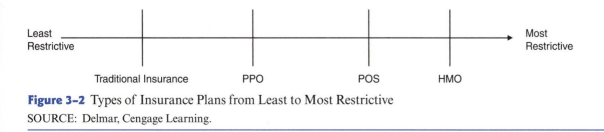

Figure 3–2 Types of Insurance Plans from Least to Most Restrictive
SOURCE: Delmar, Cengage Learning.

and screenings. Some even provide services such as smoking cessation programs and discounts on health club memberships.

Although the phrase "health maintenance organization" seemed new to most consumers and health care providers in the 1980s, the idea of paying for services on a fixed fee or capitated basis appears throughout U.S. medical history. It became most prominent, however, during the 1940s, with the development of New York's Health Insurance Plan (HIP) on the East Coast, and Kaiser Permanente on the West Coast. Expansion of the HMO approach was modest, even slow, until the 1970s, when the costs of health care began to soar and when these costs became a concern both to government and to the business community. The federal government took the initiative in 1973, with passage of the Health Maintenance Organization Act. The act provided financial incentives (by providing start-up money) for developing what then became known as HMOs. The act also instituted regulations requiring firms of twenty-five or more employees who offered health insurance to employees to include an HMO option if it was available in the firm's area. The act also preempted state legislation prohibiting HMOs, and granted federally qualified status (certification that the HMO met a minimum package of benefits) to encourage Medicare and Medicaid populations to enroll in HMOs. In the HMO approach, the government saw a way to control rising costs of health care, a sizable portion of which it paid for through Medicare and Medicaid. The HMO approach thus shifted the risk arising from increased costs caused by heavy utilization from the government to the provider of services.

Despite subsidies, HMO growth was slow, but HMO enrollment had increased by the 1980s (see Table 3–8), in part because of the continued rising cost of health care. Even as federal subsidies ended, HMOs began to develop all over the country, spurred on by the prevailing idea that costs could be controlled through competition and utilization control. Like the government earlier, businesses found HMOs appealing because they seemed like a good way to hold down rising costs; no longer would the employer pay without limit. If costs rose above the limit, the HMO would be responsible for absorbing the costs. Declining hospital bed occupancy (explained in the section "Paying Hospitals" later in this chapter) and a large supply of physicians gave the HMOs the necessary leverage to compete for business, offering employers lower costs and offering hospitals and doctors an assured flow of patients in return for greatly reduced fees.

HMOs promised lower health care costs based on the efficiency of delivering services in a coordinated and comprehensive fashion. Initial cost reductions came mainly from a reduction in inpatient and specialty care, not from a reduced quality of care. As the HMOs competed with one another for their share of the market, some critics feared HMOs would begin to curtail services to keep their costs low. They would not openly ration care but would more subtly ration by making patients wait for appointments, ordering fewer diagnostic tests, reducing the amount of nonemergency surgery, and signing up only those employee groups that appeared to be young and healthy.

More than 27 percent of the population belonged to HMOs in 1998. Enrollment in HMOs peaked in the mid-1990s at just

TABLE 3–8 **Distribution of Health Plan Enrollment (by Percentage) for Covered Workers, by Plan Type**

Year	Conventional	HMO	PPO	POS
1988	73	16	11	--
1998	14	27	35	24
2000	8	29	42	21
2002	4	27	52	18
2004	5	25	55	15
2006*	3	20	60	13

*In 2006, nearly 4 percent of covered workers were enrolled in high-deductible health plans combined with health savings accounts (HDHP/HSAs).

SOURCE: Created by Camille Barsukiewicz, based on Chart 8 from Employer Health Benefits 2006 Annual Survey (#7527) The Henry J. Kaiser Family Foundation, September 2006.

above 30 percent but has since declined to about 20 percent in 2006 (Kaiser Family Foundation 2006). In 2006, the highest concentrations of enrollees are in the West, Northeast, and large metropolitan areas. The number of HMOs grew so rapidly during the 1980s that many did not have the management skills or the number of enrollees necessary to survive. Many of the HMOs merged or disappeared during the late 1980s, resulting in fewer HMOs with a steady but slower growth in the number of people enrolled. HMOs caused a restructuring of the way health care is marketed, delivered, and financed in almost every metropolitan area of the country. There are many varieties of HMOs, but they can be categorized into four major types:

1. Staff model HMOs employ physicians directly, provide care through central offices, and pay physicians by salary (the insurer and the health care provider are one).

2. Group model HMOs contract with one independent, multi-specialty group practice to provide physician services. The HMO pays the group practice a negotiated per capita rate, and the group practice determines what each physician will be paid—typically a salary plus incentive payments. The HMO sends all of its patients to that group, and the group sees only the HMO's patients.

3. Network model HMOs resemble the group model. The only difference is that the HMO contracts with more than one independent multispecialty group practice. The group practices that contract with the HMO may be **single-specialty** or **multispecialty groups**.

4. Individual practice association (IPA) involves individual physicians in solo practice or with group practices banding together to contract their services to HMOs. Payment schemes vary from capitation to fee for service, as well as variations on these types of payment. Unlike the other HMO models, IPA physicians usually provide services in their own offices and see other patients in addition to their HMO patients. (CDC 2007)

No study has shown one model to be superior to the others, but the IPA model seems to be the most predominant in number of plans, number of people enrolled, and percentage of HMO enrollees. The group and staff models, although once the icons of HMOs, have been declining in strength over the years. The structure of HMOs is changing and becoming more diversified, as indicated by the number of mixed HMO plans and number of enrollees in those plans. HMOs are a continually changing mix of nonprofit and for-profit organizations.

The initial reduction in health care expenditures for HMO members was due mainly to a reduction in hospital admissions and a greater reliance on outpatient services, not a reduction in physician services. However, many of those initial reductions have since stabilized, and employers are not saving as much money as they had hoped. Employers continue to press to keep costs down without sacrificing quality. Even though HMO premiums continue to increase more than employers expected, employers are still turning to HMOs, often by passing more of the premium cost to employees if the employees opt for fee-for-service plans.

Membership in HMOs typically offers some advantages for enrollees, such as a predictable cost for health care, broader coverage for more routine care (for example, physical examinations), and no claim forms to fill out and submit. Disadvantages often cited are the requirement of choosing a physician affiliated with the HMO, the need to obtain approval before hospitalization or specialty care, and the difficulty of securing payment for care that an individual with insurance receives when outside of the home geographic area.

Physicians may find HMOs advantageous because they offer a guaranteed income if in a staff, group, or network model; those in an IPA model may appreciate the possibility of expanding their patient base. Disadvantages for physicians that are often cited include some loss of autonomy, minimal input into quality assurance and utilization review criteria (except in the IPA model), possible alteration of referral patterns, increased outside influence on treatment decisions, and possible reduced earnings.

Although studies have shown lower hospital utilization rates for HMOs, the results are not altogether persuasive on two accounts. First, some critics believe that many HMOs have enrolled groups that are not representative of the population, that they have sought younger groups of enrollees who would tend to be healthier, and have avoided those groups from which high utilization could be expected—principally the poor and the elderly. Second, many believe that some of the reduced utilization may stem from rationing—for example, not doing elective surgery that would serve only to improve quality of life. HMOs are increasing their enrollments; however, they are facing increasing competition from another type of managed care: preferred provider organizations.

Preferred Provider Organizations (PPOs)

Preferred provider organizations (PPOs) are primarily a phenomenon of the 1980s, and have grown dramatically from about 10 percent of health plan enrollees in 1988, to 60 percent in 2006 (Kaiser Family Foundation 2006). A PPO is an arrangement in which a limited number of health providers—physicians, hospitals, and others—agree to provide services to a defined group of people at a negotiated fee-for-service rate, which is usually discounted from the normal rate. People enrolled in PPOs have incentives to use the preferred providers because the costs of provider services are fixed and, except for routine office visits, they are typically paid for in full (or at least at 80 percent of the fee). If an enrolled person goes to a provider outside the network (a nonpreferred provider), the PPO makes a lesser payment to the provider (typically only 70 percent) and the patient must pay the balance.

PPOs have attracted enormous interest as a way to contain costs while retaining the patient's choice of physician and retaining the fee-for-service type of payment. PPOs may be sponsored by insurance companies (including Blue Cross and Blue Shield plans), employers, hospitals, or physicians. Some hospitals and physicians have joined together to form **physician-hospital organizations (PHOs)** in response to economic competition and as a mechanism for capturing and securing a share of the market, lest they lose patients. PHOs form their own preferred provider networks to contract with insurance companies or directly with employers to provide care to groups of consumers at a discounted rate, rather than waiting for insurance companies to come to them to contract for a PPO. The PHO is usually an affiliation for contracting purposes only, rather than a complete merger of organizations.

The success of PPOs depends on the recruitment of cost-effective physicians and hospitals. The competition must be strong enough for these providers to be willing to negotiate discounted rates for PPO members. PPOs, like HMOs, also depend upon management activities to keep costs down. These activities may include prior authorization for hospital admission (precertification), concurrent and retrospective utilization reviews, and mandatory second opinions for surgery.

Physicians like the PPOs' feature of maintaining fee-for-service, office-based medical practices. Many physicians see PPOs as a way to compete with HMOs. As suggested earlier, physicians see an opportunity to enlarge their patient base or to preserve their current patient base. PPOs do not restrict physicians to a single insurance plan. Most physicians have participation agreements with more than one PPO and with other types of plans in addition to the PPO.

In a PPO, physicians lose some of their autonomy as in an HMO, but they must accept some controls. External utilization review may leave physicians with less opportunity to influence the design and operation of reviews. Fee schedules are usually discounted, so physicians must see more patients to maintain the same level of income; however, many physicians view the PPO as a better option than participation in an HMO.

PPOs appeal to patients because they allow freedom of choice of physician or hospital for care. If patients prefer to use a provider outside the network, they bear some share of the costs. Admittedly, the additional cost may effectively deter them from exercising that option, but that is the purpose of the PPO concept.

Point-of-Service Plans

Point-of-service (POS) plans, sometimes called open-ended HMOs, are the most recent model of managed care and are somewhat of a hybrid of the HMO and PPO concepts. This model requires insured individuals to choose a primary care physician (PCP) who manages their overall care. The PCPs provide as much care as possible and appropriate, make referrals to specialists, and provide preventive services. Insured individuals pay only a co-payment for the PCP's services and referred services. However, unlike HMO members, individuals with insurance have the option of seeking the care of a specialist without a referral or choosing doctors and hospitals outside of the network of providers if they are willing to pay a portion of the costs. POS plans differ from PPOs in the low cost that individuals with insurance pay for staying with care provided and referred by the PCP. Enrollment in POS plans grew to a high of 24 percent in 1998 (see Table 3–8). This model of managed care is most attractive to consumers because of its greater range of provider choice and its willingness to pay some of the costs of providers outside the network. However, the premium cost for a POS plan is greater than that for other managed care models, reflecting the fact that greater flexibility comes at a greater cost. Enrollment dropped to 13 percent in 2006, perhaps a reflection of those higher premium costs (Kaiser Family Foundation 2006).

Managed Care Trends

Managed care plans continue to grow at the expense of traditional forms of health insurance. All insurance forms are in intense competition and are altering the plans they offer to respond to the demands of health care purchasers. The future for managed health care delivery systems will probably be a combination of the positive features of both PPOs and HMOs (as seen in the point-of-service plans). The traditional, unrestricted, fee-for-service system of payment plays a very small role today—only

3 percent of health plan enrollees used such a system in 2006. Even the most flexible of health plans contains some discounted payments to providers, some utilization review, and some restrictions to beneficiaries as to what services will be covered.

The initial influx of managed care resulted in contention and litigation because vital professional and public interests were at stake. Antitrust issues were raised with increased frequency as physicians were excluded from participation in some HMOs and PPOs, and as complaints arose over what were claimed to be anticompetitive practices and price fixing. Patients questioned the managed care organization's refusal to provide access to certain treatments, or denial of care. Over the years, states and, in some instances, the federal government, have passed legislation to protect patient rights. The early practice of HMOs allowing women only twenty-four hours in the hospital after giving birth has now been changed to a minimum of forty-eight hours. Gag rules, limiting the physician's ability to tell patients about the full range of treatments available if the HMO does not cover a specific treatment, have been outlawed. Most states have specific policies regarding patients' rights to petition HMOs regarding denied services. With the advent of more flexible managed care plans, HMOs have been forced to be more patient-friendly to remain competitive. The major objection to HMOs from patients continues to be the limitation in choice of physicians.

NEW APPROACHES TO INSURANCE

Universal Health Coverage

The United States is the only industrialized nation without some type of universal health care coverage. The number of individuals without insurance is a consistent statistic pointed out during various census reports. When polled, most Americans admit to concern about the uninsured population and express an interest in universal coverage. The problem, however, is finding agreement on how to achieve universal coverage.

The proposals for universal coverage range from market-based competitive models such as vouchers for people who are poor to purchase health insurance in the open market, to employer mandates, to single-payer systems. None has garnered enough political support to overhaul the current patchwork system of health care coverage.

Health Savings Accounts

The same legislation that created Medicare Part D (Medicare Prescription Drug Improvement and Modernization Act of 2003) also provided for **health savings accounts (HSAs)**. The HSAs allow people with high-deductible health care insurance

---

EXHIBIT 3–1

May 11, 2007

Big Business Wants Universal Health Care

BYLINE: Rowland Nethaway

DATELINE: Waco, Texas

After demonizing universal heath care for generations, many traditional opponents are admitting that the fragmented U.S. health care model needs a universal solution.

The United States has long been the only industrialized nation on the planet that does not offer some form of universal health care.

For years, reform efforts to offer U.S. citizens universal health care coverage were accused of peddling socialized medicine or were communist stalking horses.

The collapse of the Berlin wall and the emergence of a global capitalist marketplace have made it difficult for political opponents of universal health care to oppose a concept embraced by free-trade nations around the world.

Another long-standing argument used by universal health care opponents has been that U.S. health care is superior to the health care provided in other nations.

That argument is difficult to sustain in view of consistent reports that American citizens have a lower life expectancy than practically every developed nation, including those with universal health care systems.

The United States has a higher infant mortality rate than most nations while also spending more than any other nation on health care, about 15 percent of the nation's gross domestic product.

(continues)

EXHIBIT 3-1 (Continued)

Arguments against universal health care have been eroded by the Department of Veterans Affairs government-run single-payer health care system for the nation's veterans, which was established in 1930.

In 1965, Congress approved the Medicare health insurance program administered by the government for people older than 65.

At the same time, Congress approved the Medicaid health insurance program for citizens with low incomes and resources.

While the Medicare entitlement program is funded entirely at the federal level for seniors, the Medicaid entitlement program is a joint federal-state health care system that provides health insurance coverage to low-income children, seniors and people with disabilities.

For all other Americans, health care coverage either is supplied by employers or left to the citizens to fend for themselves in America's high-priced health care system.

Because of rising health care costs, more and more employers are finding it difficult to provide health care coverage for their workers, who are forced to pay ever-higher premiums and co-pays for the same coverage.

Approximately 46 million Americans, or 15 percent of the U.S. population, do not have any health care coverage. That number continues to grow.

Because of burdensome costs, uninsured citizens often attempt to avoid doctors, hospitals and clinics for as long as possible. As a consequence, when they do get sick, they often require more extensive treatment. Their medical bills can bankrupt hard-working families and drive up health care costs for everyone else.

It is becoming more difficult for the opponents of universal health care to make the argument that the U.S. system provides superior health care when more and more Americans are choosing to be treated for even the most difficult procedures overseas in India, Singapore, Thailand and other places for one-fifth the cost charged in the United States. These overseas medical facilities meet or exceed U.S. accreditation standards.

There are signs of cracks in the high-priced lobbying effort that keeps the dysfunctional U.S. health care system in place.

The new Coalition to Advance Healthcare Reform has launched an effort to lobby for universal health care insurance and a competitive effort to curb the escalating costs of medical care.

The new coalition includes many of the nation's largest employers such as Safeway, General Mills, PepsiCo, Pacific Gas and Electric Co., Eli Lilly and Company, drugstore chains and health insurance companies.

This may be an example of crisis management, but it is still welcome.

Rowland Nethaway is senior editor of the Waco Tribune-Herald.

Copyright 2007 Cox Enterprises, Inc.

Discussion Questions

This article summarizes many of the issues presented in this chapter. Employment-based insurance has left many without health insurance. Many have debated the issue of "universal coverage"—health insurance for every American. However, finding a system of universal health care that will satisfy everyone has been impossible thus far. President Barack Obama has backed the concept of "universal coverage," and taken bold steps to make it a policy in the United States. However, at the time this book was written, he faced opposition from many political sectors, and it remained to be seen if it would come to fruition.

1. Review the arguments for and against Obama's proposed solution.

(usually referred to as "catastrophic coverage") to establish savings accounts strictly for the purpose of paying for health care services. The money can be set aside on a "pretax basis," which means the amount is set aside from income before calculating income taxes. An individual's employer can even contribute to the HSA. The amount placed in the HSA is not taxable as long as it is used for health care services. If the money is not used at the end of a year, it simply accumulates for future health care expenses. Once people begin receiving Medicare, they can no longer contribute to HSAs (because Medicare provides first-dollar coverage), but can continue to draw on the balance for services Medicare does not cover (U.S. Department of the Treasury 2007a).

Employers can establish **high-deductible health plans (HDHPs)** with an HSA. The maximum deposits allowed into an HSA for 2007 were $2,700 for individual plans and $5,450 for family plans. The HDHP may begin to pay after a deductible of those same limits or higher. People with HDHPs and HSAs would pay for medical expenses out of the HSA (and may have to add some out-of-pocket payments) until meeting the deductible of the HDHP.

Proponents of HSAs believe that health care costs will be reduced because consumers will be more discriminate in their spending when they are using their own money (from the HSA) and will realize the full cost of care rather than paying a small co-pay or coinsurance and having the insurance company pay the remainder. Employers will benefit from the reduced cost of the HDHP (much lower than a first-dollar insurance plan) and the freedom to decide how much to contribute to the HSA. Participants in the HSA benefit in that they can use funds for health care providers of their own choosing rather than being limited to a panel of providers an insurance company has secured. They also benefit from being able to accumulate funds not used in one year for future years.

Opponents of HSAs say that they only attract young, healthy people and make traditional health insurance more expensive for everyone else. People with low incomes do not have excess income to contribute to HSAs and will be left with only the HDHPs. Because of the cost of primary care, these people will wait until they are acutely ill to access care.

According to the U.S. Department of the Treasury (2007b), HSAs covered 438,000 people in 2004. That number grew to 3.2 million in 2005, and is projected to reach 14 million in 2010.

METHODS OF PAYING FOR HEALTH CARE SERVICES

Just as the types of health insurance have changed over time, the methods by which insurance plans pay for services have also changed, although no insurance company has one plan or one method of payment. Paying for health care will be discussed in the sections that follow, without a specific type of insurance in mind, although readers will be able to recognize how certain types of payments are attached to certain insurance plans, or how they at least historically began that way.

Paying Hospitals

In the early years of hospital insurance, hospitals were paid at cost. The hospital simply kept an account of the costs involved in caring for patients; added a small amount for uncompensated care, medical education, and new construction; and billed the insurance plan. The insurance plan in turn paid the hospital's full charges. The problems are obvious. Hospitals had no incentive to operate efficiently. In fact, the more services provided and the longer the patient stayed, the more the hospital got paid. Health care expenditures rose rapidly.

In an effort to stem the rise in cost of hospital care, many approaches were taken. Some insurance companies reimbursed hospitals on the basis of average costs—based on area providers. Hospitals were compared to one another and paid an average of their combined costs, often based on a daily rate. These rates were eventually negotiated in an attempt to lower the daily rate. However, this approach did little to contain costs because hospitals still had the incentive simply to keep patients longer (even after they were well enough to be discharged) to recoup some costs.

Because the federal government is responsible for a large portion of hospital costs under Medicare and Medicaid, it is the driving force in attempts to contain increasing hospital costs. Dissatisfied with **retrospective** cost-based reimbursement, in 1972, the government began conducting several demonstration projects to evaluate a wide variety of alternative payment systems. After ten years of research, a prospective payment system (PPS) was chosen as a viable alternative to the retrospective cost-based reimbursement for Medicare patients. In 1983, Congress amended the Social Security Act to provide Medicare payment for inpatient hospital services under a prospective payment system in which payment is made at a predetermined, specific rate for each discharge according to the patient's treatment classification in one of almost 500 **diagnosis-related groups (DRGs).** The DRG takes into account the patient's principal diagnosis, principal surgical procedure (if there is one), any complicating conditions (comorbidities), and type of discharge (see Table 3–9). Each DRG is assigned a weight relative to the standard (1.00), and each hospital is assigned a fee for the standard. Payment becomes a simple formula: weight x standard = payment. The legislation still provided for capital-related costs and adjustments, such as urban or rural location, teaching hospitals, low-income case mix, and outlier cases.

TABLE 3-9 Sample Inpatient Hospital DRGs, Fiscal Year 2005

DRG	Condition	National Average Payments	National Average Charges
105	Heart valve operations	$38,528	$115,221
159	Hernia operations in adults with complications or preexisting conditions	$8,548	$27,198
303	Kidney and bladder operations for cancer	$15,173	$44,624
359	Uterus and ovary operations	$4,855	$15,084
515	Insertion of heart defibrillator	$35,116	$97,306

SOURCE: CMS. 2006c. Health care consumer initiatives, hospital inpatient. Retrieved May 22, 2007, from www.cms.hhs.gov/HealthCareConInit/02_Hospital.asp.

The transition to this PPS was made in a four-year phase-in period until 1988, when prospective payment went into full effect. The results were dramatic. DRG payment means a single payment to the hospital for the care of the patient regardless of the costs incurred. If the hospital incurs greater cost for the care of the patient than provided by the DRG, the hospital must bear the cost. If the hospital provides care to the patient at less than the DRG payment, the hospital still retains the full payment. DRGs were truly an incentive for hospitals to operate more efficiently.

It is important to note that other conditions changed somewhat in accord with the implementation of DRGs. Technology facilitated the move of many previously considered inpatient procedures to an outpatient setting. New medications made the medical management of many conditions preclude or delay surgical intervention. Coupled with DRGs, these broader environmental conditions changed the face of hospital care. Beginning in the mid-1980s, hospitals saw dramatic decreases in patient length of stay and in occupancy rates. Many hospitals responded by developing more outpatient services, converting inpatient beds to short-stay units, and developing market plans to stay financially viable. Many of these efforts resulted in vertical integration and horizontal integration within organizations. DRGs were a significant cause of these dramatic changes, along with the competition that managed care structures introduced.

Medicare introduced DRGs into hospital compensation methods. However, it did not take long for other third-party payers to adopt this method. It made sense—force hospitals to run more efficiently by shifting the cost risk to them. It also made sense for other third-party payers to protect themselves. On a cost basis, hospitals might simply have shifted any losses incurred from serving Medicare patients to the payers who were still paying at cost.

Payment by diagnostic category has become the norm for hospitals. Managed care organizations negotiate similar flat-rate payments. Prospective payment is also spreading to other service areas that previously remained under cost plus reimbursement or daily rates. The Balanced Budget Act of 1997 brought prospective payment systems to hospital outpatient services, certain community mental health services, home health care services, and rehabilitation services. Hospitals branched out to provide some of these services to protect themselves from losses of inpatient revenues, but now even that avenue seems to be closing (Balanced Budget Act 2000).

The outpatient prospective payment system (OPPS) consists of groups of services known as ambulatory payment classification (APC) groups, based on services that are similar clinically and require similar resources. Actual procedures are isolated from ancillary procedures; for example, laboratory tests or imaging might be paid for separately from surgery. However, actual surgical procedures include such things as anesthesia, supplies, and recovery rooms. The outpatient prospective payment system went into effect on July 1, 2000 (CMS 2006b).

With the early introductions of prospective payments, there were many questions about quality of care. Terms like *quicker and sicker* defined the fear that patients were going to be discharged from hospitals before they were well enough to go home, resulting in them simply returning to the hospital in a short time, even sicker than the first time around. This did not prove true. However, it was obvious that costs were simply being diverted to home health agencies, which were now seeing more patients than ever because patients required some additional care after hospital discharge. Nursing homes saw an increase in patients of shorter stays, who spent rehabilitation periods in a less expensive setting than the hospital prior to going home. Costs for home health care and skilled nursing home care rose—resulting in the introduction of DRG payments for these services several years later. However, the Balanced Budget Refinement Act of 1999 included provisions to adjust payments and protect against certain losses (budget-neutral provisions).

Paying Physicians

Physicians and hospitals are paid separately (for example, Blue Cross pays hospitals, Blue Shield pays physicians). This is true even when physicians perform services within the hospital. When a patient is admitted to a hospital, the hospital receives a facility fee and physicians receive separate payment for their services (surgical fee, consult, and so on). When we think of physician payments, however, we ordinarily think about payment for office-based care. Early forms of health insurance paid physicians on a fee-for-service basis. Physicians had their own fee schedules for various office visits and procedures and simply charged the fee amount to patients or the insurance plan. The more patients the physician saw, and the more procedures the physician performed, the greater the physician's income.

In time, many of the Blue Shield plans (as well as commercial insurance and eventually Medicare) developed contracts with "usual, customary, and reasonable" (UCR) allowances. These were schedules for payment for physician services based on the physician's history of charges (usual), the prevailing charges for physicians in the same specialty in the same locality (customary), and reasonable charges (the maximum the insurer was willing to pay). For each type of service, the insurer would pay the least of the usual, customary, or reasonable charges for that particular physician.

Enrollees covered under UCR payment schedules would not incur the cost of the physician's service if the patient used a physician who agreed to accept the insurance plan's UCR payments as full payment (such a physician is called a participating physician, referring to the physician's contract to participate in the insurance

plan). If the physician is not a plan participant, then the payment is an indemnity payment (cash payment to a patient), and the physician may charge whatever deemed appropriate. The patient is responsible for sending the payment to the physician, including any amount beyond what the insurance plan has provided. Although the UCR system kept the amount of payment per visit or procedure down, it did very little to reduce the number of visits or procedures performed. Just as in full fee-for-service payment, the incentive to overserve remained.

Until the early 1990s, Medicare paid physicians through the UCR system. Increasing costs, however, led Medicare to investigate alternative payment methods, just as it had with hospital costs in the 1980s. Medicare's answer to physician payment was the **resource-based relative value scale (RBRVS),** which was based on three main factors:

1. Total work performed by the physician for each service

2. Practice costs, including the cost of malpractice insurance

3. Cost of specialty training to perform the service

The relative-value scale is based on a model that a Harvard research group developed, and relates the value of each medical procedure to others, a dollar conversion factor and a geographic factor (see Figure 3–3). RBRVS redistributes money among physicians by increasing the amount paid for cognitive services (listening, diagnosing, explaining, and advising patients) and decreasing the amount paid for invasive procedures (for example, surgery) and diagnostic tests distributed through the Medicare fee schedule used to pay for physician services. Thus, income from Medicare patients increased for primary care physicians whereas surgeons' fees decreased. The decrease for surgical and other specialized care is not a statement that these services are any less important because of RBRVS, but historically the services had been overvalued in relation to other medical procedures. Payment according to RBRVS began in 1992, and was phased in over a five-year period (AMA 2006). Some insurance companies are following Medicare's lead and are also using the RBRVS to revise their payments to physicians.

When first introduced, RBRVS was quite controversial. Specialists feared a drastic reduction in income, which did happen in selected specialties. Primary care practitioners never quite saw increases in their income as they were projected, but they did see some improvements. Perhaps the most difficult aspect of RBRVS was the concept of "evaluation and management" (E and M) codes—the method used to bill Medicare for office visits and

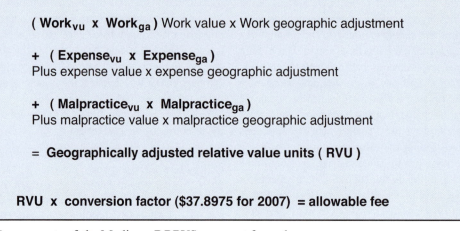

(**Work$_{vu}$ x Work$_{ga}$**) Work value x Work geographic adjustment

+ (Expense$_{vu}$ x Expense$_{ga}$)
Plus expense value x expense geographic adjustment

+ (Malpractice$_{vu}$ x Malpractice$_{ga}$)
Plus malpractice value x malpractice geographic adjustment

= Geographically adjusted relative value units (RVU)

RVU x conversion factor ($37.8975 for 2007) = allowable fee

Figure 3–3 Components of the Medicare RBRVS payment formula
SOURCE: Delmar, Cengage Learning.

consultations with patients. The evaluation and management codes take into account whether a patient is new to the physician or is an established patient, the extent of medical history taken during the visit, the extent of the examination, and the amount of medical decision making on the part of the physician necessary to determine a patient diagnosis and treatment plan. Obviously, these are very subjective criteria, and folding them all into an appropriate billing code is a difficult task, to say the least. How to document all of this information to substantiate the chosen billing level is another difficulty. The use of evaluation and management coding is still being discussed, and clear regulations governing their use were not issued until 2002. It is also important to note that, although RBRVS was designed to balance the discrepancy between primary care practitioners' and specialists' payments, it did nothing to limit the incentive to overtreat. The more procedures a physician performs, the more the physician gets paid.

Another type of physician payment is the discounted fee for service (mentioned in the discussion of PPO plans earlier in this chapter). Discounted fee for service is simply a negotiated fee scheduled between the physician and the insurance plan. The physician agrees to a reduced fee schedule in return for a potential increase in patients covered by the insurance plan (or in some cases, an assurance that the physician will not lose patients because of enrollment in the insurance plan).

A physician payment plan introduced by managed care is capitation. As mentioned previously, capitation is a fixed pay-

ment per patient per month. In return for the capitated payment, physicians agree to provide a negotiated range of services. The monthly payment remains the same whether or not the patient requires any care that month. In other words, if a physician agrees to accept a panel of 100 patients at $40 per month per patient, the physician receives $4,000 per month. That $4,000 remains the same whether the physician sees no patients that month or sees all 100 patients every day that month. The physicians are at financial risk for the range of services to which they agreed. Under capitation, it is in the physician's best interest to keep the panel of patients as healthy as possible. This is the built-in incentive in managed care for preventive services. It is also, unfortunately, an incentive to undertreat, in direct opposition to the incentive to overtreat that is built into fee-for-service medicine.

Pay for Performance

Although reducing costs has been the focus of the past changes in health care payment methods, recent efforts have targeted quality of care. CMS is collaborating with various quality organizations such as the Joint Commission and the Agency for Healthcare Research and Quality to develop a set of pay-for-performance initiatives. Pay for performance is based on increased payments to providers who meet and are willing to publicly report on specific performance standards and treatment outcomes, especially regarding the treatment of Medicare patients with chronic conditions (CMS 2005c). Pay for performance is in its early stages of implementation and evidence of its effectiveness remains to be seen. However, it may be the one means of payment for health care services that neither incentivizes overtreatment or undertreatment. Quality of care, performance standards, and treatment outcomes will be discussed further in Chapter 11.

SUMMARY

Health care insurance has a long and complicated history, but it is generally recognized that employment-based insurance had its beginning during World War II. Price and wage freezes provided employers the opportunity to attract and retain employees by providing employer-paid benefits as an incentive. Since then, the United States has relied on employment-based insurance as the major avenue to pay for health care costs.

A wide variety of health insurance products have evolved over time. Whereas Blue Cross and Blue Shield once predominated as an indemnity form of insurance product, we now see PPOs, HMOs, and POS plans in a variety of health insurance companies. Added to the mix are health benefits plans underwritten by employers, especially those doing business in multiple states.

Paying for health care services has also had a long and complicated history. Hospitals, nursing homes, physicians, and other health care providers have all been paid differently. Containing costs has been the major focus in health care delivery for a very long time, particularly with the growth of the Medicare and Medicaid programs and the government's involvement as a third-party payer. Cost became a significant issue because the government's resources are limited, mainly by the taxes it imposes. Raising taxes to pay increased costs is never a popular option. Therefore, cost containment has come in the form of prospective payments for hospitals, nursing homes, and ambulatory care facilities, as well as reduced fee schedules for physicians and other Part B providers.

Government is not the only entity concerned with costs. Employers and insurance companies also face dilemmas caused by increased health care costs. Insurers must absorb these costs and face decreased profits or pass on these costs through higher premiums for their insurance products. Employers must incorporate the rising cost of health care into their own costs, consider raising premiums for their products or services to cover that cost, or pass the increased cost on to employees through shared premium payments.

Managed care made a significant impact on the delivery and cost of health care while bringing with it new considerations and conflicts, mainly regarding choice and access to care. New approaches to health care coverage have come in the form of health savings accounts and high-deductible health plans. Concern over the growing numbers of individuals without insurance has spawned debates over methods to provide universal coverage to all citizens and residents; however, the overriding struggle in health care today is the pressure to contain costs while improving the quality of care, and it remains to be seen if both goals can be met.

ACTIVITY-BASED LEARNING

Insurance Project

As a new employee, you have been given the following information regarding three insurance plans your employer offers. Option 1 is a form of PPO plan that gives you the option of seeking services from participating providers for little or no cost or seeking services from nonparticipating providers for additional out-of-pocket expense to you. Option 2 is an HMO providing coverage for services from participating providers and no coverage for services outside the network of providers. Option 3 is a POS plan that requires you to choose a primary care physician from a panel of participating providers but allows you to see providers outside your plan for an increased cost to you (see Exhibit 3–2). You must choose your health insurance plan for an extended time period. You will not be able to change plans until the next enrollment period (on January 1 of the following calendar year).

Scenario 1

Choose a health plan assuming you are in your mid-twenties, newly married, and planning on having your first child in the near future. You and your spouse seem to be relatively healthy at the present time (the male has a family history of heart disease, the female a family history of breast cancer). You each have your own family physician, and the female spouse has heard about a wonderful obstetrician/gynecologist she would like to see, should she become pregnant.

Scenario 2

Choose a health plan assuming you are in your late forties with a spouse and three children. One child is about to enter college away from home, the second is in high school, and the third is

EXHIBIT 3–2 Plan Choices and Out-of-Pocket Payments

Benefit	Option 1—PPO		Option 2—HMO	Option 3—POS	
	In Network	Out of Network	In Network	In Network	Out of Network
Office visit, PCP	20/80 coinsurance	30/70 coinsurance	$20 co-pay	$20 co-pay	30/70 coinsurance
Office visit, specialist	20/80 coinsurance	30/70 coinsurance	$25 co-pay	$25 co-pay	30/70 coinsurance
Diagnostic services	$0	30/70 coinsurance	$0	$0	30/70 coinsurance
OB/GYN	20/80 coinsurance	30/70 coinsurance	$20 co-pay	$20 co-pay	30/70 coinsurance
Pap test	$ 0	30/70 coinsurance	$0	$0	30/70 coinsurance
Mammogram	$0	30/70 coinsurance	$0	$0	30/70 coinsurance
Delivery including pre- and post-visits	20/80 coinsurance	30/70 coinsurance	$0	$0	30/70 coinsurance
Emergency room	20/80 coinsurance	30/70 coinsurance	$50 co-pay	$50 co-pay	30/70 coinsurance
Ambulance	20/80 coinsurance	30/70 coinsurance	$50 co-pay	$50 co-pay	30/70 coinsurance
Inpatient mental health or drug and alcohol rehab	20/80 coinsurance	50/50 coinsurance	14-day limit	14-day limit	50/50 coinsurance
Outpatient mental health or drug and alcohol rehab	20/80 coinsurance	50/50 coinsurance	$25 co-pay 30 visits	$25 co-pay 30 visits	50/50 coinsurance
Durable medical equipment	$0	$0	$0	$0	$0
Prosthetics	$0	Not covered	$0	$0	Not covered
Orthotics	$0	Not covered	$0	$0	Not covered

(continues)

EXHIBIT 3-2 (Continued)

Rehabilitation	Max 60 days	30/70 coinsurance	Max 45 days	Max 45 days	30/70 coinsurance
Hospice	$0	20/80 coinsurance	$0	$0	20/80 coinsurance
Skilled nursing facility	365 days max	20/80 coinsurance	365 days max	365 days max	20/80 coinsurance
Prescription drugs	Not covered	Not covered	$20 co-pay	$20 co-pay	Not covered
Chiropractic care	20/80 coinsurance	Not covered	$20 co-pay	$20 co-pay	50/50 coinsurance
Employee cost	$95/month single	$350/month family	$50/month single $200/month family	$70/month single	$275/month family

12 years old. The college-age child is very active in sports, you are concerned that the high school student may be anorexic, and the 12-year-old has a long history of allergies. You and your spouse are relatively healthy; the occasional flu, sprains, and screening exams for your age group are expected.

Questions

• Which health insurance plan would you choose under each scenario?

• Why did you make each choice?

Your choice of health plans need not be the same for both situations, but you must give specific reasons why you chose the same, or different, health insurance plans for each of the scenarios.

Because these are theoretical situations, you do not have some of the basic information you would otherwise have, such as a list of participating providers. Such information might influence whether or not you would have access to providers with whom you are familiar and whether or not you would incur additional expenses for some services you felt were important to you. You will therefore need to make some basic assumptions about those options. It would be helpful to

report those basic assumptions in your response as it relates to how you made your insurance plan choice. Perhaps an interesting way to approach this is to think in terms of the worst-case scenario.

A QUESTION OF ETHICS

• In the discussion of payment to physicians, we see that fee-for-service structures can be an incentive for overtreatment (the provision of unnecessary services). Conversely, we see that capitation payments can be an incentive to underserve (withhold necessary services). From an ethical standpoint, which method of payment is more appropriate, in your opinion?

• Despite various government programs, over 45 million people remain without health insurance. Is it society's responsibility to provide health care services to all?

• Should there be limits to the amount of medical care provided, and should those limits be applied only to those who cannot pay? In other words, is a two-tiered system of health care appropriate—basic health care for the poor and full-coverage health care for those who can pay?

REFERENCES

1. AMA. (2006). Overview of RBRVS. Retrieved from www.ama-assn.org

2. Anderson, O. (1975). *Blue Cross since 1929: Accountability and the public trust.* Cambridge, MA: Ballinger.

3. Balanced Budget Act of 1997. (2000). Health Hippo: Balanced Budget Act of 1997. Retrieved from http://hippo.findlaw.com/Budget.html

4. CDC. (2007). NCHS definitions, health maintenance organization, National Center for Health Statistics. Retrieved from www.cms.hhs.gov

5. CMS. (2007a). Fact Sheets, Details for: Medicare outlines steps to help dual eligibles move to comprehensive Medicare drug coverage. Retrieved from http://www.cms.hhs.gov

6. ——. (2007b). Fiscal year 2004 national MSIS tables, Medicaid Statistical Information System State Summary FY2004. Retrieved from www.cms.hhs.gov/MedicaidDataSourcesGenInfo/Downloads/msistables2004.pdf

7. ——. (2006a). Participation rates as percentage of physicians, by specialty, selected periods. Data Compendium. Retrieved from www.cms.hhs.gov/DataCompendium/18_2006_Data_Compendium.asp

8. ——. (2006b). Ambulatory surgical center (ASC) payment. Retrieved from www.cms.hhs.gov/ASCPayment/06a_CMS1506fc.asp

9. ——. 2006c. Health care consumer initiatives, hospital inpatient. Retrieved May 22, 2007, from www.cms.hhs.gov/HealthCareConInit/02_Hospital.asp

10. ——. (2005a). Medicaid program, general information, technical summary. Retrieved from www.cms.hhs.gov/MedicaidGenInfo/03_TechnicalSummary.asp

11. ——. (2005b). Medicaid at-a-glance, 2005: A Medicaid information source. Retrieved from www.cms.hhs.gov/MedicaidDataSourcesGenInfo/Downloads/maag2005.pdf

12. ——. (2005c). Press Release. Medicare pay for performance (P4P) initiatives. Retrieved from www.cms.hhs.gov/apps/media/press/release.asp

13. ——. (2000). Ensuring Medicaid coverage to support work. Press Release. Retrieved from www.cms.hhs.gov/pf/printpage.asp?ref=http://www.cms.hhs.gov/apps/media/press/release.asp

14. Cunningham, P., Staiti, A., & Ginsburg, P. (2006). Physician acceptance of new Medicare patients stabilizes in 2004–2005. Tracking Report #12. Washington, DC: Center for Studying Health System Change, January 2006.

15. DeNavas-Walt, C., Proctor, B. D., & Smith, J. C. 2008. U.S. Census Bureau, current population reports, P60-235. *Income, poverty, and health insurance coverage in the United States: 2007.* Washington, DC: U.S. Government Printing Office.

16. Fuchs, V. (1974). *Who shall live? Health, economics, and social choice.* New York: Basic Books.

17. Hawley, P. R. (1949). *Non-profit health service plans.* Chicago: Blue Cross Commission and Blue Shield Commission.

18. Health Insurance Institute. (1978). Source book of health insurance data 1977–78. Washington, DC: Health Insurance Institute.

19. Kaiser Family Foundation and Health Research and Educational Trust. (2006). Employer health benefits annual survey, 2006. Retrieved from www.kff.org/insurance/7527/upload/7527.pdf

20. Medicare. (2008). *Medicare and you.* Retrieved from www.medicare.gov/Publications/Pubs/pdf/10050.pdf

21. ——. (2007). *Your Medicare coverage.* Retrieved from www.medicare.gov/Coverage/Home.asp

22. Menzel, P., & Light, D. (2006). A conservative case for universal access to health care. *Hastings Center Report, 36*(4), 36–45.

23. Oregon Health Plan. (1998). The prioritized list—An overview. Retrieved from www.oregon.gov/DHS/healthplan/priorlist/main.shtml

24. U. S. Department of Labor. (2007). Frequently asked questions about portability of health coverage and HIPAA. Retrieved from www.dol.gov/ebsa/faqs/faq_consumer_hipaa.html

25. U. S. Department of the Treasury. (2007a). Office of Public Affairs. About HSAs. Retrieved from www.treas.gov/offices/public-affairs/hsa/about.shtml

26. U. S. Department of the Treasury. (2007b). Office of Public Affairs. Fact Sheet, Dramatic Growth in HSAs. Retrieved from www.treas.gov/offices/public-affairs/hsa/pdf/factsheet-dramatic-growth.pdf

Chapter 4

Health Status and Health Care Utilization

CHAPTER OBJECTIVES

After reading this chapter, readers should have an understanding of the following:

- The major causes of death and disability in developed countries of the world
- The major causes of death and disability in the United States
- Utilization rates of various types of health care in the United States
- Theories of health care utilization
- Disparities in access to health care services across demographic groups in the United States

INTRODUCTION

Many complete books have been written about health status and health care utilization. It is not the objective of this chapter to give a complete picture of either. However, this chapter will highlight some indicators to help readers get a full picture of the U.S. health care system and its functions. Who seeks health care services and why people seek services are factors that determine costs, access, quality, and equity in health care delivery. However, the "who" and the "why" are often difficult to pinpoint—particularly the "why."

This chapter presents some of what we do know and also highlights what we still struggle to learn.

HEALTH STATUS IN THE UNITED STATES

Although the United States spends a larger portion of its gross domestic product (GDP) on health care than any other developed nation in the world, its health indicators fall short in many areas. The World Health Organization (WHO) statistics on **mortality** indicate that the United States is not ranked highest in **life expectancy** and prevention of infant mortality, two strong indicators of the health of a nation (see Table 4–1). Many developed countries rank higher and yet spend less per capita on health care (see Table 4–2). Canada and the United Kingdom, often referenced in the discussion

TABLE 4-1 Life Expectancy and Infant Mortality for Selected Countries, 2007

Country	Life Expectancy at Birth		Infant Mortality Rate (per 1,000 live births)
	Males	Females	
Australia	79	84	5
Austria	77	82	4
Canada	78	83	5
Cuba	75	79	5
Finland	76	82	3
France	77	84	4
Germany	76	82	4
Greece	77	82	4
Iceland	79	83	2
Israel	78	82	4
Italy	78	84	4
Japan	79	86	3
Netherlands	77	81	4
New Zealand	77	82	5
Norway	77	82	3
Singapore	78	82	2
Spain	77	84	4
Sweden	79	83	3
Switzerland	79	84	4
United Kingdom	77	81	5
United States	75	80	7

SOURCE: World Health Organization. 2007. World Health Statistics. Geneva, Switzerland: WHO Press.

of universal health care, each have lower mortality and higher longevity rates and spend less per capita than the United States. The reasons for higher mortality may be based on genetics, environment, lifestyle, or the health care system itself. We have no clear answers at this time to explain the discrepancies.

Despite mortality rates higher than other developed countries, the mortality rate in the United States has been decreasing almost steadily since the early 1900s (Minino et al. 2006). Life expectancy reached a record high of 77.9 years for the total U.S. population in 2004, reflecting increases for white and black males and females. Infant mortality rates decreased in all categories. However, rates for black infants are still much higher than for white infants (see Table 4–3).

Causes of Death

The Centers for Disease Control and Prevention (CDC) reports that the ten leading causes of death for 2004 were the same as

TABLE 4-2 Health Care Spending for Selected Countries, 2004

Country	Health Expenditures as % of GDP	Government Expenditures on Health as % of Expenditures on Health	Per Capita Expenditures on Health (in U.S. dollars)
Australia	9.5	67.5	$3,123
Austria	7.5	67.6	3,683
Canada	9.9	69.9	3,038
Cuba	7.3	86.8	230
Finland	7.4	76.5	2,664
France	10.0	76.3	3,464
Germany	11.1	78.2	3,521
Greece	9.9	51.3	1,879
Iceland	10.5	83.5	4,413
Israel	8.9	68.2	1,534
Italy	8.4	75.1	2,580
Japan	7.9	81.0	2,823
Netherlands	9.8	62.4	3,442
New Zealand	8.1	78.3	2,040
Norway	10.3	83.7	5,405
Singapore	4.5	36.1	943
Spain	7.7	71.3	1,971
Sweden	9.4	85.2	3,532
Switzerland	11.5	58.5	5,572
United Kingdom	8.0	85.7	2,900
United States	15.2	44.6	6,096

SOURCE: World Health Organization. 2007. World Health Statistics. Geneva, Switzerland: WHO Press.

those for 2003, with the seventh and eighth causes exchanging ranks. Diseases of the heart, **malignant neoplasms** (cancer), and cerebrovascular diseases (stroke) lead the list (see Figure 4–1). In 2004, deaths from all causes totaled 2.4 million. Diseases of the heart and malignant neoplasms accounted for 1.2 million deaths or half of all deaths in 2004 (Minino et al. 2006). Of course, the ten leading causes of death are for all ages. When broken down by age group, the leading causes of death change. Accidents, including automobile accidents, are the leading cause of death in a large age group—age 1 to 44. Congenital malformations are the second leading cause of death in 1- to 4-year-olds and the third leading cause of death for 5- to 14-year-olds. In 15- to

TABLE 4–3 U.S. Total Deaths, Age-Adjusted Death Rates, Life Expectancy at Birth, and Infant Mortality Rates, by Race and Sex; Final 2003 and Preliminary 2004

Measure and Sex	All Races[1,2]		White[2]		Black[2]	
	2004	2003	2004	2003	2004	2003
All deaths	2,398,343	2,448,288	2,059,949	2,103,714	284,877	291,300
Age-adjusted death rate[3]	801.0	832.7	787.4	817.0	1,019.3	1,065.9
Male	955.1	994.3	937.4	973.9	1,258.4	1,319.1
Female	680.1	706.2	668.6	693.1	849.6	885.6
Life expectancy at birth[4]	77.9	77.5	78.3	78.0	73.3	72.7
Male	75.2	74.8	75.7	75.3	69.8	69.0
Female	80.4	80.1	80.8	80.5	76.5	76.1
Infant mortality rate[5]	6.76	6.85	5.65	5.72	13.65	14.01

[1]Includes races other than white and black.
[2]Race categories are consistent with the 1977 Office of Management and Budget Standards.
[3]Age-adjusted death rates are per 100,000 U.S. standard population.
[4]Life expectancy at birth stated in years.
[5]Infant mortality rates are deaths under 1 year per 1,000 live births in specified group.

SOURCE: National Center for Health Statistics. 2006, June 28. National Vital Statistics Reports, Vol. 54, No. 19, Table A.

1. Diseases of the heart
2. Malignant neoplasms (known commonly as cancers)
3. Cerebrovascular diseases (any disorder that causes a lack of blood flow)
4. Chronic lower respiratory disease
5. Accidents (unintentional injuries)
6. Diabetes mellitus (adult onset or Type II diabetes)
7. Alzheimer's disease
8. Influenza and pneumonia
9. Nephritis, nephritic syndrome and nephrosis (diseases of the kidney)
10. Septicemia (serious infection of the blood stream)

Figure 4–1 Leading Causes of Death in the U.S. in 2004

SOURCE: National Center for Health Statistics. 2006, June 28. National Vital Statistics Report, Vol. 54, No. 19, Table B.

24-year-olds, homicide and suicide are the second and third leading causes of death. Heart disease, cancer, and cerebrovascular diseases begin to appear in the 25- to 44-year-old category, but become even more prevalent in those over 45.

Infant mortality rates are calculated by dividing the number of infant deaths in a specific year by the number of live births in that same year. Neonatal deaths are defined as deaths of infants fewer than 28 days of age. However, causes of death are reported for total infant deaths. The leading causes of death for infants are congenital malformation, deformations and chromosomal abnormalities, and disorders related to short gestation (prematurity) and low birth weight (see Figure 4–2). These two categories are responsible for 37 percent of all infant deaths (Minino et al. 2006).

Morbidity

An important indication of the health status of a population, in addition to death rates, is morbidity. **Morbidity** is defined as the state of being diseased or the prevalence of disease (Answers.com 2007). Looking at mortality and morbidity is akin to considering the quantity and quality of life in a population. Increasing longevity is a benefit, but not necessarily desirable if those additional years are filled with disease and pain. Therefore, both mortality and morbidity reflect the health status of the population.

The Centers for Disease Control and Prevention (CDC) conducts the National Health Interview Survey. Along with other information, the respondents are asked, "Would you say that your health in general is excellent, very good, good, fair, or poor?" (CDC 2007). This self-reported information gives a better indication of health status than mortality rates alone. As would be expected, the percentage of people reporting "excellent/very good" health status decreases as age increases, and the percentage of people reporting "poor/fair" health status increases as age increases (see Table 4–4). Income also seems to play a part in how well people feel. Generally speaking, individuals who are poor and near-poor report poorer health status than individuals who are nonpoor. The relationship between income and health is a focus of much research and is confounded by such issues as access to health care, environmental factors, genetics, and so on.

The National Health Interview Survey also provides data on the types of **chronic conditions** that contribute to health status (see Table 4–5). As people age, a larger percentage reports dealing with chronic conditions. Asthma is the one exception in which the percentage of people reporting the condition remains somewhat stable across age categories (CDC 2007). Chronic diseases such as heart disease, cancer, pulmonary disease, and diabetes develop later into the causes of death as seen in Figure 4–1. The percentage of people reporting various chronic diseases varies by race and ethnicity (see Table 4–6), as does the percentage of people reporting poor to excellent health status (see Table 4–7).

---

1. Congenital malformations, deformations and chromosomal abnormalities
2. Disorder related to short gestation and low birth weight, not elsewhere classified
3. Sudden infant death syndrome (SIDS)
4. Newborn affected by maternal complications of pregnancy
5. Newborn affected by complications of placenta, cord, and membranes
6. Accidents (unintentional injuries)
7. Respiratory distress of newborn
8. Bacterial sepsis of newborn
9. Neonatal hemorrhage
10. Intrauterine hypoxia and birth asphyxia

Figure 4–2 Ten Leading Causes of Infant Mortality in U.S. for 2004

SOURCE: National Center for Health Statistics. 2006, June 28. National Vital Statistics Reports, Vol. 54, No. 19.

TABLE 4-4 U.S. Health Status of All Genders and All Races/Ethnicity in Percentage by Age and Income, 2000–2005

Health Status	Fair/Poor				Good				Excellent/Very Good			
Income	All	Poor	Near Poor	Nonpoor	All	Poor	Near Poor	Nonpoor	All	Poor	Near Poor	Nonpoor
All Ages	9.2	20.8	14.5	6.2	23.8	30.0	28.4	20.9	67.0	49.2	57.1	72.9
0–17	1.8	4.1	2.4	0.9	16.0	27.7	20.6	10.7	82.1	68.2	77.1	88.4
18–44	5.6	12.7	8.5	3.4	22.1	30.5	28.0	18.8	72.3	56.8	63.5	77.9
45–64	14.6	42.4	28.4	9.2	28.8	30.0	33.6	27.9	56.6	27.6	38.0	62.9
65+	26.3	42.3	33.7	20.4	35.8	33.0	36.3	36.1	37.9	24.7	30.0	43.5

SOURCE: National Center for Health Statistics. National Health Interview Survey, Office of Analysis and Epidemiology, Centers for Disease Control and Prevention. The survey is a continuous national survey of the civilian noninstitutionalized population of the United States (self-reported health status).
This survey is a continuous national survey of the civilian noninstitutionalized population of the United States (self-reported health status).

TABLE 4-5 Chronic Conditions among U.S. Adults, by Age, Genders, Races/Ethnicity, Income, and Location, 2003–2005

Age / Condition (percentage reporting)	18–24	25–44	45–64	65+	65–74	75+
Heart disease	3.0	4.6	12.9	31.7	27.1	36.8
Coronary heart disease	0.4	1.1	6.9	21.6	18.5	25.1
Heart attack	*	0.4	3.7	11.6	10.1	13.3
Hypertension	2.6	9.0	30.5	52.0	49.4	54.8
Stroke	*	0.5	2.3	9.2	6.8	11.9
Cancer, all	0.8	2.3	8.0	21.0	18.6	23.7
Cancer, breast	*	0.2	1.4	4.1	3.5	4.7
Cancer, colorectal	*	0.1	0.4	2.4	1.6	3.3
Cancer, lung	*	*	0.2	0.9	0.9	1.0
Cancer, prostate	*	*	1.0	8.6	6.2	11.8
Cancer, skin	*	0.4	2.3	5.5	5.1	6.1
Chronic obstructive pulmonary disease	2.8	3.4	6.1	9.6	9.8	9.4
Asthma	7.5	6.3	7.1	6.8	7.5	6.1

(continues)

TABLE 4-5 (Continued)

Age	18–24	25–44	45–64	65+	65–74	75+
Condition (percentage reporting)						
Arthritis	3.5	9.4	29.3	50.0	46.5	54.0
Diabetes	0.9	2.5	9.9	17.0	18.2	15.6

*Unreliable data

SOURCE: National Center for Health Statistics. National Health Interview Survey, Office of Analysis and Epidemiology, Centers for Disease Control and Prevention. The survey is a continuous national survey of the civilian noninstitutionalized population of the United States (self-reported health status).

TABLE 4-6 Chronic Self-Reported Conditions for U.S. Adults, by Selected Race/Ethnicity, 2003–2005

Race/Ethnicity	All	White Non-Hispanic	Black Non-Hispanic	Hispanic	American Indian Alaskan Native
Condition (percentage reporting)					
Heart disease	11.5	12.2	9.9	8.2	12.8
Coronary heart disease	6.2	6.4	5.6	5.4	6.3
Heart attack	3.3	3.4	2.7	2.6	2.7
Hypertension	21.9	21.2	31.0	19.6	24.8
Stroke	2.5	2.4	3.4	2.3	3.9
Cancer, all	7.0	8.0	3.9	3.4	6.6
Cancer, breast	1.2	1.3	.8	.6	*
Cancer, colorectal	.5	.6	.5	.3	*
Cancer, lung	.2	.3	.1	.1	*
Cancer, prostate	1.8	1.8	2.6	1.2	*
Cancer, skin	1.8	2.3	.1	.1	*
Chronic obstructive pulmonary disease	5.2	5.7	4.7	3.3	5.9
Asthma	6.8	7.1	7.7	4.9	8.7
Arthritis	21.5	22.6	21.4	16.5	26.9
Diabetes	7.0	6.2	10.8	9.5	13.4

*Unreliable data

SOURCE: National Center for Health Statistics. National Health Interview Survey, Office of Analysis and Epidemiology, Centers for Disease Control and Prevention. This survey is a continuous national survey of the civilian noninstitutionalized population of the United States (self-reported health status).

TABLE 4–7 U.S. Health Status of People over 65 Years of Age, by Income and Race, 2000–2005

Health Status		Fair/Poor				Good				Excellent/Very Good			
	Income	All	Poor	Near-Poor	Nonpoor	All	Poor	Near-Poor	Nonpoor	All	Poor	Near-Poor	Nonpoor
65+	Ethnicity												
	All	26.3	42.3	33.7	20.4	35.8	33.0	36.3	36.1	37.9	24.7	30.0	43.5
	White	24.8	40.0	32.2	19.6	35.9	33.0	36.6	36.0	39.4	27.0	31.3	44.4
	Black	40.3	51.5	43.9	30.4	35.5	33.0	35.1	37.4	24.2	15.5	21.1	32.3
	American Indian/ Alaska native	38.3	56.2	40.7	30.1	33.8	*	*	35.2	27.9	*	*	34.6
	Asian	29.3	43.2	39.0	22.9	36.6	33.9	35.7	37.5	34.1	22.9	25.2	39.7
	Native Hawaiian and other Pacific Islander	*	*	*	*	*	*	*	*	*	*	*	*
	Multiple race	33.9	29.4	48.8	27.2	34.1	34.1	23.7	39.8	32.0	36.5	27.4	33.0
	Hispanic	39.0	49.4	43.4	29.3	33.2	29.0	32.1	36.6	27.8	21.6	24.5	34.1
	Puerto Rican	41.6	57.3	42.3	28.6	34.9	*	36.7	39.5	23.5	*	21.0	31.9
	Mexican	40.1	49.1	45.4	29.6	34.0	30.4	32.5	37.7	25.9	20.6	22.2	32.7
	Non-Hispanic white	23.7	37.8	31.1	19.2	36.1	34.1	37.0	36.0	40.2	28.1	31.9	44.8
	Non-Hispanic black	40.5	51.9	43.8	30.7	35.3	32.7	35.1	37.2	24.1	15.5	21.1	32.

*Unreliable data

SOURCE: National Center for Health Statistics. National Health Interview Survey, Office of Analysis and Epidemiology, Centers for Disease Control and Prevention. The survey is a continuous national survey of the civilian noninstitutionalized population of the United States (self-reported health status).

A recent concern regarding chronic diseases is the prevalence of both males and females of all races who are overweight or obese (see Table 4–8). Of primary concern is the fact that some 15 percent of children are overweight. People who are overweight have a greater risk for diabetes, heart disease, high blood pressure, joint disorders, and other related diseases. In addition, individuals who are overweight have an increased risk of premature death. There is also much social stigma placed on obesity, therefore people who are overweight (particularly young people) may suffer from low self-esteem and depression (Thompson 2004). Although much work is being done on the causes of overweight and obesity, today's prevalent models are based on lifestyle, genetics, and environment.

Much research is being done to determine the cause of the variations in health status. There are many models of health determinants. However, they all include individual lifestyle, neighborhood or community, living conditions, work conditions, genetics, social relationships, health care, income, and culture in some way (Dahlgren and Whitehead 1991; Evans and Stoddart 1990; Institute of Medicine 2000).

Eliminating health care disparities is the second of two major objectives of Healthy People 2010 (U.S. Department of Health and Human Services 2000). This applies to "all segments of the population including differences that occur by gender, race or ethnicity, education or income, disability, geographic location, or sexual orientation" (ibid.). The first goal is "to help individuals of all ages increase life expectancy and improve their quality of life" (ibid.). Access to health care services, one of twenty-eight goals, addresses both of these objectives (although it is not the only factor influencing both objectives). If there are barriers to access based on population differences, life expectancy and quality of life are affected.

TABLE 4–8 Overweight/Obesity among U.S. Adults, Percentage by Race and Gender, 2004

Weight Status	Healthy Weight			Overweight*			Obese**			Severely Obese***		
	All	Male	Female	All	Male	Female	All	Male	Female	All	Male	Female
Race/ Ethnicity												
All	32.3	28.4	36.1	34.6	41.0	28.4	31.3	29.4	33.1	4.9	3.2	6.6
Non-Hispanic white	33.9	27.9	39.8	33.8	40.8	27.0	30.5	30.3	30.7	4.5	3.2	5.8
Non-Hispanic black	24.4	31.1	18.9	31.8	35.9	28.4	42.0	30.8	51.1	9.4	4.4	13.4
Mexican American	26.5	26.5	26.6	39.3	44.7	33.1	33.9	28.6	39.8	4.5	2.4	6.8

*Body mass index (BMI) greater than or equal to 25.0 kg/m² and less than 30.0 kg/m²
**BMI greater than or equal to 30.0 kg/m²
***BMI greater than or equal to 40.0 kg/m²

SOURCE: National Center for Health Statistics. 2003–2004. National Health and Nutrition Examination Survey, Centers for Disease Control and Prevention.

TABLE 4–9 Percentage* of U.S. People Receiving Prenatal Care by Date of First Prenatal Visit, by Race and Age during Pregnancy, 2002–2004

Prenatal Care	First Trimester								
Maternal Age	**All**	**<18**	**10–14**	**15–17**	**18–19**	**20–24**	**25–29**	**30–34**	**35–39**
Race/Ethnicity									
All	83.8	64.6	48.6	65.4	72.7	78.8	85.6	85.5	85.4
White/non-Hispanic	88.9	71.1	55.3	71.6	77.7	83.5	90.6	90.4	89.8
Black/non-Hispanic	76.1	58.6	42.7	59.8	68.8	74.2	78.3	77.0	78.6
Native American or Alaskan native	69.9	56.2	45.4	56.8	63.3	69.3	72.4	70.3	71.6
Hispanic	77.1	64.2	52.1	64.8	69.8	74.5	78.7	77.9	78.9

*Percentage is based on three-year averages.

SOURCE: National Center for Health Statistics. Health data for all ages. Office of Analysis and Epidemiology, Centers for Disease Control and Prevention. This survey is a continuous national survey of the civilian noninstitutionalized population of the United States (self-reported health status).

HEALTH CARE UTILIZATION

Just as morbidity and mortality among various groups of people are different, health care utilization between and among various demographic groups are also different. Table 4–9 shows that a higher percentage of white non-Hispanic women receive prenatal care in their first trimester than do Hispanic, black, or American Indian and Native Alaskan individuals.

In all categories, a higher percentage of individuals considered poor and near-poor than nonpoor report having no regular source of health care (see Table 4–10). Having a regular source of care (often seen as having a primary care physician) may be an indication of what may be referred to as "future orientation." Those who are future-oriented plan ahead and, in the case of health care, partake in preventive care. Individuals who are poor or near-poor are less likely to be future-oriented; they are unable to spend time and money on checkups for illnesses that may or may not become a reality down the road. For these people, time and money are scarce and are spent on issues of current need.

In all categories, individuals who are non-Hispanic whites report a lower percentage of not having a regular source of care than any other racial or ethnic groups. Although the lack of future orientation should also apply to poor whites, the lack of trust in health care providers is not as strong as it may be among minorities. Because we are looking at people in the United States, people 65 and over are not surprisingly most likely to have a regular source of care primarily because of the Medicare system of payment for health care services.

At first glance, it may seem that being white and nonpoor are the keys to receiving care. However, much more enters into each individual's decision to seek health care services. Many researchers have studied the factors that influence health care utilization (Aday and Andersen 1974; Becker 1974; Gish 1990; Greenlick 1968; Pescosolido 1992; Rosenstock 1966), resulting in a number of health behavior models. Two of the most prominent models (modified by many others) come from Andersen and Rosenstock.

Rosenstock (1966) and Becker (1974) offer the health belief model. The model proposes that care is sought if individuals (1) perceive themselves to be susceptible to a particular health

40+	All	<18	10–14	15–17	18–19	20–24	25–29	30–34	35–39	40+
				Late or None						
88.5	3.6	8.3	15.0	8.0	5.9	4.7	3.2	3.2	3.3	2.6
92.2	2.2	6.0	13.3	5.8	4.0	3.2	1.8	1.9	2.0	1.6
81.2	5.9	9.8	17.0	9.2	7.0	6.1	5.4	5.7	5.5	5.3
73.8	7.9	11.9	18.1	11.6	9.3	7.9	7.4	7.8	7.5	7.2
81.6	5.4	9.0	13.4	8.7	7.3	6.1	4.9	5.2	5.0	4.3

TABLE 4-10 Percentage of People without a Regular Source of Health Care, by Race or Ethnicity, Age, and Income, 2003–2005

Race/Ethnicity		All	White Non-Hispanic	Black Non-Hispanic	Native American/ Alaska Native	Asian	Hispanic
Age	Income						
All	All	12.8	10.3	13.6	15.9	14.3	23.1
	Poor	21.1	17.1	18.9	17.8	24.1	29.9
	Near-poor	18.4	15.2	16.0	20.0	20.5	27.1
	Nonpoor	9.7	8.6	10.3	12.5	11.1	16.9
0–17	All	5.4	3.2	6.2	7.3	7.5	11.3
	Poor	9.9	7.4	7.7	*	12.6	14.2
	Near-poor	7.7	4.7	6.5	*	14.4	13.3
	Nonpoor	3.1	2.2	4.8	*	4.2	6.9
18–44	All	22.1	18.1	22.2	26.9	21.8	37.4
	Poor	33.2	26.7	28.9	36.4	34.8	46.9
	Near-poor	31.0	26.0	26.2	33.3	30.0	43.3
	Nonpoor	17.1	15.3	17.7	19.1	17.1	28.1

(continues)

TABLE 4-10 (Continued)

Race/Ethnicity		All	White Non-Hispanic	Black Non-Hispanic	Native American/ Alaska Native	Asian	Hispanic
Age	Income						
45–64	All	10.3	8.8	11.9	11.8	13.8	20.6
	Poor	21.2	18.0	21.7	*	30.5	29.1
	Near-poor	16.8	14.8	15.0	*	20.5	26.2
	Nonpoor	8.0	7.4	7.8	12.0	10.8	15.0
65+	All	3.7	3.3	4.7	*	*	7.3
	Poor	6.2	5.6	5.7	*	*	10.1
	Near-poor	4.0	3.5	5.8	*	*	6.9
	Nonpoor	3.2	3.0	*	*	*	5.8

*Unreliable data

SOURCE: National Center for Health Statistics. National Health Interview Survey, Office of Analysis and Epidemiology, Centers for Disease Control and Prevention. This survey is a continuous national survey of the civilian noninstitutionalized population of the United States (self-reported health status).

problem; (2) see this problem as a serious one; (3) are convinced that treatment or prevention activities are effective but not overly costly either in terms of money or effort; and (4) receive a prompt or cue to seek health care services.

The model may be more understandable if it is broken down into each of the four areas and considered in terms of examples. An individual may have a family history of diabetes (contributing to perceived susceptibility toward diabetes) and may have watched a family member go through the associated problems of diabetes (that is, the person sees it as serious). The individual then must decide if prevention (good diet, exercise, and regular checkups) is worth the time, effort, and monetary commitment. The cue to seek services may be as simple as hearing the symptoms on a radio spot or as specific as experiencing the early symptoms. Beliefs are difficult to modify, and that is why people still smoke even though many educational programs have spread the word about the dangers of smoking. Some people just don't believe they are susceptible to illness, or they feel like giving up smoking is too big a price to pay for prevention.

Andersen (1995) initially developed a model of health services utilization based on predisposing factors, enabling factors, and need (see Figure 4–3). Predisposing factors determining the use

of health services include demographics—age, gender, and race or ethnicity—which are **immutable factors** (they cannot be changed). Social structure—education, occupation, and location—is also an immutable factor on a short-term basis. The last component of predisposing factors is health beliefs. Beliefs, as mentioned previously, are difficult to change, especially if they are cultural beliefs such as distrust of medical care.

Enabling factors are **mutable factors** (they are changeable), and include personal and community components. Personal factors such as income and insurance status can be changed and often are through social welfare programs. The community can provide health services resources such as health care facilities and transportation. Need is determined by personal perceptions (similar to the health beliefs model). Predisposing factors, enabling factors, and need combine to formulate the decision to seek health care services.

HEALTH DISPARITIES

There are significant health care disparities between nonminorities and racial and ethnic minorities. The causes of these disparities are complex and involve many factors described in the following report from the Institute of Medicine.

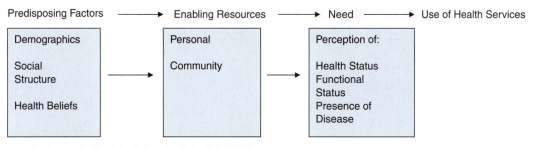

Figure 4–3 Andersen's Health Behavior Model (1968)

SOURCE: Andersen, R. 1995. Revisiting the behavioral model and access to medical care: Does it matter? *Journal of Health and Social Behavior* 36:2.

Racial and ethnic minorities tend to receive a lower quality of health care than nonminorities, *even when access-related factors, such as patients' insurance status and income, are controlled.* The sources of these disparities are complex, are rooted in historic and contemporary inequities, and involve many participants at several levels, including health systems, their administrative and bureaucratic processes, utilization managers, health care professionals, and patients. Consistent with the charge, the study committee focused part of its analysis on the clinical encounter itself, and found evidence that stereotyping, biases, and uncertainty on the part of health care providers can all contribute to unequal treatment. The conditions in which many clinical encounters take place—characterized by high time pressure, cognitive complexity, and pressures for cost containment—may enhance the likelihood that these processes will result in care poorly matched to minority patients' needs. Minorities may experience a range of other barriers to accessing care, even when insured at the same level as

whites, including barriers of language, geography, and cultural familiarity. Further, financial and institutional arrangements of health systems, as well as the legal, regulatory, and policy environment in which they operate, may have disparate and negative effects on minorities' ability to attain quality care.

Institute of Medicine. 2003. *Unequal Treatment: Confronting Racial and Ethnic Disparities in Healthcare*

Health behavior and health care utilization models shed some light on the disparities in health care utilization but do not answer all of the questions regarding variation. Table 4–9 shows that white women are more likely to receive prenatal care than minority women. Table 4–11 indicates that, although infant deaths have decreased between 1980 and 2004, black infants consistently have a higher death rate than white infants. Leading causes of death have already been discussed. However, there are differences in death rates (per 100,000) between people of various racial or ethnic backgrounds (see Table 4–12). The

TABLE 4–11 Infant Mortality Rates by Race for Selected Years, 1980–2004

Deaths per 1,000 Live Births							
Year	**1980**	**1990**	**2000**	**2001**	**2002**	**2003**	**2004**
Race							
All	12.6	9.2	6.9	6.8	7.0	6.9	6.8
White	10.9	7.6	5.7	5.7	5.8	5.7	5.7
Black	22.2	18.0	14.1	14.0	14.4	14.0	13.8

SOURCE: National Center for Health Statistics. 2006. Health United States, 2006, with Chartbook on Trends in the Health of Americans. MD: Hyattsville.

TABLE 4–12 U.S. Death Rates per 100,000 People for Selected Diseases by Race and Gender, 2005

	All		White Non-Hispanic		Black		Native American/Native Alaskan		Asian/Pacific Islander		Hispanic	
	Male	Female	Male	Female	Male	Female	Male	Female	Male	Female	Male	Female
Diseases of the heart	260.9	172.3	262.2	170.3	329.8	228.3	173.2	115.9	141.1	91.9	192.4	129.1
Cerebrovascular disease	46.9	45.6	44.8	44.4	70.5	60.7	31.3	37.1	41.5	36.3	38.0	33.5
Malignant neoplasms	225.1	155.6	227.3	159.1	293.7	179.6	147.6	105.9	133.0	94.5	152.7	101.9
Lower respiratory disease	51.2	38.1	54.7	42.5	44.1	22.8	34.9	25.5	22.5	9.7	25.1	15.4
HIV	6.2	2.3	3.0	.6	28.2	12.0	4.0	1.5	1.0	*	7.5	1.9
Motor vehicle injuries	21.7	8.9	22.0	9.4	22.5	7.6	34.3	15.4	9.6	5.9	21.3	7.8
Homicide	9.6	2.5	3.5	1.8	37.3	6.1	11.3	4.0	4.4	1.6	12.1	2.4

*Unreliable data

SOURCE: National Center for Health Statistics. 2007. Health United States, 2007, with Chartbook on Trends in the Health of Americans. MD: Hyattsville.

EXHIBIT 4–1

July 20, 2007

Tests of ER Trainees Find Signs of Race Bias in Care: Study Seeks Root of Known Disparity

The Boston Globe

Stephen Smith GLOBE STAFF

Deeply imbedded attitudes about race influence the way doctors care for their African American patients, according to a Harvard study that for the first time details how unconscious bias contributes to inferior care.

Researchers have known for years that African Americans in the midst of a heart attack are far less likely than white patients to receive potentially life-saving treatments such as clot-busting drugs, a dramatic illustration of America's persistent health care disparities. But the reasons behind such stark gaps in care for heart disease, as well as cancer and other serious illnesses, have remained murky, with blame fixed on doctors, hospitals, and insurance plans.

In the new study, trainee doctors in Boston and Atlanta took a twenty-minute computer survey designed to detect overt and implicit prejudice. They were also presented with the hypothetical case of a 50-year-old man stricken with sharp chest pain; in some scenarios, the man was white, while in others he was black.

"We found that, as doctors' unconscious biases against blacks increased, their likelihood of giving [clot-busting] treatment decreased," said the lead author of the study, Dr. Alexander R. Green of Massachusetts General Hospital. "It's not a matter of you being a racist. It's really a matter of the way your brain processes information is influenced by things you've seen, things you've experienced, the way media has presented things."

Specialists predict that the novel study, appearing on the website of the Journal of General Internal Medicine, will result in considerable soul searching in the medical profession, rethinking of medical school curriculum, and refresher courses for veteran doctors.

"Years of advanced education and egalitarian intentions are no protection against the effect of implicit attitudes,"

said Dr. Thomas Inui, president of the Regenstrief Institute Inc. in Indianapolis, which studies vulnerable patient groups. "When do they surface? When we're involved with high-pressure, high-stakes decision making, when there's a lot riding on our decisions but there isn't a lot of time to make them, that's when the implicit attitudes that are not scientific rise up and grab us."

Green said he cannot explain why implicit bias would cause doctors to deprive patients of potentially life-saving therapy, and other researchers said they do not know how big a factor unconscious prejudice is in the far-reaching problem of disparities.

The best way to combat those impulses is by acknowledging them, specialists said, suggesting that medical personnel take a test to measure unconscious bias, such as one at implicit.harvard.edu.

"The great advantage of being human, of having the privilege of awareness, of being able to recognize the stuff that is hidden, is that we can beat the bias," said Mahzarin R. Banaji, a Harvard psychologist who helped design a widely used bias test.

Dr. JudyAnn Bigby, Massachusetts secretary of health and human services and a specialist in health care disparities, said the study demonstrates the importance of monitoring how hospitals and large physician practices provide care to patients of different races.

But Inui and other specialists said that even conquering doctor bias will not be enough to eliminate health care disparities.

A succession of studies during the past decade has demonstrated graphically the scope of disparities and the complexity of the problem, which touches on issues from poverty to geography to genetics.

Black patients in the process of having a heart attack, for example, are only half as likely as whites to get clot-busting medication, and they are much less likely to undergo open-heart surgery. Similarly, African American women receive breast cancer screenings at a rate substantially lower than white women. Fewer black babies live to celebrate their first birthdays: In Massachusetts, the

(continues)

EXHIBIT 4-1 (Continued)

mortality rate for black infants is more than double the rate for white babies.

Health care disparities emerged as a national issue with the 2002 release of a landmark study titled "Unequal Treatment" that was commissioned by Congress and produced by the Institute of Medicine. In Boston, the city health department released a sweeping blueprint for addressing disparities two years ago, with Mayor Thomas M. Menino describing the issue as the most pressing health problem confronting the city.

"Most physicians are now willing to acknowledge that important disparities exist in the health care system," said Dr. John Ayanian, a health care policy specialist at Brigham and Women's Hospital who was not involved with the new research. "There's still a barrier, though, to many physicians acknowledging that disparities may exist in the care of their own patients."

It was during a lecture three years ago by Banaji that Green came up with the idea of measuring the unconscious bias of physicians by using a test Banaji had helped develop.

Green and his colleagues decided to test residents at Massachusetts General, the Brigham, and Beth Israel Deaconess Medical Center in Boston, as well as at an Atlanta hospital. Residents were told that the study was evaluating the use of heart attack drugs in the emergency room, but not that it was also examining racial bias; 220 trainee doctors were counted in the results.

The residents were first given a narrative describing a male patient who shows up in the emergency room complaining of chest pains. Accompanying the narrative was a computer-generated image of the patient, either a black or white man shown in a hospital gown from the chest up, wearing a neutral facial expression.

The doctors were asked if, based on the information provided, they would diagnose the man as having a heart attack and, if so, whether they would prescribe clot-busting drugs called thrombolytics, commonly used in community hospitals to stabilize patients having heart attacks, and how likely they were to give those drugs.

Study participants were also asked questions designed to determine if they were overtly biased. Answers showed they were not.

Last, the residents took Banaji's "implicit association test," which is based on the concept that the more strongly test takers associate a picture of a white or black patient with a particular concept, say cooperativeness, the faster they will make a match. White, Asian, and Hispanic doctors were faster to make matches between blacks and negative concepts and slower to make matches between blacks and positive ones. The small number of African American physicians in the study were as likely to show bias against blacks as against whites.

The researchers then compared the implicit association test scores with the decisions about whether to provide the clot-busting medicine and found that doctors whose ratings of African Americans were most negative were also the least likely to prescribe the drug to blacks.

Another study, scheduled to be presented by a Johns Hopkins medical researcher in October, reaches similar results.

"At the end of the day, even among very well-intentioned people, implicit biases can be both prevalent and in some situations can impact clinical decisions," said Dr. Amal Trivedi, a health care disparities specialist at Brown Medical School who was not involved in the study. "What this study can do is raise awareness of that finding."

Discussion Question

The study suggests subconscious bias. Although we might know of people who are openly biased, bias could be unintentional in health care delivery, harboring a set of stereotypes toward people who are different from us.

1. Is it worth additional study of bias as a cause of health care disparities?

---

greatest differences are between black and white individuals. In fact, Hispanic, Asian, and Native American individuals have lower death rates from heart disease, malignant neoplasms, lower respiratory disease, and cerebrovascular disease than white individuals (see Table 4–6). Are all of these differences due to diet, genetics, and lifestyle?

TABLE 4-13 Breast Cancer Death Rates and Incidence Rates, by Race/Ethnicity for Selected Years

	1990	2000	2003	2005
Race	**Deaths per 100,000 Resident Population**			
White, non-Hispanic	33.2	26.3	25.2	23.4
Black	38.1	34.5	34.0	32.8
Native American/ Native Alaskan	13.7	13.6	14.0	15.2
Asian/Pacific Islander	13.7	12.3	12.6	12.2
Hispanic	19.5	16.9	16.1	15.0
	Number of New Cases per 100,000 Population			
White, non-Hispanic	138.9	147.4	134.0	132.7
Black	116.5	119.1	119.7	118.8
Native American/ Native Alaskan	65.3	88.8	81.6	85.9
Asian/Pacific Islander	86.9	91.4	88.0	92.5
Hispanic	88.2	93.6	81.9	83.9

SOURCE: National Center for Health Statistics. 2007. Health United States, 2007, with Chartbook on Trends in the Health of Americans. MD: Hyattsville.

An illustration of health disparities is evident when reviewing breast cancer statistics. Incidence rates (number of new cases per year) are greater among white females than all other minorities, yet death rates from breast cancer are higher in black females than all other minorities (see Table 4–13). Although the incidence of breast cancer is higher for white females, they also have a higher survival rate than black females (see Table 4–14). The cancer may not be detected as early in black females, or early treatment may not be offered. These discrepancies between black and white cancer survivors are cause for concern, and the issues surrounding detection, treatment, and survival are in dire need of research.

TABLE 4-14 Five-Year Relative Breast Cancer Survival Rates for White and Black Females for Selected Years

	1990–1992	1993–1995	1996–2003
Race	**Percentage of Patients**		
White	86.7	87.9	90.3
Black	71.7	72.8	77.9

SOURCE: National Center for Health Statistics. 2007. Health United States, 2007, with Chartbook on Trends in the Health of Americans. MD: Hyattsville.

SUMMARY

Health status and health care utilization are dependent on many factors. The United States has a very diverse population and is the only industrialized nation without universal health care. We believe we have one of the most advanced health care systems in the world, and yet we have higher death rates than many other countries both with and without universal health care coverage. However, universal health care coverage may not erase all the disparities in health status and health care utilization.

Finding a way to pay for health services is not the only factor that influences people to seek care or to follow treatment plans when care is provided. Health beliefs, access to care, transportation, education, and other factors play a part in determining an individual's decision to seek care. As a diverse nation, we may have to devise diverse methods of providing care and motivating preventive behavior.

ACTIVITY-BASED LEARNING

Much of the data provided in the tables in this chapter are derived from data basis developed by government agencies. Analyzing the data takes time and results in delayed publication of information. Each table has a "source" line indicating from where the data came.

- Go to www.who.int/whosis/en/ to view the WHO Statistical Information System. Is there a more recent publication than the "World Health Statistics 2007"? Browse through available tables. How does the United States compare in the many mortality, morbidity, and other measures that the World Health Organization provides?

Perhaps the most disturbing statistics available are those on infant mortality. Research the issue of infant mortality in the United States, according to various regions of the country. Does this shed any light on the possible causes of high infant mortality rates?

A QUESTION OF ETHICS

- Are health care disparities an issue of ethical health care delivery?
- Should we expect people of different ethnic and racial backgrounds to have the same longevity and incidence of diseases?

REFERENCES

1. Aday, L., and Andersen, R. (1974). A framework for the study of access in medical care. *Health Services Research, 9*, 208–220.

2. Andersen, R. (1995). Revisiting the behavioral model and access to medical care: Does it matter? *Journal of Health and Social Behavior, 36*, 1–10.

3. Answers.com. (2007). Morbidity. Retrieved from www.answers.com/topic/morbidity

4. Becker, M. (1974). *The health belief model and personal health behavior*. San Francisco: The Society for Public Health Education.

5. Dahlgren, G., and Whitehead, M. (1991). Policies and strategies to promote social equity in health. Stockholm, Sweden: Institute for Futures Studies.

6. Evans, R., and Stoddart, G. (1990). Producing health, consuming healthcare. *Social Science and Medicine, 31,* 1347–1363.

7. Gish, O. (1990). Some links between successful implementation of primary health care interventions and the overall utilization of health services. *Social Science and Medicine, 30,* 401–405.

8. Greenlick, M. (1968, Winter). Determinants of medical care utilization. Health Services Research, 296–315.

9. Institute of Medicine. (2003). Unequal treatment: Confronting racial and ethnic disparities in healthcare (B. Smedly, A. Stith, & A. Nelson, Ed.). Washington, DC: National Academies Press.

10. Institute of Medicine. (2000). Promoting health: Intervention strategies from social and behavioral research. Washington, DC: National Academies Press.

11. Minino, A., Heron, M., & Smith, B. (2006). Deaths: Preliminary data for 2004, *CDC national vital statistics report, 54* (19).

12. Centers for Disease Control and Prevention (CDC). (2007). National Health Interview Survey. Health data for all ages. Office of Analysis and Epidemiology, National Center for Health Statistics. Retrieved from http://www.cdc.gov.nchs/nhis.htm

13. Pescosolido, B. (1992). Beyond rational choice: The social dynamics of how people see help. *American Journal of Sociology, 97,* 1096–1138.

14. Rosenstock, I. (1966). Why people use health services. *Milbank Memorial Fund Quarterly, 44,* 94–124.

15. Thompson, B. (2004). Notes and comments—The obesity agency: Centralizing the nation's fight against fat. *American Journal of Law & Medicine, 30,* 543.

16. U.S. Department of Health and Human Services. (2000, November). *Healthy People 2010.* 2nd ed. With Understanding and Improving Health and Objectives for Improving Health. 2 vols. Washington, DC: U.S. Government Printing Office. Retrieved from www.healthypeople.gov/document/tableofcontents.htm#partb

Chapter 5

Medical Education

CHAPTER OBJECTIVES

After completing this chapter, readers should have an understanding of the following:

- The history of medical education
- The difference between undergraduate and graduate medical education
- How medical education is financed
- The determination of physician competency through licensing and certification
- Current trends in medical education

INTRODUCTION

Physicians today are vastly different from practitioners in seventeenth- and eighteenth-century America. Today's physicians pursue a rigorous course of study and clinical practice under the close supervision of faculty who are typically at the forefront of the health professions. Not only must today's physicians pass courses in a premedical curriculum at a college or university and courses the medical school offers, but they must also complete a year of general residency and pass the licensing exam. Nearly all physicians, moreover, now undertake at least three years of additional supervised specialty training in a nationally accredited residency training program after completing their basic medical education. In most states, physicians must also participate in approved continuing medical education programs to maintain licensure.

Although state law does not require certification in the physician's area of expertise, most hospitals, managed care organizations, and insurers do require certification, as well as licensure and continuing education. The end result are people licensed by the state government, certified by a specialty board, and competent to diagnose and treat most illnesses while knowing when to refer patients for specialty care.

Licensure and certification do not guarantee that all physicians are excellent and and will provide the best possible medical care, or that diagnostic and treatment errors are not made. However, such licensure and certification do provide that most physicians are competent and that patients have some grounds for assessing competency. Licensure and/or accreditation have been benchmarks in the past, whereas new methods for assuring quality of care have been elusive.

MEDICAL TRAINING AND KNOWLEDGE IN COLONIAL AMERICA

In colonial times, women in the family treated most of the sick at home. They used medicinal herbs, relied on family and friends for advice, and later used medical guides that were specifically published for laypeople. During that period, people with little or no training could also treat the sick and be regarded as physicians. Most "physicians" were trained under an apprenticeship system, with no organized method for testing the competence of those practitioners or their students. No effective organizations or formats existed to attest, by the granting of a license, to physicians' competence (Packard 1963).

In the traditional British categorization of practitioners, physicians typically held university medical degrees and practiced what we would call internal medicine. An **apothecary** was not a medical doctor but was trained as an apprentice to learn to dispense drugs. However, people frequently sought medical advice from apothecaries as they do from today's pharmacists (Colonial Williamsburg Foundation 2007). Surgeons (known as chirurgeons) were also trained through apprenticeships.

These distinctions became blurred in colonial America, for very few physicians came to the New World. According to William Smith's 1758 *History of New York,* America had no medical schools to train them (Packard 1963). Furthermore, all the colonies had only one hospital, the Philadelphia Hospital, and it had been open for only a few years. The first medical school was established in 1756, at the College of Philadelphia (later, University of Pennsylvania). The second medical school was at King's College (later, Columbia University), founded in 1768. By the time of the Revolutionary War, neither school had made significant medical manpower contributions to the total number of medical practitioners in the colonies.

Some of the early practitioners without medical degrees were simply learned men[1]—ministers, planters, lawyers, teachers—who could apply knowledge from a smattering of books they read. Those who aspired to practice medicine apprenticed with established physicians for a number of years. During a training period, apprentices would watch, assist, and read their preceptors' books. Upon completing the training, physicians would give the apprentice a signed testimonial that constituted the certificate of proficiency. Some physicians in colonial times, however, may not have had any qualifications other than "an interest in the sick and assurance enough to hang out a shingle" (Corner 1965).

With the opening of the Pennsylvania Hospital (described in Chapter 8), a significant new pattern of training began to develop. Physicians not only began to take their apprentices with them to the hospital to assist, but they also began to allow other students to follow them as they examined and treated their hospital patients.

By 1773, the hospital administration had decided to regulate this system so that aspiring physicians could pay a fee to the hospital and be formally apprenticed to the institution for five years. The institution granted a certificate to apprentices upon completing the apprenticeship. In 1765, the University of Pennsylvania established a medical department, and the hospital apprentices attended lectures. This practice continued until 1824, when the hospital required future residents to be regular graduates from the medical college before taking up their hospital appointments (Packard 1963).

NINETEENTH-CENTURY MEDICAL EDUCATION

Only four medical schools—Harvard University (founded in 1783), Dartmouth College (founded in 1797), the College of Philadelphia, and King's College—had been established by 1800. These schools were not like medical schools of today. Sometimes only three or four (or less) faculty members were available. Corner (1965) tells us that Dartmouth "appointed the formidable Harvard graduate Nathan Smith to be a one-man medical faculty. For ten or twelve years he alone ably taught all the courses" (p. 57). The science and art of medicine were extremely limited in what they could offer in the way of cures. However weak the first schools were, they marked an important forward step. Stevens (1971) notes that "the foundation of the medical school in Philadelphia . . . was a part of the movement by university trained physicians to organize and rationalize medicine on a European model and to institute recognizable

---

[1]At this point, the use of the word *men* is appropriate, for medicine was a male domain. Female involvement in "medical" matters was confined to midwifery, and to the extent that some of them received formal training, formal training was frequently provided by medical practitioners. The first female medical school graduate was from the Geneva Medical College around 1850. See "Women in American Medicine," by R. H. Shryock, 1950, *Journal of the American Medical Women's Association* 5(9) (reprinted in Shryock 1966).

educational standards" (p. 17). Men with European medical training dominated the early medical faculties at Philadelphia, Harvard, Columbia, and even at Dartmouth. As the number of medical schools grew, and as more and more U.S. medical graduates went abroad to Edinburgh, London, Paris, and other cities of Europe, many returned and gravitated to the medical school faculties, and they championed reform.

Three local physicians in Castleton, Vermont, established the first proprietary medical school in 1818 (Stevens 1971). In Boston, among the better private schools were the Tremont Street School—established in 1838 by four physicians, including Oliver Wendell Holmes—and the University of Massachusetts Medical School in Boylston (Packard 1963). The Tremont Street School flourished and offered lectures in embryology and anatomy, surgical pathology, chemistry, **auscultation** and percussion, and microscopic anatomy. The faculty consisted mostly of moonlighting Harvard faculty, something that is notable, because faculty members rarely relied solely on medical school income in those days.

In medicine, as in most other endeavors, those who are most expert initiate the effort to raise standards and elevate the level of practice (Stevens 1989). The effort was evident in medicine as medical professionals were involved in founding university medical schools, establishing early medical societies, and initiating medical journals. All of these steps were designed to share knowledge, communicate, improve the quality of practice, and establish a profession in which standards and esteem were comparable to those of European colleagues.

As the decades advanced in the nineteenth century, more medical practitioners were educated in medical schools. A decreasing percentage came from the apprenticeship system. In the absence of a strong licensing mechanism, the measure of a physician's competence came to rest on the standard of whether or not the physician had graduated from a medical school with a doctor of medicine (MD) degree.

This new standard encouraged the development of a large number of new medical schools—some at universities that were ill-equipped to support and nourish them, and a great many freestanding schools with no university ties. Many schools were located in rural areas with no hospital or other clinical facilities.

The notion of university-based medical education came to the United States primarily from Scotland. Physicians trained at University of Edinburgh strongly influenced the structuring of the schools at Philadelphia and Columbia. University-based medical education was also dictated by the absence of strong hospitals in colonial America that could provide the setting for excellence. In England, however, a number of medical schools grew up around such long-established hospitals as Guy's and St. Thomas's, from which came the acceptable model of free-standing and hospital-based schools in the nineteenth-century United States.

Some of the new nonuniversity schools were good and had reputable faculties. Some of the schools were weak and were allegedly set up to make money because each student directly paid professors in most (good and bad) schools for attendance at lectures. Even the quality of education at the "better" schools left much to be desired. Medical science was rather primitive, with a very limited understanding of the causes or options in the treatment of disease.

During the 1870s, Harvard increased its length of training from two to three years, instituted written exams, and then required a college degree or the passing of a qualifying exam for admission. In 1892, the training was lengthened to four years. In 1893, Johns Hopkins University launched its pioneering effort in medical education with a four-year curriculum. This curriculum became the model used to reform all medical education.

THE AMERICAN MEDICAL ASSOCIATION AND ITS INFLUENCE ON MEDICAL EDUCATION

The American Medical Association (AMA) was founded in 1847, with a primary goal of improving medical education. At the organizational meeting in Philadelphia, the Committee on Medical Education was established (Johnson 1947). Reform was difficult because many of the AMA's members were stakeholders in the very educational institutions the AMA sought to revamp.

In 1876, twenty-two medical schools organized the Association of American Medical Colleges (AAMC) as part of the effort to improve the quality of medical education. This new organization struggled over issues to establish higher standards and higher graduation requirements in particular (Coggeshall 1965). Both the AMA and the AAMC thus encountered the problem that besets all representative bodies: To continue to exist, the organization had to retain the support of its constituency. Progress was made, but with incremental steps so as not to lose the constituency.

The AAMC was persuaded to support a four-year curriculum in 1894. The organization played an important role, increasingly so from the 1890s on, but clearly it did not have enough clout to bring about the necessary reform by itself. At this point, the AMA began to play a significant role.

In 1901, the AMA was restructured to become a more representative body by lessening the influence of medical educators in its governing House of Delegates. In 1904, the House of Delegates acted on a report of the Committee on Medical Education and created a new Council on Medical Education. The council's functions were to report annually on the existing conditions of medical education, suggest means and methods by which the AMA could favorably influence medical education, and act as the AMA's agent in its efforts to elevate medical education (Johnson 1947). The council still exists, and its annual report, published in the *Journal of the American Medical Association* (Barzansky and Etzel 2004), offers a definitive account of the current state of medical education.

However, even before the council's work began, leadership in the AMA was making progress. Beginning in 1902, the *Journal of the American Medical Association* (JAMA) published medical school failure statistics on state board licensing examinations, a form of exposure that could not help but embarrass and lead to institutional reform. In 1907, the assessment grouped schools into four classes determined by percentage of failure. The council subsequently decided to rate each school on the basis of not only the state board exam performance but also on such factors as entrance requirements, medical curriculum, laboratory facilities, hospital facilities, faculty quality, library, and research. The resulting scores would place each school in one of three categories: Class A (acceptable), Class B (doubtful), and Class C (unacceptable). Each school was visited, and the findings were reported.

The classifications were not published; however, each school was notified of its standing. The result of the report was a great wave of improvement in medical education, from changes in curriculum to school mergers (Johnson 1947).

THE FLEXNER REPORT AND REFORM

In 1905, the Carnegie Foundation had set out to investigate all of the professions (law, medicine, and theology). The Carnegie Foundation when contacted by the Council on Medical Education, was impressed by the efforts being made to improve medical

education and by the large amount of data available, and agreed to conduct an independent investigation. Abraham Flexner of the foundation began the study of medical education in 1909. Flexner was not a physician, but an educator, and his study was mainly an educational survey. He identified the following five factors that would provide him with conclusive data as to the quality of a school:

1. Entrance requirements
2. The size and training of the faculty
3. The financial resources and expenditures of the institution
4. The quality and adequacy of the laboratories provided for instruction in the first two years
5. The relations between the medical school and hospitals

He secured the data through interviews with the dean and the faculty and through observation of the facilities, particularly laboratories and equipment (Flexner 1940).

The Carnegie Foundation published Flexner's formal report, *Medical Education in the United States and Canada*, in 1910. Though controlled in language, the report provided a candid, searing critique of medical education in both the United States and Canada. It named schools, their assets, and their liabilities, and it offered a prescription for each school, for each state and region, and for the country as a whole. Where schools were no more than business ventures, Flexner said so. Some medical schools, such as Dartmouth, were recognized for excellent preclinical training but criticized for a lack of opportunities in clinical training. Still others received high praise (Flexner 1910).

The **Flexner report** caused some schools to close and some to consolidate. Some allegedly closed before the report's publication to escape the criticism (Flexner 1940). In all, Flexner recommended that the number of schools be reduced from 155 to 31. By 1920, the number of schools was down to 85. By that time, however, the need for more than 31 schools was apparent because of population increase and new knowledge that permitted more treatment for patients.

The report, coming from an independent body, strengthened the hand of medical reformers in the AMA, AAMC, state medical societies, and, importantly, state licensing boards. Licensing legislation in the states mandated more rigorous control. The AMA's Council on Medical Education, moreover, leaned on people in state societies, even before the Flexner study, to ensure that reform-minded people were appointed to state licensing

EXHIBIT 5–1

From the 1910 Flexner report, *Medical Education in the United States and Canada,. . .*

The University of Buffalo Medical Department, organized in 1846.

Despite the university charter, the University of Buffalo is a fiction. Schools of medicine, law, dentistry, and pharmacy are aggregated under the designation; but they are to all intents and purposes independent schools, each living on its own fees.

Entrance requirement: Admission is on the basis of the Regents' Medical Students Certificate, being the equivalent of a high school education.

Laboratory facilities: The school has a conventionally adequate equipment for anatomy, ordinary laboratories for chemistry, bacteriology, and pathology, a meager outfit in physiology,—it having been found that the students cannot profitably do much experimental work themselves,—nothing for pharmacology. The "whole time" teachers have in the main other duties besides teaching in medicine: the professor of pathology and bacteriology is registrar, the chemist officiates in the pharmacy department, the anatomist in the dental department. There is a small museum, but a good library of 8,000 volumes, current German and English periodicals, with a librarian in charge.

Clinical facilities: For clinical teaching, the school relies mainly on the Buffalo General Hospital close by. It has access to some 200 beds, used for demonstrative teaching in the wards. Records are made by interns. Students do no clinical laboratory work in connection with special patients, the teaching in clinical microscopy being separately given at the college. Infectious diseases are didactically taught. Clinical obstetrics is imperfectly organized. Besides the Buffalo General Hospital, a weekly clinic is held at the County Hospital, four

miles distant, four clinics at the Sisters' Hospital, one and a half miles away, etc.

Despite the size of the city, the college dispensary is wretched. It has an attendance of perhaps 3,000 during the college year, skin, eye, and ear cases mainly. A definite statement is impossible because there are no systematic records. The rooms are ill equipped. Records consist of brief pencil notes in separate books, usually without index. The work is hastily and superficially done, and its influence on the students, so far as it goes, must be thoroughly bad. The catalogue states, however, that as attendance in the dispensary is obligatory, each student "will secure an unusually thorough training in the taking and recording of histories."

From www.smbs.buffalo.edu
Date of visit: October, 1909.

Today, the University of Buffalo is part of the larger State University of New York (SUNY) system. Since 1987, it has been known as the School of Medicine and Biomedical Sciences and trains both future physicians and future medical scientists. It continues to affiliate with the hospitals mentioned in the Flexner report as well as many others (Children's Hospital of Buffalo, the VA Hospital, and Millard Fillmore Hospitals, to name a few). The School of Medicine and Biomedical Sciences is accredited by the Liaison Committee on Medical Education, the Accreditation Council for Continuing Medical Education, and the Accreditation Council for Graduate Medical Education.

Discussion Questions

1. In your opinion, was the Flexner report on the University of Buffalo complementary or critical?
2. How did the Flexner report on the University of Buffalo influence the future of its School of Medicine?

---

boards. Many boards began to set new requirements, which included increasing the length of medical training and providing students with modern laboratories, libraries, and clinical facilities (Stevens 1971).

The increased leverage provided by the work of the AMA and the AAMC was evident in their increased coordinated efforts. This led, in 1942, to the establishment of the **Liaison Committee on Medical Education (LCME)**, which developed

educational program guidelines, inspected schools, and became the official accrediting body for medical schools.

The final leverage for reform came from foundations and individuals whom the foundations could persuade. Flexner's influence here was a critical factor. Shortly after his report, he joined the General Education Board, a Rockefeller charity that poured enormous sums into medical education (Flexner 1940). The monies went to the better schools and to those that showed promise of moving in the direction laid out in Flexner's report. University medical schools usually had a better academic reputation and a more solid financial base than proprietary schools, and therefore they acquired the new money that became available for medical education. Because of this influx of money, universities gained control of medical education (Ludmerer 1985).

MODERN MEDICAL EDUCATION

Today, medical education typically begins with premedical education consisting of four years of study that result in a baccalaureate degree from a college or university. Most premedical students major in the sciences, although they can, in fact, major in almost any academic program, as long as they take the specified science and other courses required by the medical school to which they apply for admission.

Many students are attracted to medicine because it is a prestigious, well-paying profession. Competition for entrance to medical school is very intense. Between 2003 and 2004, 125 U.S. and 17 Canadian medical schools were fully accredited to award an MD degree. Over 42,000 people applied to medical schools in 2007. Of these, 44.6 percent were accepted (AAMC 2007a). Once accepted, students are seldom dismissed for poor academic standing. Usually they are allowed to repeat all or part of the academic year if they are in academic difficulty. The AMA's Council on Medical Education reports data on medical school application and admissions.

The number of medical school applicants and students increased during the 1980s through the mid-1990s. Between 1997 and 2002, there was a steady decrease in applicants and enrollment until 2004. Since then, applications and enrollments have again been on the increase. The change in the number of applicants is reflected among female applicants, male applicants, and groups considered to be underrepresented. Since 1994, the number of applications submitted per person has continued to be between eleven and twelve, reflecting a continuing recognition on the part of applicants of the difficulty of being admitted (Barzansky and Etzel 2004).

Women made up 48.3 percent of the total first-year medical school enrollment in 2007, and 48.6 percent of all medical school students. The percentage of female medical school students has consistently been rising, notably since the 1970s. Minority group members made up about 37 percent of the total medical school enrollment in 2007 (AAMC 2007a).

Of those matriculating since 1995, the average premedical grade point average has been over 3.6, with a high of 3.65 in 2007. Medical school admission is based, however, on a number of factors, in addition to grade point average. These include performance on the Medical College Admission Test (MCAT), which nearly all accepted applicants take, as well as on recommendations and interviews. The MCAT is an objective test that measures knowledge of science (biology, chemistry, and physics), ability to solve science problems, analysis and reading skills, and quantitative skills. In 1991, the MCAT was modified to strengthen the evaluation of skills such as critical thinking, verbal reasoning, and communication, which have become more important because the vast expansion and change in medical knowledge requires physicians to rely less on rote memory. The MCAT includes two nonscientific essays to help assess these skills. Beginning in January 2007, all MCAT exams were computerized. This allows for multiple testing times (from two to twenty-two times a year), fewer questions, and a shortened time period to receive scores (about thirty days after testing (AAMC 2007b).

Another weighted factor in medical school admission is the report from the student's premedical advisers. In many schools, this confidential report is a committee report, which serves to minimize risks of bias. Applicant interviews are also considered important in asserting personality factors that tests and recommendations may not reveal.

Nearly all leaders in medical education endorse the desirability of a broad liberal education in the arts, humanities, and social sciences, in addition to study in the biological and physical sciences during the premedical years. They recognize that such an education can enhance patient communication, improve understanding of the influence of social and economic problems on disease and convalescence, and enable physicians to acquire an understanding of the past that will help them contribute constructively to changes in society.

Although students typically hold a baccalaureate degree, they are considered undergraduates in medical school; hence, undergraduate medical education refers to medical schools and the training of physicians who will, upon graduation, be awarded a doctor of medicine (MD) or doctor of osteopathy (DO) degree.

Graduate medical education refers to formalized post-MD or post-DO training in an approved residency. Postgraduate or continuing medical education refers to formalized training on a short-course or short-term basis for physicians who have completed a period of graduate medical education; it generally includes refresher courses or intensive courses to develop new skills.

UNDERGRADUATE MEDICAL EDUCATION

The typical medical school program lasts four years. A few universities today integrate their premedical and medical school programs and require less time to earn an MD degree. The Liaison Committee on Medical Education (LCME) accredits the programs that award MD degrees. The U.S. Secretary of Education and the Council on Postsecondary Education recognize accreditation by the LCME, adding to its legitimacy (LCME 2006). The **American Osteopathic Association (AOA)** accredits osteopathic medical schools. The U.S. Secretary of Education and the Council on Postsecondary Education also acknowledge the AOA's legitimacy in this role.

Medical School Curriculum

Although the structure of medical education has not changed significantly for almost fifty years, new ways of teaching are being introduced to cope with the vast amount of information and the changing way in which medicine is practiced. The first two years of medical school have changed little; they are devoted largely to the basic medical sciences (anatomy, physiology, biochemistry, histology, pharmacology, microbiology, and so on). During the final two years, students rotate through clinical clerkships, in which they acquire clinical skills and give general medical care. Students are assigned patients on whom they conduct histories, physical examinations, and some laboratory tests. The students are actively involved in the diagnosis and treatment of these patients under the supervision of the resident and faculty.

The clinical experience ranges from **primary care** to **tertiary care** in a variety of inpatient and outpatient settings. Usually students do clerkships in internal medicine, obstetrics and gynecology, pediatrics, psychiatry, and surgery. Most schools allow students some elective courses or other clerkships during the final year. Medical school graduates are not expected to become experts in all subjects and are not prepared for immediate independent, unsupervised practice; instead, they are prepared to enter a program of graduate medical education.

Most medical schools now require courses to facilitate a humanistic approach—courses designed to improve physician–patient relationships, to enhance communication skills, and to grapple with social and ethical issues (Robinson 1999). The AAMC has stressed the need to address the humanistic aspect of medicine, health care quality improvement, informatics, genetics, pain management, and a wide range of other topics, in addition to the basic sciences (AAMC 2007c).

The Institute for Healthcare Improvement (IHI) established an education collaborative to improve care through new approaches in health professions education. Twenty medical schools have joined with schools of nursing, pharmacy, and health administration to venture into the areas of "vertically integrated undergraduate curricula, interprofessional learning, redesigned residency programs, the development of exemplary clinical settings where optimal patient care and education take place in a seamless fashion, practice-based learning and improvement throughout the entirety of one's professional career, and the creation of an academic base to facilitate these goals" (IHI 2007).

Whatever the curriculum, most medical schools require that students take Steps 1 and 2 of the **United States Medical Licensing Examination (USMLE)**. The USMLE was established by the National Board of Medical Examiners (NBME) and the Federation of State Medical Boards of the United States (FSMB). The examination has three parts, the third of which assesses the knowledge and understanding of biomedical and clinical science necessary for the unsupervised practice of medicine. It consists of computer-based case simulation and is the basis for state licensing and insurance.

OSTEOPATHIC MEDICINE

According to the American Osteopathic Association (AOA), there are currently over 61,000 DOs (doctors of osteopathy) in the United States. Osteopathic medicine represents an approach to medical practice that views the overall health of patients, including their home and work environment, and also advocates the value of osteopathic manipulative treatment "to relieve pain, restore range of motion, and enhance the body's capacity to heal" (AOA 2007). An **osteopath** is a physician, licensed in all fifty states to practice medicine and surgery.

Osteopaths are trained in essentially the same way and in most of the same specialties as **allopathic physicians** (physicians trained in the medical schools). Individuals must graduate from an osteopathic medical school (there are currently twenty-three in the United States). Applicants typically have a four-year undergraduate degree, take the MCATs, and go through a personal interview to assess their interpersonal communications skills. Similar to applicants in medical schools, the number of osteopath applicants decreased beginning in 1996, and then began increasing in 2003 (see Table 5–1). The curriculum emphasizes preventive medicine and holistic patient care. After completing the osteopathic medical school curriculum, DOs serve a one-year rotating internship. Many DOs then choose residency training if they wish to practice a medical specialty, either through osteopathic or allopathic residency placement (American Association of Colleges of Osteopathic Medicine 2007a).

As a school of medicine, osteopathy developed following the civil war under the leadership of a former army physician, Andrew Taylor Still. On the basis of the role that the musculoskeletal system plays in the body's effort to resist and overcome illness and disease, Still believed that manual manipulation was useful in stimulating the body's ability to fight disease (American Association of Colleges of Osteopathic Medicine 2007b). Because his theories received little support from the established schools, Still branched off and opened the first osteopathic school in 1892. Others followed. Flexner included osteopathic schools in his 1909 study, and his report resulted in reform also in osteopathic medical education.

For many years, osteopaths were unable to secure licenses in some states and were given limited licenses in others. Today, however, they are licensed in all states, with the same rights and responsibilities as MDs. In some states, osteopaths are licensed by an MD medical board; in some, by a joint MD-DO board; and in others, the osteopaths have their own licensing boards (see Table 5–2).

In 1970, the AMA granted membership to osteopathic physicians and granted a voting seat in its House of Delegates to the AOA in 1996.

Approximately 64 percent of actively practicing osteopaths are in primary care fields (AOA 2006), whereas the percentage of allopathic physicians in primary care fields is only about 47 percent (National Center for Health Statistics 2006).

Osteopathic physicians are very different from chiropractors. Osteopaths are licensed physicians; chiropractors, although licensed, are not physicians. Chiropractors use manipulative procedures and physiotherapy, and are permitted to take X-ray films for diagnostic purposes. However, their range and scope of treatment options are more limited than those of physicians.

COST OF MEDICAL EDUCATION

The cost of training physicians is high, and tuition in most schools covers only a small portion. Nationally, tuition and fees constitute less than 4 percent of revenue for school and university activities. The greatest source of revenue for medical schools comes from practice plans (revenue from patient care), which amounted to nearly 36 percent of total revenue for 2001–2002. Grants and hospital support also provide significant portions of medical school income (about 32 percent). Revenue proportions differ for public and private organizations, as well as for nonprofit and for-profit organizations. However, osteopathic medical schools derive a higher percentage of their revenue from tuition, mainly because they do not receive as much research funding, contracts, and hospital revenue (American Medical Student Association 2007). Because of the varied sources of funds and differing accounting practices, determining exactly what training a single physician costs is difficult.

TABLE 5–1 Number of Applicants, First-Year Enrollees, Total Enrollment, and Graduates from Schools of Osteopathic Medicine, 2004–05 and 2005–06

Academic Year	Applicants	Entering Class	Total Enrolled	Graduates
2004–05	46,750	3,646	12,525	2,756
2005–06	51,099	3,908	13,406	2,849

SOURCE: Annual Osteopathic Medical School Questionnaires, 2004–05 and 2005–06 academic years. Retrieved from www.aacom.org/resources/bookstore/2006statrpt/Pages/default.aspx. Reprinted with permission from the American Association of Colleges of Osteopathic Medicine. All rights reserved.

TABLE 5–2 State Medical and Osteopathic Boards

Alabama	Medical Board
Alaska	Medical Board
Arizona	Separate Medical and Osteopathic Boards
Arkansas	Medical Board
California	Separate Medical and Osteopathic Boards
Colorado	Medical Board
Connecticut	Medical Board
Delaware	Medical Board
District of Columbia	Medical Board
Florida	Separate Medical and Osteopathic Boards
Georgia	Composite State Board of Medical Examiners
Hawaii	Medical Board
Idaho	Medical Board
Illinois	Board of Professional Regulation
Indiana	Medical Board
Iowa	Medical Board
Kansas	Board of Healing Arts
Kentucky	Medical Board
Louisiana	Medical Board
Maine	Separate Medical and Osteopathic Boards
Maryland	Board of Physician Quality Assurance
Massachusetts	Medical Board
Michigan	Separate Medical and Osteopathic Boards
Minnesota	Medical Board
Mississippi	Medical Board
Missouri	Board of Registration for the Healing Arts
Montana	Medical Board
Nebraska	Medical Board
Nevada	Separate Medical and Osteopathic Boards
New Hampshire	Medical Board
New Jersey	Medical Board

(*continues*)

TABLE 5-2 (Continued)

New Mexico	Separate Medical and Osteopathic Boards
New York	Medical Board
North Carolina	Medical Board
North Dakota	Medical Board
Ohio	Medical Board
Oklahoma	Separate Medical and Osteopathic Boards
Oregon	Medical Board
Pennsylvania	Separate Medical and Osteopathic Boards
Puerto Rico	Medical Board
Rhode Island	Medical Board
South Carolina	Medical Board
South Dakota	Joint Board
Tennessee	Separate Medical and Osteopathic Boards
Texas	Medical Board
Utah	Separate Medical and Osteopathic Boards
Vermont	Separate Medical and Osteopathic Boards
Virginia	Medical Board
Washington	Separate Medical and Osteopathic Boards
West Virginia	Separate Medical and Osteopathic Boards
Wisconsin	Medical Board
Wyoming	Medical Board

SOURCE: Administrators in Medicine (AIM), National Organization for State Medical & Osteopathic Board Executive Directors. Retrieved from www.aimmembers.org/boarddirectory/.

For a great many years after World War II, federal monies, in the form of research contracts and grants, fueled expansion in medical education. The monies did not come to the deans of the medical schools but to the individual researchers. Medical schools reflected the universities of which they were a part; the rewards of promotion and salary increases went to those who brought in the most grant money and to those who published. Relatively small amounts of grant money went directly for support of medical education; most went to research.

Change occurred during the early 1960s. There was a widely perceived physician shortage, and Congress responded by passing the Health Professions Education Assistance Act of 1963. The primary purpose of the act was to increase the supply of professional health care personnel. The legislation provided direct federal assistance to medical schools in the form of construction grants, student loans, and financial distress grants. In 1965, the law was amended to provide direct institutional support for operating expenses on the condition that schools expand their enrollments to eliminate the physician shortage.

The Comprehensive Health Manpower Training Act of 1971 greatly increased support for operating costs, and established a "capitation grant" of $2,500 per student for the first three years and $4,000 per student for the last year of medical school. However, schools that received capitation grants were required to emphasize training of primary care physicians. Emphasis was also placed on training physician assistants, improving geographic maldistribution, and increasing enrollment of minorities (Health Services and Research Administration 2005). As a result, the financial condition of medical schools greatly improved, and their enrollments increased by 50 percent, from 31,491 between 1962 and 1963 to 47,546 between 1972 and 1973.

For the first time, the 1971 Comprehensive Health Manpower Training Act required that institutions carry out certain programmatic activities in addition to increasing student enrollment as a condition for receiving capitation grants. To qualify for grants, institutions had to present a plan to implement projects in at least three of nine categories described in the legislation. Categories included promoting interdisciplinary training, establishing a team approach for providing health services, and establishing programs in drug use and abuse and nutrition, among others. This was the first time the federal government had intervened in the internal program decisions of medical schools. The legislation also expanded student loan and scholarship opportunities, and provided grants to initiate, expand, or improve professional training programs in family medicine. When the legislation expired in 1974, the physician shortage was perceived to have disappeared, but the legislation was renewed in 1976, placing emphasis on specialty and geographic distribution problems. Again in 1992, the Health Professions Education Extension Amendments provided funding for primary care education and a focus on filling the needs of **medically underserved communities (MUCs)**. In 1998, the programs were again reauthorized under the Health Professions Education Partnerships Act, allowing for more flexibility in redesigning grants and establishing the Advisory Committee on Training in Primary Care Medicine and Dentistry to evaluate the review and make recommendations regarding activities supported by the act (Health Services and Research Administration 2005).

As in all other areas of health care delivery, medical education programs struggled to cope with the cost-containment efforts of the 1980s and 1990s. Graduating medical students carry heavy educational debt. Loans accounted for approximately 65 percent of how students pay for medical school (AAMC 2005). In 2004, average debt of medical graduates was $100,000 for those attending public schools and just under $140,000 for those attending private schools. The AAMC projects those figures could go up to $120,000 for public and $160,000 for private schools. Yet, estimated future earnings for physicians are uncertain as the health care delivery system continues to undergo change. Since the mid-1990s, average physician income has been relatively stable at just under $200,000 (AAMC 2005).

THE DEVELOPMENT OF MEDICAL SPECIALTIES

Most physicians in the colonial and postcolonial periods were general practitioners as the state of medical science was rather primitive. Surgical practice was limited, until 1846, by the absence of anesthesia. Physicians who did develop special skills or interests and became known for them remained primarily general physicians, practicing their specialties (such as obstetrics or surgery) only on occasion. Shryock (1966) reminds us that this was the age of bleeding and purging, and surgery was limited largely to trauma cases.

During the first half of the nineteenth century, a growing number of U.S. physicians went to France for advanced study. During this period, French investigators were effectively proving the errors of bleeding and purging, as well as the ineffectiveness of many drugs then in common use. Their investigations pointed to specific pathology in different locations and systems of the body, there being no single or simple explanation for disease. These findings made the notion of specialization appealing to those physicians whose interest was excited by special health problems.

Specialties did not begin to make headway until the 1860s. Resistance to specialties was at times vigorous, and the issues were complex. Fishbein (1947), in his history of the AMA, summarized issues pertaining to specialization in a report at the association's 1866 meeting. Many of those same issues persist to this day:

- Should a patient go first to the general practitioner or directly to the specialist?
- Will the specialist treat the whole patient?
- Will the surgeon operate because that is what a surgeon is taught to do?
- Does specialty practice lead to unnecessary procedures?
- Will people study specialty medicine for the sake of the higher fees paid to specialists?
- Don't we want the best medical care, and isn't the specialist the best?

Some of the early specialty groups were the American Ophthalmological Society (1864), the American Otological Society (1868), the American Gynecological Society (1876), the American Association of Obstetricians and Gynecologists (1888), and the American Pediatric Society (1888). There were also state and local specialty societies—some established before the national body, some later. Specialty journals followed. In many cities, the specialty was advanced by the presence of specialty hospitals and clinics. In most large cities today, one can find specialty hospitals still thriving or only recently merged with other hospitals.

In the late nineteenth and early twentieth centuries, these specialty hospitals and clinics became the foci for training in those specialties because, generally speaking, the most outstanding practitioners were affiliated with those institutions. However, some outstanding specialists did practice and train others in the more generally oriented hospitals.

The Development of Standards in Graduate Medical Education

At the turn of the twentieth century, there was no standard for what constituted adequate training in a specialty. Courses were offered by medical societies, hospitals, specially founded schools, and universities. The programs of study lasted anywhere from a few weeks to three years. Flexner (1910) described the postgraduate school as "established to do what the medical school failed to accomplish. . . . The postgraduate school was thus originally an undergraduate repair shop. . . . Urgency required that in the shortest possible time the young physician already involved in responsibility would acquire the practice technique which the medical school had failed to impart" (pp. 174–77).

The "repair shop" to which Flexner referred was also the rationale for the internship in the later part of the nineteenth century. Over time, the **internship** became standard practice, requiring an additional year of supervised training to give medical graduates (still, in a sense, students) that extra bit of on-the-job training necessitated by the medical schools' adoption of the Harvard practice of not requiring an apprenticeship before medical school. This need for additional training also motivated many physicians to go abroad. As Stevens (1971) notes, the internship tended to emphasize either medicine or surgery and thus became an introductory phase of specialization.

With the advent of anesthesia, antiseptic techniques, new instrumentation, and new technology learned from the civil war battle casualties, as well as from European research, a new era

began. Hospitals grew in number because people could now go to them for general and specialty surgeries with less fear of pain and more assurance that they would survive the encounter and improve as a result of it.

The American College of Surgeons (ACS), which was established in 1912, set specific requirements in an effort to improve the skills of physicians it accepted into fellowship. Stevens (1971) notes that "prerequisites included a one-year internship, three years as an assistant, fifty case abstracts, visits to surgical clinics, and for graduates of 1920 and after, two years of college before medical school" (p. 92). This suggested a pattern for certifying specialists. Clearly, the ACS requirements raised standards to improve surgical practice. Though the college could not license surgeons, it could pass professional judgment by approving of accomplishments and behavior of surgeons.

All these developments by the ACS were important, but not enough. The next step was to inspect the places in which internships were provided—that is, the general and specialty hospitals around the nation. Both the AMA and the ACS moved on this front. The AMA began to pay attention to the internship at the time it established its Council on Medical Education. The council surveyed hospitals that were offering internships and published its first list of approved internship hospitals in 1914. At about the same time, the ACS began to think about establishing hospital standards for surgical practice. In 1916, it received a Carnegie grant for this purpose. The first list of hospitals that the ACS felt met its standards was ready in 1919, but the conditions encountered in its survey were so bad that the college suppressed the list. In 1924, the Council on Medical Education began to approve hospitals for residency (specialty) training programs. At that time, a key requirement was that the hospitals must first have approval for internship programs.

By the mid-1960s, nearly all medical school graduates were taking three or more years of residency (specialty) training after an internship. The growth of the specialties was a direct result of new knowledge and new technology, enabling physicians to do more than ever before to help people in need. As with internships, residency programs proliferated into hospitals of all types and sizes.

For the second time in its history, the AMA assumed a leadership role and commissioned the Citizens Commission on Graduate Medical Education to examine the medical education process. This time, the mandate was to examine graduate medical education—the internship and the residency—and to make recommendations to improve this part of a physician's formal training. The Millis Commission's report, *The Graduate Education of Physicians,* was issued in 1966 (Citizens Commission on Graduate Medical Education 1966). Among key recommendations was a call for the elimination of the independent internship, meaning that no internship be approved unless it is linked with and part of an approved residency training program. The first year of each residency program, however, should be one that gives the resident a broad clinical experience. The commission further recommended that this change in the nature of the internship should not mean an additional year of residency training.

Another key recommendation related to the role of hospitals. The commission felt that hospitals as a whole had to play some role in residency programs in terms of providing resources and facilitating cooperation between other hospital departments and services. It recommended that accreditation of residency training programs be given to institutions rather than to the individual services involved. There were many other recommendations, but these are the ones of most concern in this discussion.

The Millis report is an excellent example of a health policy plan. Although not completely implemented, it led to considerable discussion within the medical profession and to positive reforms in line with the spirit of the report. In late 1970, the AMA's House of Delegates endorsed the concept that the first year of graduate medical education be in a program approved by the appropriate residency review committee (which each specialty board had) rather than by the AMA's Council on Medical Education. Thus, in effect, the AMA said that it would no longer review and approve internships, and that internships would have to be integrated with residency training programs. In fact, since 1975, the AMA has ceased the use of the term *internship* in its Directory of Residency Training Programs.

Modern Graduate Medical Education

Graduate medical education today consists of a period of supervised training for a medical specialty in an approved clinical setting following graduation from medical school. Hospitals provide the large majority of graduate medical education opportunities, but ambulatory settings are beginning to play a more important role.

Graduate medical education includes training in specialties and subspecialties (the residency) and training preliminary to the **residency** program (a one-year general residency or the transitional year). Accreditation of graduate medical education programs is granted by the Accreditation Council for Graduate

Medical Education (ACGME), which is jointly sponsored by the American Medical Association, the Association of American Medical Colleges, the American Board of Medical Specialties, the Council of Medical Specialty Societies, and the American Hospital Association. Accreditation is based on an evaluation of both the institution and the program it provides (ACGME 2007a). Recent studies of medical education have called for more resident training to take place outside of the hospital with ambulatory patients, more emphasis on training primary care physicians, increasing minority participation, and providing cultural competency training (Ebert and Ginsberg 1988; Council on Graduate Medical Education 2000).

In 2004, there were over 4,602 active residency training programs in the United States. The largest number of programs was in internal medicine followed by family practice, and then pediatrics. From 1999 to 2007, the total number of residency slots and positions filled rose slowly. The number of residents on duty is smaller than the number of residency slots approved. This may be a result of an imbalance of specialties providing residencies with the specialties that medical school graduates desire (National Resident Matching Program 2007).

Securing a Residency and Becoming a Specialist

The National Resident Matching Program (NRMP) is a computerized service that matches resident applicants with approved hospital training programs. The aim is to meet the desires of the hospitals and the would-be residents to the greatest extent possible. Additional aims are to eliminate, if possible, pressures and special inducements that tend to skew the distribution of residents, leaving some hospitals with many unfilled slots and other hospitals oversubscribed (National Resident Matching Program 2006).

The NRMP was introduced when twice as many positions were available each year as there were graduating seniors. By the 1980s, that ratio had changed because of the increased number of U.S. and international medical school graduates applying for residencies.

In 2007, a total of 27,944 applicants participated in the NRMP, competing for 24,685 positions offered by 4,602 programs (National Resident Matching Program 2007). For the 1999–2000 training year, first-year residents received an average annual stipend of $43,265, which represents an increase of approximately 3.2 percent over the previous year. For the second year of graduate medical training, the average base salary was

$45,005, also indicating an increase of about 3.2 percent over the previous year (AAMC 2007d).

Traditionally, resident physicians have worked long hours while gaining the clinical experience necessary to practice medicine. However, the number of hours residents should be on duty is controversial and was questioned in 1987, when the state of New York investigated the number of hours residents worked following mishandling of an emergency case. The residents involved had been on duty for an extended period of time. New York set rules to govern the working hours of residents to minimize the risk of future mishaps that might be attributable to residents being too tired to think clearly. The rules require an average eighty-hour workweek and shifts limited to twenty-four hours followed by sixteen hours off (Whang et al. 2003). Some program faculty objected because the rules could interfere with continuity of care. Additional controversy revolves around increased costs of training with limitations on work hours. However, in 2003, the ACGME implemented duty hour restrictions across all residency programs. Similar to those in New York State, they consisted of a limit of eighty hours per week averaged over a four-week period, one day in seven free from all clinical and educational activities, also averaged over a four-week period, and other on-call restrictions (ACGME 2007b). The results of such work-hour limitations are still difficult to determine. Reed et al. (2007) indicate that work-hour limitations do improve the well-being of residents but also put additional work-hour pressures on senior residents and faculty. Effects on patient outcomes are still to be determined.

Prior to the 1990s, resident training focused largely on acute care in the tertiary care setting, reinforcing the physician's decision-making skills, the use of large regimens of diagnostic tests over a short period of time, and wide variations in treatment planning based on the customs and training of the faculty involved. The setting of the inpatient acute care facility also fostered specialty training rather than primary and preventive care (family practice, pediatrics, internal medicine, and so on). Since the mid-1980s, much of the delivery of health care has been moving from the inpatient to the ambulatory setting. Prospective payment and new technology have reduced lengths of stay, promoted less-invasive techniques, and encouraged prevention over intervention. The 1997 Budget Reconciliation Agreement provided incentives to train physicians in ambulatory sites by making direct medical education and indirect medical education payments available to such sites (Young and Coffman 1998).

The time required for training in a specialty varies with the specialty (see Table 5–3). The training program is known as the residency in a particular clinical area. The person being trained is a graduate of a medical school and is known as a resident although in residency. The AMA publishes the Graduate Medical Education Directory, which spells out the general requirements for approval and accreditation of residency programs. It also describes the specific requirements that apply to the respective specialties and gives listings with contact information for accredited programs. Each accredited residency program is responsible for providing the training as specified in the Essentials section.

Specialty Boards

To become a specialist in a particular medical area today, physicians must pass a qualifying examination administered by a specialty board (following medical school, the general residency, and the specialty residency). The appropriate specialty board then certifies physicians as diplomats (diploma holders) of that specialty. The various boards are legitimized by their sponsors: the specialty society (or societies) in that area and the appropriate specialty section of the AMA.

The number of specialty boards stood at twenty-four in 1995. These boards are responsible for certifying specialists in more than 130 specialties and subspecialties (American Board of Medical Specialties 2006a). Application for the development of a specialty board is submitted to the Liaison Committee for Specialty Boards (LCSB), a joint creation of the AMA's Council on Medical Education and the American Board of Medical Specialties (ABMS). The ABMS is a coordinative body representing the twenty-four existing approved specialty boards, with five cooperating or associate members who are there for liaison purposes: the American Hospital Association, the Association of American Medical Colleges, the Council of Medical Specialty Societies, the Federation of State Medical Boards of the United States, and the National Board of Medical Examiners. The ABMS was established in 1933, as the Advisory Board for Medical Specialties when there were only four existing certifying boards, but the trend toward establishing specialty certifying boards was clearly established. The board was reorganized, and its name was changed to the American Board of Medical Specialties in 1970. The major purposes of the ABMS are to represent approved specialty boards, resolve problems that arise among specialty boards, deal with the approval of new specialty boards and types of certification, and prevent duplication of effort among boards.

TABLE 5-3 Length of Training in Some Specialties and Their Recertification Requirements

Residency Program	Years of Specialty Training	Recertification Period
Family practice	3	7
Emergency medicine	3	10
Pediatrics	3	7
Internal medicine	3	10
Obstetrics/gynecology	4	6
Pathology	3–4	10
General surgery	5	10
Neurological surgery	5	N/A
Orthopedic surgery	5	10
Otolaryngology surgery	5	10
Urology	3–4	10
Anesthesiology	3	10
Dermatology	3	10
Neurology	5	10
Nuclear medicine	3	10
Ophthalmology	3	10
Physical medicine	3	10
Psychiatry	4	10
Radiology, diagnostic	4	10
Radiation oncology	4	10

SOURCE: Data from the American Board of Medical Specialties (2008) and individual specialty boards.

Specialty certification in the United States is voluntary. Certification in a medical specialty is separate and distinct from the license to practice medicine in a state. There are no legal requirements for licensed physicians to seek specialty board certification to offer specialty services. Even though certification is not a form of licensure, it is required for certain appointments, such as hospital medical staff privileges, participation in health care insurance programs, and participation in managed care plans. Therefore, the majority of physicians choose to become board-certified in their specialty.

In 1973, the ABMS adopted a policy urging voluntary, periodic recertification of medical specialists by all member boards. In 1980, the ABMS issued guidelines to assist member boards with the recertification process. Most boards require recertification within a ten-year period, although family practice and pediatrics require recertification in seven years. Most boards require a written examination. A smaller number require oral exams or other forms of assessment. The ABMS also calls for publication of members' certification status in the ABMS directory. In 1998, ABMS proposed the move from recertification exams to a maintenance of certification process (MOC) for continuous professional development throughout specialists' careers. Many of the medical organizations (including the AMA) supported the proposal for implementation by 2005 (American Board of Medical Specialties 2006b). The focus areas of MOC are (1) patient care, (2) medical knowledge, (3) practice-based learning and improvement, (4) interpersonal and communications skills, (5) professionalism, and (6) systems-based practice.

Although MOC still requires an examination, it also requires physicians to participate in ongoing education and evaluation of the quality of their practice through comparison of data against benchmarks.

Graduate Medical Education Financing

The cost of graduate medical education (GME) involves resident salaries, the administration of programs, the cost of having more complicated cases, and the increased cost of patient care associated with the hospital's teaching function (increased use of diagnostic services and length of stay). As a result, the cost per case at teaching hospitals is higher than at comparable nonteaching hospitals (Bajaj 1999b).

Until recently, financing GME was not a major problem. Patient care revenues support about 80 percent of residents' training costs, but now costs are rising rapidly and are paid for largely by government programs. Private insurance companies do not directly support medical education, and decreased payments for patient care have ended the type of cost shifting that once allowed for indirect support of GME built into higher patient charges. Federal and state governments, which were willing to subsidize GME when there was a shortage of physicians and when funds were more plentiful, are now searching for ways to reduce their support. Medicare is now the major source of funds for GME. It subsidizes GME indirectly with adjustments to the diagnosis-related group (DRG) payments to teaching hospitals. Direct GME payments to hospitals under Medicare were once based on the hospital's cost of training. Since 1985, direct GME payments have been capitated and are linked to a "per resident" amount (Bajaj 1999a). Reimbursement to

hospitals from Medicaid is hardly adequate to cover essential patient care, and yet government is looking for ways to contain costs in that area also.

GME funding is also coming under scrutiny because of a perceived imbalance in the physician-population ratio and an oversupply of specialists and undersupply of primary care physicians. Medicare has changed its funding policies to take the first step toward curtailing an overabundance of physicians. The new rules cap the number of residency slots Medicare will fund, permits payments to nonhospital providers, and provides incentives for facilities to reduce the number of residents they train (Martin 1998). Prior to 1997, Medicare payments to HMOs included an adjustment for medical education but contained no requirements for the HMO to provide medical education. The new legislation decouples GME payments from HMO payments (Young and Coffman 1998).

MEDICAL LICENSING

In the second half of the nineteenth century, many states established or reestablished licensing boards. However, not all states at the turn of the twentieth century required passing a state board licensing examination to practice medicine in that state. In 1873, Texas was the first state to establish a state board of medical examiners. By the turn of the twentieth century, thirty-seven states required credentials of some sort for licensure, and twenty-three of these states required more than a diploma. Some states also began to recognize the credentials and licenses of certain other states on a reciprocal basis; hence, the practice of reciprocity came into being (Womack 1965).

Practices for governing the qualifications for medical practice differed widely. The need for some kind of national standard was apparent to many, but bringing this about was not easy. As with so many efforts at change, resistance is often encountered. In 1912, The Federation of State Medical Boards of the United States was formed. Despite initial disagreements over aims of the federation, all medical (MD) boards as well as nine osteopathic examining boards and the medical boards of some Canadian provinces were members by 1978.

During the early part of the twentieth century, some in the AMA were interested in national licensure, but this never became a strong movement because of constitutional concerns over the question of states' rights. This is a nice way of stating two related points of view: concern over federal bureaucratic control of the right to practice and concern by state boards about

Requirement	Time of Testing
Steps 1 & 2 USMLE	During Medical School* for U.S. and Canadian Medical School graduates; prior to entering residency for International Medical Graduates
Step 3, USMLE	After completion of Medical School and general residency (internship)
General Residency	After medical school graduation (for 1 year)
Specialty Residency	After general residency; length determined by specialty board.
Board Certification	Testing after completion of specialty residency

*Includes Allopathic and Osteopathic Schools.

Figure 5–1 Licensing and Certification of Physicians

their rights (self-preservation). Many people involved believed that the state boards were better able to assess competence to practice medicine. The idea, then, of some kind of national examining system as a means for comparing medical graduates from different schools gained acceptance, and this led to the formation of the **National Board of Medical Examiners (NBME)** by 1915.

The AMA's endorsement of the NBME came in 1916, and, with that, endorsement of the NBME was fully legitimized. Despite the significant advances brought about through the NBME examinations, state variation in some structuring of examinations prompted concern. These variations posed very real problems in terms of facilitating reciprocity of licenses among states.

The state boards began a move toward improving the situation by creating one national test. The Federation of State Medical Boards (FSMB) developed the **Federation Licensing Examination (FLEX)** from NBME questions. FLEX was accepted by all state boards for medical licensure until 1994. Each state administered the exam, which the NBME graded and the federation recorded for reference purposes. The grade was then reported to the appropriate state boards. All states had set the pass level at the FLEX-weighted average of 75, although individual states differed about the number of times FLEX could be taken.

FLEX was taken by graduates who wished to practice in the few states where the NBME was not accepted, by a few medical school graduates who did not have an NBME certificate, and by international medical graduates. The great majority of medical school graduates took the NBME examinations (the "national boards") to receive licensure.

Finally, in 1992, after nearly a century of debate about a national licensing system, the FSMB and the NBME together introduced the United States Medical Licensing Examination (USMLE), a single, uniform examination for medical licensure. The USMLE replaced the NBME examinations and FLEX. No other national examination was available after 1994.

The USLME is a three-step examination. Steps 1 and 2 can be taken during undergraduate medical school and are often folded into the curriculum as a measure of performance or criteria for advancement. Students take Step 3 after completing medical school and in conjunction with practicing in a particular state. Most states require completion of the one-year general residency in addition to undergraduate medical school to obtain licensure (USMLE 2007). Since spring of 1999, the USMLE has been administered on computer, reflecting the introduction of technology into more areas of education and evaluation (see Figure 5–1).

CONTINUING MEDICAL EDUCATION

Lifelong learning is essential for members of the medical profession (as for many other professions). Many physicians pursue their continuing medical education informally by reading journals, having conversations with colleagues, and attending presentations or discussions at medical staff or medical society meetings. Many states require participation in continuing medical education for license renewal; state medical societies require it for membership; and specialty societies require it for membership and recertification. In an age of quality assurance, continuing medical education is only one of the tools used to measure physicians' abilities. As previously mentioned, more emphasis has been placed on reexamination for recertification in specialties. Competitive forces have brought about new evaluation methods such as outcomes measurement and adherence to standards of care. In many specialties, benchmarks are available to physicians to compare their patient outcomes to the outcomes of other physicians in similar practices.

INTERNATIONAL MEDICAL GRADUATES

The United States has always attracted graduates of foreign medical schools, who come for a variety of reasons: to escape wars, religious persecutions and other repressions, as well as to seek new opportunities for adventure, economic well-being, and so on. In the eighteenth and nineteenth centuries, these physicians often provided a level of expertise very much needed in this land. Following World War II, Americans began to experience a new wave of physician immigration: graduates of European schools who sought to establish a new life in the United States, in large measure because of the dislocations resulting from the war or of the economic chaos that reigned in the postwar period. As Europe was reconstructed, the flow of physicians waned.

A new group of physicians began to come to the United States to establish new lives and to obtain advanced training; some came under the guise of obtaining advanced training, but hoped to stay. During the 1950s and 1960s, the flow from Asia did not contribute much to the permanent physician supply in the United States, because our immigration laws were weighted heavily against Asians and Africans. Changes in 1968 and 1970, however, opened the gates to immigration from all countries. Physicians came in large numbers from a former U.S. colony (the Philippines), from newfound military allies (South Korea, Thailand, Iran, and Taiwan), and from India and Pakistan. Americans welcomed them because they helped fill the physician shortage experienced as a result of a rapidly growing population, hospital expansions, and expansions due to research and technological advances that enabled physicians to help people in ways that were not previously feasible.

The **international medical graduates (IMGs),** formerly called foreign medical graduates (FMGs), provided medical services in three important areas: residencies providing patient care in teaching hospitals that were unable to fill their residency positions with U.S. medical graduates; patient care for the medically underserved areas of the inner city; and specialties such as pathology and institutional psychiatry that have not tended to attract U.S. medical graduates. The unknown quality of the foreign schools raised legitimate questions about the adequacy of their student training and their graduates' competence. The language barriers caused communication problems between physicians and patients, as well as between IMGs and their American colleagues.

Canadian physicians, however, are not considered foreign-trained. Because of the similarities between the U.S. and Canadian educational systems and the medical school accreditation process, graduates of approved Canadian schools are considered eligible to be examined by all state boards on the same basis as U.S. graduates, and about half the states grant reciprocity.

For a long time, it was relatively easy for IMGs to come to the United States for graduate medical training and to remain in this country for an indefinite period of time. Many foreign medical graduates took the medical knowledge and language reading ability test that the **Educational Commission for Foreign Medical Graduates (ECFMG)** developed in the 1950s. The test was administered in many overseas locations, but it was advisory only and not legally binding. The failure rates were disturbingly high. IMGs could also enter the United States with or without ECFMG certification and take positions in places that did not attract enough U.S. medical graduates (for example, state mental hospitals and inner-city indigent hospitals). Then, in 1974, the Coordinating Council on Medical Education reported an increasing concern that the United States had become overly dependent on IMGs to provide medical services, especially in hospitals. The report also stated that the IMGs coming from so many different countries, cultures, and educational institutions were not screened vigorously enough and might jeopardize the health and safety of the patients they treated. In testimony before a congressional committee in 1974, the variety of practices that were occurring and the serious questions about the quality of care many of the IMGs were discussed. Because of the physician shortage in certain areas, some states issued temporary licenses (American Medical News 1977b).

The data and the official reports that focused on the IMG problem, along with the emerging realization that there could be an excess supply of physicians by the 1980s, resulted in amendments to the Health Professions Educational Assistance Act of 1976. The amendments placed restrictions on the number of IMGs entering and remaining in the United States. In addition, the legislation mandated that IMGs who wished to enter the United States as immigrants on the basis of their medical skills and qualifications would have to pass Parts 1 and 2 of the NBME examination, or their equivalent, and be competent in written and oral English. The visa qualifying exam (VQE) was subsequently developed and certified as equivalent. Failure rates were high—80 percent for 1977 and 1980. IMGs performed better on the clinical portion than on the part testing basic medical science knowledge.

In 1984, a new test, the **Foreign Medical Graduates Examination in Medical Sciences (FMGEMS)**, replaced the VQE for ECFMG certification. ECFMG certification is necessary for graduates of foreign medical schools who want to be licensed and practice in the United States. At the present time, IMGs who are not U.S. citizens are required to pass either the FMGEMS or the new USMLE (basic science and clinical components), as well as an English-language proficiency test, to become certified. To be eligible to take the basic science portion of the FMGEMS, applicants must have completed at least two years at a medical school listed in the *World Directory of Medical Schools*. To take the clinical portion, applicants must have graduated from such a school.

About half of the IMGs today are U.S. citizens who were unable to gain admission to a U.S. or Canadian medical school and so took their training in foreign countries. Virtually all of these IMGs plan to practice in the United States. The exact number of those studying abroad is not known, but fewer are now accepted in residency programs. In 1984, 1,831 U.S. citizen IMGs (USIMGs) were accepted in residency programs in the United States, but only 929 were accepted in 1990—a 61 percent decrease. This decrease is due in large part to the efforts of U.S. medical organizations and the government to limit the numbers of both USIMGs and IMGs because of uncertainty about the adequacy of their training and a desire to prevent an oversupply of physicians (Whitcomb 1995).

As stated earlier, American and international students who complete their undergraduate medical education in a foreign country must pass the FMGEMS or Parts 1 and 2 of the USMLE before entering an accredited residency program in the United States. All of these measures are designed to discourage U.S. citizens from seeking medical undergraduate education abroad,

to restrict the number of alien IMGs, and to assure the quality of IMGs who train and practice in the United States.

In the current atmosphere of questioning whether the United States has too many physicians, training of IMGs is under scrutiny. Because Medicare is the primary source of funding for graduate medical education, the government has a critical stake in how many residents are trained. Throughout the 1990s, efforts were made to develop policy that would reduce the overall numbers of physicians being trained, redistribute the emphasis in training from specialization to primary care practice, and develop ways to attract physicians to underserved areas after training. Under such policy considerations, the practice of training IMGs who return to their respective countries after training is questioned. Yet, historically, IMGs have filled a very real void in hospitals and clinics that have not attracted U.S. medical graduates. As Medicare funding for residency training slots is withdrawn, hospitals may still find maintaining and filling those slots with alternatively funded IMGs desirable, rather than give up their residency training programs. Such an approach would simply skew the ratio of IMGs to U.S. medical graduates even further. In 2006, IMGs accounted for 26 percent of the 104,879 medical residents (AMA 2007). Of the total 902,053 physicians in the United States in 2006, 228,665 (25.3 percent) were IMGs (ibid.).

SUMMARY

Medical education has undergone massive changes over the years. It has evolved from apprenticeship to a highly complex system of academic, clinical, and continuing education. Prospective medical students must complete a bachelor's degree and maintain high academic standing to be considered for medical school. The medical school may be training in allopathic or osteopathic medicine. Many professional organizations and government bureaus oversee the process of medical education. Those who have the stamina to complete the rigorous training are not then left to their laurels. The oversight process continues through licensing and credentialing.

The content of medical education is also changing. Medical students must learn business skills and computer skills in addition to receiving scientific and clinical training. Many medical schools have incorporated more "caring" into their training by offering electives in "spirituality and medicine," ethics, cultural competency, and interpersonal relationship training to enhance the patient–physician relationship.

Organizations such as the Institute for Healthcare Improvement have made it a priority to change medical education to make it more reflective of prevention, patient-centered care, and high-quality care.

Graduate medical education has also undergone changes. The health care delivery organization rather than a specific service is the point of certification. Residencies vary in length by the specialty of training. Board certification, although not required for licensing, is required for many other areas of practice such as hospital privileges, insurance participation, and managed care participation. Once a lifetime certification, board certification is now renewable through examination.

Many of the changes in medical education and certification are attempts to ensure the quality of medical delivery, but they are not a guarantee of the quality of care physicians may render. Other efforts at quality assurance will be introduced in later chapters.

ACTIVITY-BASED LEARNING

Research your library or online resources for a copy of the Flexner report. Find a report on a medical school that sounds familiar to you (perhaps has the name of a familiar city or state in its name). What did the report say in regard to the school? Does this medical school still exist?

Consider the physicians with whom you have contact (family physician, specialist, or acquaintance). Determine if the physician is board-certified. When was the physician certified? Has there been recent recertification?

A QUESTION OF ETHICS

The high cost of a medical education, as well as the time that must be devoted to the entire training process, makes medicine as a profession available to only a select group of people.

- Does the medical education system inherently exclude certain populations, such as the poor and minorities?

- What changes could be instituted to make medicine as a profession available to a more diverse population?

It is generally believed that U.S. citizens who attend foreign medical schools do so because they are not accepted to U.S. medical schools.

- Should U.S. government funds be used to support the residency of American-born IMGs?

- Should U.S. government funds be used to support the residency of foreign-born IMGs?

IMGs often fill residencies and later practice medicine in areas that are not attractive to U.S. medical graduates, such as poor urban areas.

- Is this a commentary on the quality of care provided to the poor?

- What should be done (if anything) to attract more U.S. medical graduates to positions in these areas if they are not filled by IMGs?

REFERENCES

1. AAMC. (2007a). *Facts—Applicants, matriculants, and graduates*. Retrieved from www.aamc.org/data/facts/

2. AAMC. (2007b). *Computerized MCAT exam.* Retrieved from www.aamc.org/students/mcat/cbt.htm

3. AAMC. (2007c). *Number of U.S. medical schools teaching selected topics, 2004–2005*. Retrieved from http://www.services.aamc.org/currdir/section2/04_05hottopics.pdf

4. AAMC. (2007d). *2006 AAMC survey of housestaff stipends, benefits and funding*. Retrieved from http://www.aamc.org/data/stipend/2006_hssreport.pdf

5. AAMC. (2005). *Medical educational costs and student debt*. Washington, DC. Retrieved from www.brynmawr.edu/healthpro/documents/MedSchoolDegt05.pdf

6. ACGME. (2007a). *The ACMGE at a glance*. Retrieved from www.acgme.org/acWebsite/newsRoom/newsRm_acGlance.asp

7. ACGME. (2007b). *Duty hours language*. From www.acgme.org/acWebsite/dutyHours/dh_Lang703.pdf

8. AMA. (2007). International medical graduates in the U.S. workforce: A discussion paper. Retrieved from www.ama-assn.org/ama1/pub/upload/mm/18/img-workforce-paper.pdf

9. AOA. (2007). *Frequently asked questions*. Retrieved from www.osteopathic.org/index.cfm?PageID=faq_cons#dodef

10. AOA. (2006). *Fact sheet 2006: Osteopathic physicians*. Retrieved from www.osteopathic.org/pdf/ost_factsheet.pdf

11. American Association of Colleges of Osteopathic Medicine. (2007a). *Osteopathic Specialty Colleges*. Retrieved from http://www.aacom.org

12. American Association of Colleges of Osteopathic Medicine. (2007b). *Osteopathic medical education*. Retrieved from http://www.aacom.org

13. American Board of Medical Specialties. (2006a). About ABMS member boards. Retrieved from www.abms.org/About_ABMS/member_boards.aspx

14. American Board of Medical Specialties. (2006b). *Maintenance of certification*. Retrieved from http://www.abms.org/Maintenance_of_Certification/

15. American Medical News. (1977, March 7).

16. American Medical Student Association. (2007). *Medical school tuition frequently asked questions*. Retrieved from www.amsa.org/student/tuition_FAQ.cfm

17. Colonial Williamsburg Foundation. (2007). Apothecary, more than a druggist. From www.history.org/Almanack/life/trades/tradeapo.cfm

18. Bajaj, A. (1999a). How Medicare calculates GME payments. (Part 1). *JAMA, 281*(20), 1958.

19. Bajaj, A. (1999b). How Medicare calculates GME payments. (Part 2). *JAMA, 281*(22), 2156.

20. Barzansky, B., & Etzel, S. (2004). *Educational programs in U.S. medical schools*, 2003–2004. *JAMA, 292*(9), 1025–1031.

21. Citizens Commission on Graduate Medical Education. (1966). *The graduate education of physicians*. Chicago: American Medical Association.

22. Coggeshall, L. T. (1965). *Planning for medical progress through education*. Evanston, IL: Association of American Medical Colleges.

23. Corner, G. W. (1965). *Two centuries of medicine: A history of the School of Medicine, University of Pennsylvania*. Philadelphia: Lippincott.

24. Council on Graduate Medical Education. (2000). *Financing graduate medical education in a changing health care environment*. Summary of Fifteenth Report. Retrieved from www.cogme.gov/rpt15.htm

25. Ebert, R., & Ginsberg, E. (1988). *The reform of medical education*. Health Affairs, 7 (2, Suppl.).

26. Fishbein, M. (1947). *A history of the American Medical Association, 1847–1947*. Philadelphia: Saunders.

27. Flexner, A. (1940). *I remember*. New York: Simon & Schuster.

28. Flexner, A. (1910). *Medical education in the United States and Canada*. Washington, DC: Science and Health Publications, Inc.

29. Health Services and Research Administration. (2005). *Evaluating the Impact of Title VII, Section 747 Programs, 5th Annual Report to the Secretary of the U.S. Department of Health and Human Services and to Congress, Advisory Committee on Training in Primary Care Medicine and Dentistry Programs*.

30. IHI. (2007). *Health professions education: General*. Retrieved from www.ihi.org/IHI/Topics/HealthProfessionsEducation/EducationGeneral/HealthProfessionsEducationGeneralHome.htm

31. Johnson, V. (1947). *The council on medical education and hospitals*. In M. Fishbein (Ed.), *A history of the American Medical Association, 1847–1947*. Philadelphia: Saunders.

32. LCME. (2006). *Overview: Accreditation and the LCME*. Retrieved from www.lcme.org/overview.htm

33. Ludmerer, K. M. (1985). *Learning to heal, the development of American medical education*. New York: Basic Books.

34. Martin, S. (1998, July 27). New Medicare residency funding rules combat oversupply. *American Medical News*, p. 8.

35. National Center for Health Statistics. (2006). *Health, United States 2006 with chartbook on trends in the health of Americans*. Hyattsville, MD.

36. National Resident Matching Program. (2006). *About the NRMP*. Retrieved from www.nrmp.org/about_nrmp/index.html

37. National Resident Matching Program. (2007). *Selected data tables 2007*. Retrieved from www.nrmp.org

38. Packard, F. R. (1963). *History of medicine in the United States*. New York: Hafner.

39. Reed, D., Levine, R., Miller, R., Ashar, B., Bass, E., Rice, T., & Cofrancesco, J. (2007). Effect of residency duty=hour limits: Views of key clinical faculty. *Archives of Internal Medicine, 167*(14), 1487.

40. Robinson, J. (1999). The new face of medical education. *JAMA, 281*(13), 1226.

41. Shryock, R. H. (1966). *Medicine in America*. Baltimore: Johns Hopkins Press.

42. Stevens, R. (1971). *American medicine and the public interest*. New Haven, CT: Yale University Press.

43. Stevens, R. (1989). *In sickness and in wealth*. New York: Basic Books.

44. USMLE. (2007). *U.S. medical licensing exam, 2007 USMLE Bulletin*. Retrieved from www.usmle.org/General_Information/bulletin/2007/overview.html?

45. Whang, E., Mello, M., Ashley, S., & Zinner, M. (2003). Implementing resident work hour limitations: Lessons from the New York State Experience. *Annals of Surgery*, *237*(4), 449.

46. Whitcomb, M. (1995). Correcting the oversupply of specialists by limiting residencies for graduates of foreign medical schools. *New England Journal of Medicine*, *333*(7), 454.

47. Womack, N. A. (1965, June 7). The evolution of the National Board of Medical Examiners. *JAMA*, *192*.

48. Young, J., & Coffman, J. (1998). Overview of graduate medical education: Funding streams, policy problems, and options for reform. *Western Journal of Medicine*, *168*(2), 428–437.

PART TWO

The Internal Environment of Health Care Delivery

Chapter 6

Professions in Health Care

CHAPTER OBJECTIVES

After completing this chapter, readers should have an understanding of the following:

- The multiple participants in the provision of direct and indirect patient care
- The differences in training and credentialing of health care service providers
- The tensions that may exist among health care service providers
- The difficulties in coordinating care among various providers, given cost and payment restrictions

INTRODUCTION

Physicians historically gained control of health care delivery through licensing and credentialing. They had the knowledge regarding diagnosis and treatment of disease and the authority (often sole authority) to act on that knowledge. Rapid changes in the health care market (managed care, cost-containment incentives, the rise in corporate medicine, the introduction of information systems technology) have drawn attention to the question of whether new forms of health care delivery reduce physician authority and raise the professional discretion of other health care providers—and whether those changes in authority are appropriate. The historic dominance of physicians in health care can be explained by the following:

- The division of labor in health care delivery that requires that all other health care professionals work under "orders" the physician gives (Friedson 1985)

- The amount of knowledge physicians have, particularly in comparison to the patients they treat (Folland et al. 2007; Phelps 2002; Starr 1982)

- The capitalist economy, which promotes the freedom of practice and economic dominance of physicians (Friedson 1985)

The free market assumes participation of consumers based on the premise of "buyers beware," whereas professions operate on the basis of the buyers believing in (or trusting) the professional (Torres 1991). This difference, referred to as **asymmetry of information**, stems from the fact that professionals are deemed to have knowledge or expertise not available to laypeople. **Professionals** possess not only complex knowledge, but also the knowledge is viewed as critical to the social welfare. Most people would agree that physicians fit the criteria of "professional." Occupations acquire professional status over time. The state becomes involved in establishing boundaries (licensing of practitioners), which other occupations cannot cross. The profession must be in continuous movement to ensure its status in legislation as competing occupations vie for control of protected areas of performance (Torres 1991).

Deprofessionalization occurs with the reduction in the knowledge gap between physicians and consumers that is fostered by the increase in consumer education and computer access to information on diagnoses and treatment. Deprofessionalization also occurs as more physicians assume salaried positions in organizations and as new professions emerge with authority to treat patients independently of physicians. Researchers and administrators employ a **macro view** of providing health care to the population, whereas practitioners employ a **micro view** of individual patients. Conflicts occur and practitioners are often limited in their freedom to choose a particular mode of care because administration controls resources. Professional standards generate constraints on clinical judgment, and practitioners are forced to justify any moves outside those standards. Computers can add a level of control by monitoring practice habits and flagging "deviant" behavior.

Other medical specialists (nurse practitioners, physician assistants, and so on) are assuming roles that physicians previously played, thus reducing physician control and autonomy. The emergence of the health care team in patient treatment often requires deferment of judgment by the physician to the team or a specific team member involved in the patient's care (Rutherford et al. 2004).

The questions of physician control and the limits of practice placed on other health care providers are not new. Struggles between the professions for areas of exclusive privileges are as old as the professions themselves. Legal practice parameters change as professions lobby state legislatures. Accepted standards of practice often change with reimbursement decisions made at the federal level by the Centers for Medicare and Medicaid Services (CMS). Although we attempt to describe the functions of various health care professionals in this chapter, we recognize that these functions are changing with time and may vary from state to state.

Countless health professionals provide direct patient care and/or work in support of those providing direct patient care. As the provision of health care changes and technology is adopted, categories of personnel also change. The health professionals discussed in this chapter do not constitute all health care professionals but are representative of the critical distinctions among health care providers.

REGISTERED NURSES (RN)

Nurses are "the hearts and hands of health care" (Friedman 1991), and they continue to be the largest group of health care professionals. Nursing is unique in that it encompasses the only group of health care professionals that is predominantly female, with only 5.8 percent being male. Although the majority of nurses still work in hospitals, nursing practice is shifting to a focus on disease prevention and modification of lifestyles. This shift in focus results in more nurses working in community clinics, doctors' offices, long-term care facilities, schools, and home health agencies. Insurance companies, peer review organizations, managed care organizations, and pharmaceutical companies are also recruiting experienced nurses. Some have their own independent practices (see Table 6–1). The nursing profession is undergoing change in educational and training programs and in the tasks that nurses perform (U.S. Department of Health and Human Services 2004).

Nursing began as a helping profession in the United States, with training programs associated with general hospitals. The pattern that developed dominated the nursing field until after World War II: Nurses were trained for three years in specialty schools associated with hospitals. On successfully completing the course of study, graduating students were awarded diplomas; on passing the state licensing examination, a nurse became a **registered nurse (RN)**. Only about 25.2 percent of RNs were graduates of hospital diploma schools of nursing in 2004. The percentage has been decreasing since the 1980s, as the number of graduates from two- and four-year college programs is rising. This changing scene will be discussed after briefly examining the various types of nursing programs (U.S. Department of Health and Human Services 2004).

Hospital diploma school programs typically had a large service emphasis; that is, the training was heavily weighted in favor of on-the-job training rather than academic training. The number of diploma programs has declined significantly from 63.2 percent in 1980, to 25.2 percent in 2004, as previously mentioned.

During World War I, a number of university nursing programs were developed that granted baccalaureate degrees instead of diplomas. On passing the same state licensing examination that diploma school graduates take, baccalaureate graduates also became RNs. Baccalaureate programs experienced a rapid rise, from 15 percent of all programs in 1960, to 31.5 percent in 2004 (Moskowitz 1999; U.S. Department of Health and Human

TABLE 6-1   **Employment Settings for Registered Nurses, 1980–2004**, in Thousands**

Setting	1980	1984	1988	1992	1996	2000	2004
Hospital	1,361	1,300	1,271	1,233	1,105	1,012	836
Public/community health*	360	402	363	250	181	167	158
Ambulatory care	278	209	179	144	159	129	103
Nursing homes	153	153	171	129	108	115	101
Nursing education	63	47	49	37	30	40	48
Other	156	81	83	56	43	21	22

*Includes school and occupational health
**The total numbers of RNs across all settings of employment may not equal the total estimated number of nurses due to incomplete information of survey respondents.

SOURCE: U.S. Department of Health and Human Services. 2006. *The registered nurse population, findings from the March 2004 National Sample Survey of Registered Nurses*, Chart 7. Health Resources and Services Administration, Bureau of Health Professions.

Services 2004). Graduates of baccalaureate programs constituted just over 34 percent of the total registered nurse population in 2004. Enrollment in these programs, as in other nursing degree programs, has fluctuated from 1980, through the turn of the twenty-first century, as health care has gone through various streamlining efforts as a result of cost containment (see Figure 6–1). Many nurses who initially receive an associate degree in nursing go on to get a baccalaureate degree. In 2004, nearly 21 percent of nurses with associate degrees received a baccalaureate degree or higher (U.S. Department of Health and Human Services 2004).

A third type of nurse training program began to develop in community colleges during the 1950s. These programs last two to two and a half years and grant an associate degree to students. On passing the same state licensing examination that diploma school and college or university graduates take, students become registered nurses. Associate degree programs have also experienced a rapid rise, from only 5 percent of all programs in 1960, to 42 percent in 2004 (Moskowitz 1999; U.S. Department of Health and Human Services 2004). As mentioned previously, many RNs from these programs eventually go on to college or university programs to also earn bachelor's degrees. In 2004, approximately 34 percent of the total number of practicing RNs held an associate degree as a terminal degree (U.S. Department of Health and Human Services 2004).

As we have illustrated, there are three basic pathways to becoming an RN. Each has an academic component, each uses hospital facilities for clinical training, and all graduates become registered by taking a common state examination that the state board of nurse examiners administers. The diploma programs and associate degree programs are credited for providing more clinical experience than the baccalaureate programs. The baccalaureate approach is distinctive in that it provides the additional educational requirements that are necessary if an RN wishes to pursue a graduate degree. Whether trained at the diploma, associate degree, or baccalaureate level, nurses have similar roles and functions in hospitals and generally receive the same salary.

There was a movement on the part of nurse leaders to close the diploma schools because they believed nurse training should be part of an educational system and not under the control of a hospital or of any other profession. Diploma schools were closing, and although professional pressures were partially responsible, the cause was primarily cost. The costs of diploma education cannot be buried in general hospital costs and covered by insurance payments. Those programs that survived were often affiliated with a college or university that offered the academic courses and supplemented the hospital training that results in an associate or bachelor's degree upon completion. The difference between the diploma and the other degrees is evident only in the fact that diploma students sit for

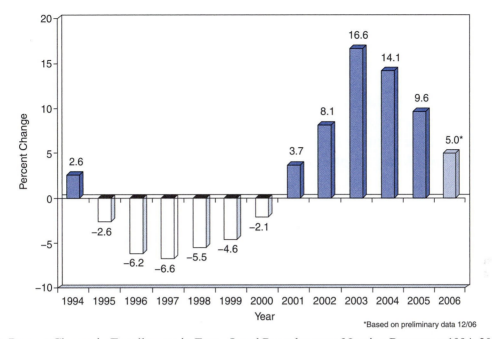

Figure 6-1 Percent Change in Enrollments in Entry-Level Baccalaureate Nursing Programs: 1994–2006

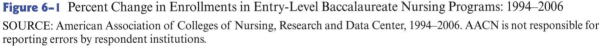

SOURCE: American Association of Colleges of Nursing, Research and Data Center, 1994–2006. AACN is not responsible for reporting errors by respondent institutions.

the state exam and licensing before completing the academic portion of training. The closing trend has somewhat diminished with the nursing shortage. Hospitals realize that the diploma program is a shorter route to a fresh supply of nurses than the baccalaureate degree and often comes with loyalty to the hospital by the graduates.

The National Advisory Council on Nurse Education and Practice (NACNEP) has since taken up the cause of professionalism in nursing. Their report to the Secretary of Health and Human Services and Congress highlights the need to increase recruitment into nursing and career enhancement to retain those already in nursing. Regarding education, NACNEP presents a model that should (1) further the achievement of its goal that two-thirds of the RN workforce should have at least a baccalaureate degree by 2010, and (2) help to develop those eligible to become faculty members (NACNEP 2003).

Although the number of people seeking baccalaureate degrees has increased, those seeking associate degrees are a much larger number. However, a more disturbing fact is that more than 40,000 qualified applicants were not admitted to nursing

school because of a shortage of faculty. Of those, more than 3,300 were applicants to graduate programs—those with the potential to fill future faculty positions (American Association of Colleges of Nursing 2007).

Nurse leaders now also recognize professional nurses as being those who earn a master's degree (12 percent of the 2004 nursing workforce) and work as specialists in a clinical area of nursing (for example, pediatrics, public health, medical-surgical nursing, intensive care) or in a health services management area; or as those who hold a doctorate (about 1 percent of the 2004 nursing workforce), not in sociology or higher education but in one of the developing doctoral programs in nursing, health administration, or health services research (U.S. Department of Health and Human Services 2004). Just as in other areas of health care delivery, professional nursing is no longer concerned only with "sick care" but also with "wellness." Others argue that nurses have a unique role that relates to helping people cope with conditions that medicine is unable to cure or help: the growing area of chronic care.

EXHIBIT 6-1

The Washington Post

August 26, 2007

Reversing a Trend, Nursing Shortages Return; Compounding the Problem: Schools Can't Find Enough Faculty and Are Turning Away Applicants

BYLINE: Lisa Rein; Washington Post Staff Writer

Maryland hospitals are short of **nurses** again after two years of declining vacancies.

The **shortages,** reported this month in a survey by the Maryland Hospital Association, result from changes in demographics and health care: Demand for **nurses** rises as people live longer and need more care. At the same time, the **nurses** of the baby boom generation are starting to retire.

"The issue is not going to go away, and we think it's going to get worse," said Catherine Crowley, the association's vice president and a specialist in workforce issues.

Maryland's 47 hospitals reported an average vacancy rate for **nurses** of 13 percent, or 2,340 positions in 2006, compared with 10 percent in 2005. Vacancies hit a high of 15.6 percent in 2001, the association said. The rate is projected to be 18 percent by 2016.

The association does not collect individual hospital data, but Crowley said facilities with the biggest nursing **shortages** are in Montgomery and Prince George's counties and in the Baltimore area. The survey analyzed vacancies in forty other positions, finding similar needs for radiographers and physical and occupational therapists, for example.

The **shortage** does not necessarily mean that patients are going without nursing care. Emergency room patients in Maryland are frequently diverted to other hospitals because of a dearth of **nurses** at the first facility, Crowley said.

There has been a chronic **shortage of nurses** and other health care workers across the country for years, as hospitals compete with high-paying technology companies. Among the solutions has been heavy recruitment from developing countries such as the Philippines.

There is, however, a growing interest in the field. Maryland has 18,000 full-time hospital-based **nurses**, compared with 14,400 in 2001, the association reports. Average salaries for full-time **nurses** have risen to $87,000.

With a new flow of young people into the profession, the problem appears to be finding experienced faculty to teach.

"The pool is expanding," Crowley said. "But we're turning away people who are qualified to be **nurses** because we don't have enough teachers."

Enrollment at Maryland's twenty-five nursing schools has jumped by about 40 percent in six years. But many applicants are turned away because the programs are short of faculty.

Enrollment in the College of Southern Maryland's nursing program has doubled in the past six years.

During that growth, school officials have struggled to recruit faculty members with college teaching experience, said Sandra Genrich, chairman of nursing and health technology for the college.

In 2001, the nursing program admitted about sixty-five students—far below its goal of eighty. Now it admits two classes of about sixty-five each year and turns away thirty to forty qualified applicants during each admissions cycle, Genrich said. Total enrollment in the program is about 235 students, she said.

The total number of faculty also has increased since 2001, but many of the new instructors are people with limited teaching experience filling part-time positions, Genrich said. In 2001, the college had ten full-time faculty and four part-time employees. Now it has seventeen full-time faculty and thirteen part-time employees.

"When we bring our new faculty on, part-time faculty in particular, they do not have any teaching experience in an academic environment," Genrich said. "The full-time faculty are spread thinner."

At Prince George's Community College, which offers a two-year degree for registered **nurses** and a one-year program for licensed practical **nurses**, faculty **shortages** have limited enrollments. The school could offer just 68 slots for 150 applicants this year, said Cheryl Dover, head of the nursing department.

(continues)

EXHIBIT 6-1 (Continued)

A state grant will add one or two positions to the seventeen-member faculty, Dover said. But several professors are in their fifties and are planning to retire in a few years. "And there's nobody coming out there to replace us when we retire," she said. The average salary for nursing faculty is $45,000 to $50,000, the association said.

To address a similar **shortage** of nursing faculty at Virginia's colleges and universities, Gov. Timothy M. Kaine (D) announced a scholarship program this summer that encourages master's and doctoral nursing students to teach at state schools after they graduate.

In Maryland, some hospitals are lending staff **nurses** to professional schools to serve as adjunct faculty, and the state loosened a requirement that all faculty have master's degrees in nursing, instead allowing that advanced degree to be in a related field.

Community College of Baltimore County is starting to recruit emergency medical technicians to become **nurses**, an effort to recognize their education in a related field.

Maryland's nursing schools are relying increasingly on computer-based coursework. However, the electronic curricula are no substitute for hands-on, clinical work, Crowley said.

Staff writer Matt Zapotosky contributed to this report.

Copyright 2007 The Washington Post

Reprinted with Permission

Discussion Question

1. The need for qualified nursing faculty is evident. What might be some of the reasons that qualified nurses do not go on for higher degrees to become nursing faculty?

Changes in health care require health professionals to function in teams, and physicians and nurses are now working in a more collaborative, rather than adversarial, environment. Change is very prominent in the large teaching hospitals, where nurses today are doing things that neither they nor physicians ever thought would be nursing functions. Nurses are performing tasks that are new, as well as some functions that physicians once did. Though the theory of nursing may not have taken such events fully into account, nursing is being operationally redefined. There is, of course, no ironclad definition of what nurses or physicians are. The terms and the things they describe are human devices applied to a world that is forever changing.

Nurses have continued to struggle to expand their role in the changing, more technological atmosphere of health care. They have taken advanced training either to specialize in a certain clinical area (for example, intensive care unit, neonatal intensive care unit, psychiatry, operating room, and so on) or to provide more independent care (for example, as nurse practitioners, nurse-midwives, and so on).

Strains between physicians and nurses continue to exist as the nursing role expands and the relationship with physicians becomes more of a collaborative partnership, with nurses being a part of the clinical decision-making process. Designed to ease some of the friction, the AMA House of Delegates adopted a statement in 1983, that nurses should not be expected to blindly follow all medical orders and that nurses may take action contrary to standing orders to protect patients in an emergency if a physician is not available. The resolution was sending a message to physicians that nurses have a responsibility to use judgment too.

In their effort to define nursing, the American Nurses Association (2007a) has released the following statement on their website:

Nursing is the protection, promotion, and optimization of health and abilities, prevention of illness and injury, alleviation of suffering through the diagnosis and treatment of human response, and advocacy in the care of individuals, families, communities, and populations.

The human response...

What defines nursing and sets it apart from other health care professions, particularly medicine with which it has long been considered part and parcel? It is nurses' focus—in theory and practice—on the response of the individual and the family to actual or potential health problems. Nurses are educated to be attuned to the whole person, not just the unique presenting health problem. While a medical diagnosis of an illness may be fairly circumscribed, the human response to a health problem may be much more fluid and variable and may have a great effect on the individual's ability to overcome the initial medical problem. It is often said that physicians cure, and nurses care. In what some describe as a blend of physiology and psychology, nurses build on their understanding of the disease and illness process to promote the restoration and maintenance of health in their clients.

Factors Affecting the Supply of Nurses

Throughout the 1980s, there were increases in the national nursing shortage. The severity of the shortage depended upon the geographic location and type of nurses needed. Although the national shortage was much discussed in the 1980s, changes in hospital reimbursements resulted in many hospitals releasing nurses in an attempt to downsize and reduce costs. The downsizing resulted in the use of other personnel, such as nursing assistants, to pick up some of what had traditionally been nurses' responsibilities. However, hospitals also found themselves working with patients who were older and more critically ill, as many of the less acute cases were handled on an outpatient basis.

The early 1990s again saw a shortage of highly skilled nurses, mainly in large urban hospitals providing high-tech care to patients who were sicker. Wages and working conditions also contributed to the shortage. The wages of hospital nurses compared poorly to the wages of female professional and technical workers in other fields. Although the starting salaries of nurses are now comparable to those of other college graduates, the maximum average salary is much lower (see Table 6–2). Women who plan to work a number of years do not find the pay raises and career

ladders in nursing that exist in many other professions women now enter. In other words, women have many more career options in which the economic rewards are greater, their contributions are better recognized, and the hours are more regular.

By the mid-1990s, there was some indication that the shortage had eased and the supply of nurses was adequate for the needs. However, early in the next decade, the shortage again became an issue and seemed to be more widespread across areas of nursing and areas of the country (Buerhaus et al. 2005). These authors noted that the reasons for the shortage seemed somewhat the same: negative perceptions of nursing as a career, undesirable working hours, low salaries, more career options for women, and so on (p. 65). Although still a problem, nursing shortages seemed to decrease in 2004, compared to 2002. Many hospitals have made huge efforts in recruiting more nurses by offering sign-on bonuses, support for additional education, higher salaries, and flexible work hours (p. 67).

In hospitals, the hours are a particular problem because of the need to have nurses available twenty-four hours a day and seven days a week. New nurses are hard-pressed to find positions that do not require evening, nighttime, weekend, or holiday hours. Those who remain in nursing have more options to work in other clinical sites, such as medical practices, managed care, ambulatory surgical centers, home care, and so on, which may not offer the same hourly wages but offer a more stable work schedule.

Just as in physician education and practice, coping with new knowledge has forced specialization in nursing. A nurse with a baccalaureate degree may undertake graduate study toward a master's degree and/or a doctorate in a variety of clinical areas to develop the needed special competence for teaching, supervision, and advanced practice. In addition to training in such clinical specialties as pediatrics, obstetrics, medical-surgical services,

TABLE 6–2 Actual and "Real" Average Annual Salaries of Full-Time Registered Nurses for Selected Years

Setting	1980	1984	1988	1992	1996	2000	2004
Actual salary	$17,398	$23,505	$28,383	$37,738	$42,071	$46,782	$57,784
Real salary*	$17,398	$19,079	$20,839	$23,166	$23,103	$23,369	$26,366

*Earnings that take into account the purchasing power of the dollar over time

SOURCE: U.S. Department of Health and Human Services. 2006. *Preliminary findings: 2004 National Sample Survey of Registered Nurses, Chart 9*. Health Resources and Services Administration, Bureau of Health Professions.

and psychiatry, a number of specialized programs have been developed, such as those for the nurse practitioner and nurse-midwife, that train nurses to work on their own in private practice or as equals on a health care team. Some of these programs are described in more detail later in this chapter.

LICENSED PRACTICAL NURSES (LPN)

Licensed practical nurses (LPNs) provide nursing care to patients under the direction of a physician, dentist, podiatrist, optometrist, or registered nurse. Their responsibilities are similar to, but more limited than, those of registered nurses. Most LPNs can take vital signs, treat bedsores, prepare and give injections, insert catheters, and the like. Their responsibilities differ by state regulations. Some states certify LPNs to administer medications and intravenous therapy after specific additional training (Bureau of Labor Statistics 2006a).

The position of LPN developed from the nursing shortage that followed World War II; hospitals began to hire LPNs in place of more expensive RNs whenever possible. However, this trend subsided as technological procedures increased and hospitals admitted patients who were sicker. LPN training takes twelve months on average to complete and is usually part of public vocational school programs, although hospitals, community colleges, or community agencies run some LPN programs. In 2004, approximately 1,200 schools offered LPN programs. In the same year, LPNs held over 7,000 jobs, over half of them

TABLE 6–3 Average Earnings of LPNs, 2004

Site of Employment	Average Annual Salary
Actual salary	$41,550
Nursing care facilities	35,460
Home health care services	35,180
General medical and surgical hospitals	32,570
Offices of physicians	30,400

SOURCE: U.S. Department of Labor, Bureau of Labor Statistics. 2006. Licensed practical and licensed vocational nurses. Retrieved from www.bls.gov/oco/ocos102.htm.

in hospitals or nursing homes. If LPNs wish to go on to other nursing programs, they must start from the beginning with no transfer or carryover credits. In 2004, the median annual salary for LPNs was $33,970. Earnings vary by location of employment (see Table 6–3).

NURSING EDUCATION APPROVAL AND ACCREDITATION AND THE NATIONAL LEAGUE FOR NURSING

Nursing programs—LPN, diploma, associate degree, and baccalaureate degree—must be approved by an agency of state government if graduates are to be permitted to take the licensing examination. The state board of nurse examiners is typically the name of the state agency that handles this. The National Council of State Boards of Nursing (NCSBN) provides two licensure examinations, the National Council Licensure Examination for Registered Nurses (NCLEX-RN) and the National Council Licensure Examination for Practical Nurses (NCLEX-PN), to state and territorial boards of nursing for nurse licensure (NCSBN 2007).

The National League for Nursing (NLN) provides a mechanism for academic accreditation over and above the state approval process. The NLN focuses principally on certifying nurse educators—for LPN, diploma, associate, baccalaureate, and advanced degrees programs. The NLN also works to foster nursing education research by providing grants for scholarships and research projects.

Graduate programs in nursing can be professionally accredited by the National League for Nursing Accreditation Council (NLNAC). Approval of graduate programs is usually beyond the scope of state government authority. Specialty subcomponents of a master's program are sometimes accredited by a nurse specialty body, in addition to being accredited by the NLNAC.

THE AMERICAN NURSES ASSOCIATION

The American Nurses Association (ANA) is a professional association for RNs that establishes and implements nursing political and legislative programs, promotes a professional and equitable work environment for nurses, and develops standards that ensure high-quality patient care. It also approves organizations for providing continuing nursing education. The ANA works to increase nurses' pay and improve their conditions of employment. It actively lobbies lawmakers and regulators whose decisions impact nursing concerns. Its current focus is on improving working conditions for nurses, particularly the stress nurses encounter under staff shortages and mandatory overtime. With the focus on cost containment, the professional organization is concerned with the quality of care rendered to patients in this nurse shortage environment (American Nurses Association 2007b).

The American Nurses Credentialing Center (ANCC) has provided certification programs for the ANA since 1973. The certification programs are similar to those in other areas of medical care, administering exams and requiring documentation regarding formal and continuing education for each level of certification. The certification process offers certification programs in such areas as adult nurse practitioner, cardiovascular nurse, gerontological nurse, advanced diabetes management, and more. AANC also accredits approvers of continuing education and providers of continuing education in nursing. ANCC accreditation is recognized by most state licensing boards (ANCC 2006).

Public Health and Community Nursing

Public health nursing, with its focus on preventing disease and promoting health in the community, offers an alternative to hospital care for those who are sick. It also provides nurses with an opportunity to work more independently than in the hospital. For the most part, public health training is generalized to enable a single well-trained nurse working in the community to recognize and cope with multiple problems that may arise in a family. Generalized training is based on the premise that people and families, rather than diseases or physical situations, should be served. There is some specialized training in such areas as industrial or full-time clinical nursing. The ANCC offers certification as a public/community heath clinical nurse specialist.

Most state health departments have separate bureaus or divisions of public health nursing, in which public health nurses are employed as advisers to local health departments, boards of education, voluntary health agencies, and other state agencies. They may also conduct in-service training and promote services that are available through the local public health nursing programs.

At the local level, public health nurses are employed by local health departments, where their primary tasks relate to disease prevention and health promotion; and by agencies such as visiting nursing associations, which are concerned primarily with rendering home nursing care to those who are sick. When employed outside of a public health department, public health nurses are frequently called community nurses. The nomenclature, however, is not precise. Some public health departments also call their public health nurses community nurses (American Public Health Association 2007).

Nurse Practitioners

An expanded role for nurses is that of the **nurse practitioner**, who is trained to serve as the regular health care provider for children and adults during health and illness. Nurse practitioners obtain medical histories, perform physical examinations, diagnose illness and disease, order laboratory tests, prescribe medications (in collaboration with physicians in some states and independently in others), provide education and counseling, and assume responsibility for medical management of cases with emphasis on primary care. Typically, nurse practitioners graduate from a two-year master's program in one of many specialty areas; however, some are educated at the doctoral level. Nurse practitioners are employed in both urban and rural areas in settings such as community-based clinics, physicians' offices, home health agencies, nursing homes and hospices, hospitals, and independent nurse practitioner offices. The most important reasons nurses give for becoming nurse practitioners are the chance to have a greater influence on patient care and the opportunity for additional learning.

Many of the 115,000 practicing nurse practitioners choose settings where populations are underserved for health care services. A large number of nurse practitioners are in rural states, and the majority practice in clinics providing direct primary care. They practice independently and have a collaborative arrangement with a physician, who cooperates in the management of patients' health care problems when necessary. Presumably, nurse practitioners functioning "interdependently" have a physician available for ready consultation and can refer patients easily (American Academy of Nurse Practitioners 2007a).

Since January 1998, Medicare has reimbursed nurse practitioners directly for independent patient care. As of 2003, Medicare will only certify master's-prepared nurse practitioners for Medicare reimbursement. Some states have extended prescription-writing privileges to nurse practitioners (American Academy of Nurse Practitioners 2007b).

Nurse-Midwives

The number of **nurse-midwives** is increasing in the United States, totaling about 7,000 in 2004. Approximately 6,000 of them are in clinical practice. The number of deliveries by nurse-midwives has also increased every year since 1975, with only a small decrease from 2003 to 2004. Certified nurse-midwives delivered over 308,000 babies in 2004—11 percent of all vaginal births that year (see Table 6–4).

Midwives delivered most newborn Americans until World War I, when medical advances and the acceptance of hospital deliveries resulted in a dramatic decline in the practice of midwifery. Early midwives were not professionally trained or licensed, but apprenticed with other practicing midwives. However, that has changed, and currently there are forty accredited nurse-midwife education programs in the United States; thirty-seven of them are graduate programs, and three are postbaccalaureate certificate programs. About 4 percent of midwives have a doctoral degree. The American College of Nurse-Midwives (ACNM) accredits the education programs (American College of Nurse-Midwives 2005).

According to the ACNM:

- Nurse-midwifery practice is legal in all fifty states and the District of Columbia.

- Thirty-three states mandate private insurance payment for services, and Medicaid reimbursement is mandatory in all states.

- Most births attended by a certified nurse-midwife occur in hospitals; only 1 percent occurs in freestanding birthing centers and 1 percent in the home.

- The primary workplace of most nurse-midwives is an office or clinic environment.

- Nurse-midwives have prescription-writing privileges in all fifty states and the District of Columbia (Pennsylvania was the last state to approve medication dispensing in July 2007).

- Visits to the nurse-midwife include annual exams, reproductive health visits, and visits outside the maternity cycle.

Nurse-midwives tend to offer personalized, family-centered, low-intervention maternity care. They have low cesarean section rates and low infant mortality rates—both an indication of quality care and a result of the fact that nurse-midwives refer high-risk cases to physician specialists.

Even though nurse-midwives have physician backup, physicians are often considerably opposed to nurse-midwives opening their own practices. In many instances, nurse-midwives and their collaborative physicians have been refused hospital privileges, and the authority to admit and care for private patients. However, a midwife-attended birth costs about 50 percent less than a physician-attended birth. This

TABLE 6–4 Births Attended by Certified Nurse-Midwives and Other Midwives in the U.S., 1997–2004

Year	Total Births	Total Births by Midwives	Births by Certified Nurse-Midwives	Births by Other Midwives
1997	3,880,894	272,201	258,227	13,974
1998	3,941,553	293,386	277,811	15,575
2000	4,058,814	314,539	297,902	16,637
2002	4,021,726	325,235	307,527	17,708
2003	4,089,950	328,153	310,342	17,811
2004	4,112,052	325,899	308,113	17,786

SOURCE: National Vital Statistics Report; Vol.47, No. 18, 1999, Table 38; Vol. 48, No. 3, 2000, Table 38; Vol. 50, No. 5, 2002, Table 38; Vol. 52, No. 10, 2003, Table 38; Vol. 54, No. 2, 2005, Table 38; Vol. 55, No. 1, 2006, Table 27.

difference in cost has led managed care organizations and clinics in underserved areas to embrace the concept of midwife deliveries. Specialists with busy obstetric practices have also recognized the value of midwife deliveries in low-risk pregnancies. Collaboration is now more common, although some stress remains over the scope of midwife practices in more competitive environments.

Certified Registered Nurse Anesthetists

Certified registered nurse anesthetists (CRNAs) became the first clinical nursing specialists in the late 1800s, as a response to the growing need surgeons had for anesthetists. Today, more than 30,000 CRNAs are providing 65 percent of the 26 million anesthetics given to patients in the United States each year (American Association of Nurse Anesthetists 2007a).

CRNA training requires registered nurses to attend an accredited nurse anesthesia education program to receive an extensive education in anesthesia. Entry into the program requires a bachelor's degree in nursing or another appropriate baccalaureate degree, a license as a registered nurse, and a minimum of one year of acute care nursing experience. CRNA programs range from twenty-four to thirty-six months of graduate course work, including both classroom and clinical experience. All nurse anesthesia education programs now offer a master's degree in nursing, allied health, or biological and clinical sciences. Upon graduation, nurses must pass a national certification exam to become CRNAs and pass a recertification program every two years thereafter (American Association of Nurse Anesthetists 2007a).

All states permit CRNAs to practice. Although CRNAs can be found in various practice settings (hospitals, freestanding surgical centers, and so on) and in various geographic areas, they are the sole anesthesia providers in more than 70 percent of rural hospitals in the United States. There is much debate about the propriety of allowing CRNAs to practice independently of physician supervision. In 1986, CMS eliminated Medicare requirements that CRNAs be supervised, saying no studies indicated negative patient outcome when CRNAs were unsupervised. The American Society of Anesthesiologists and the AMA argue that there is potential increased risk to patients. However, in the report "Quality of Care in Anesthesia," the American Association of Nurse Anesthetists (AANA) indicate, "there is no statistically significant difference between the anesthesia care provided by CRNAs working alone, CRNAs working with anesthesiologists, or anesthesiologists providing care alone" (American Association of Nurse Anesthetists 2007b).

PHYSICIAN ASSISTANTS

Physician assistants (PAs) are licensed to practice medicine with supervision by physicians. As members of the health care team, PAs "conduct medical exams, diagnose and treat illness, order and interpret tests, counsel on preventive health care, assist in surgery, and write prescriptions" (American Academy of Physician Assistants 2007, 1).

The American Academy of Physician Assistants indicates that more than 70,000 PAs were eligible to practice in the United States in 2006. More than half report that their primary specialty is one of the primary care fields: family or general practice medicine (27 percent), general internal medicine (7 percent), general pediatrics (3 percent), and obstetrics or gynecology (2 percent). Other prevalent areas of practice for PAs include general surgery and surgical subspecialties (25 percent), emergency medicine (10 percent), and the subspecialties of internal medicine (11 percent) (see Figure 6–2). More than one-third (38 percent) of all respondents work in a hospital, another 44 percent work in solo or group practice offices, about 8 percent work in some type of federally qualified health center or community health facility, and about 9 percent work for a government agency (see Figure 6–3) (American Academy of Physician Assistants 2006).

In response to a perceived doctor shortage in the mid-1960s, the PA profession was started, to increase access to medical care and to reduce the cost of the services. Dr. Eugene Stead started the first PA training program at Duke University, forming the first class in 1965. Originally, most PA programs were designed to attract hospital corpsmen or medics who were leaving the armed forces. Because many of these people had some formal training and usually a considerable amount of experience, it was felt that their talents could be effectively employed in civilian health care. Within ten years, fewer than half of PAs had a military background, and today the vast majority are men and women with no military experience.

Physician assistants are educated in intensive medical programs accredited by the Accreditation Review Commission on Education for the Physician Assistant. There are currently 130 accredited programs. Education consists of classroom and laboratory instruction in the basic medical and behavioral sciences, followed by clinical rotations in internal medicine, family medicine, surgery, pediatrics, obstetrics and gynecology, emergency medicine, and geriatric medicine. State licensure requires graduation from an accredited physician assistant

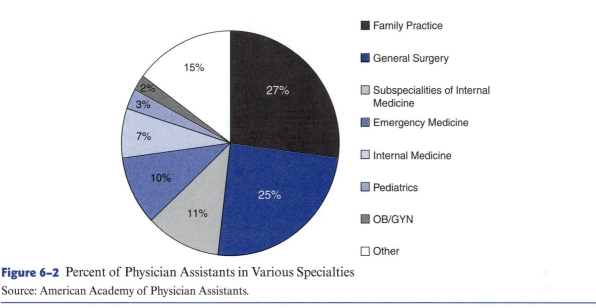

Figure 6–2 Percent of Physician Assistants in Various Specialties
Source: American Academy of Physician Assistants.

program and passage of the national certifying exam, developed by the National Commission on Certification of Physician Assistants in conjunction with the National Board of Medical Examiners (American Academy of Physician Assistants 2007).

To remain certified, PAs must take 100 hours of continuing medical education every two years and pass a recertification exam every six years. Certified PAs carry the title "PA-C." PAs are licensed to practice and have prescribing authority in all fifty states. Physicians have had mixed responses to the growth in the numbers of PAs in practice, depending largely on the degree of competition in their health care environment. Many patients view their PA as their primary care provider and have a continuing relationship with the PA. PAs are not simply seen as an occasional fill-in for the doctor. PAs refer patients to a physician

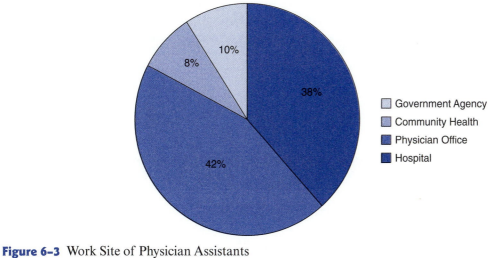

Figure 6–3 Work Site of Physician Assistants
Source: American Academy of Physician Assistants.

and/or closely consult with a physician in complicated cases; otherwise, the physician acts only in a supervisory role.

PHARMACISTS

Pharmacy is an ancient profession, certainly prominent in seventeenth-century England; the practitioners were apothecaries who ran shops and compounded various drugs and medications. Pharmacists today, however, are rarely called on to compound a drug or medication, which now comes packaged from the manufacturer. **Pharmacists** have become part of the health care delivery team, with an emphasis on more direct patient care, particularly in counseling patients about medication use, possible adverse effects, and other medication-related concerns.

More than 230,000 pharmacists practiced in the United States in 2004, with the numbers increasing annually (Bureau of Labor Statistics 2006b). Pharmacists are the third largest group of health care professionals, exceeded only by physicians and nurses. Most pharmacists entering the workforce today choose to practice in community pharmacies, and a substantial number take positions within the pharmaceutical industry. This trend has left a shortage of pharmacists available to work in the hospital setting. Community pharmacists make higher salaries than hospital pharmacists and spend more time on patient care functions.

Hospital pharmacy is an expanding area. Pharmacists and hospitals are responsible for systems of total control of drug distribution, designed to ensure that each patient receives the appropriate medication in the correct form and dosage at the correct time. They are also an authoritative source of drug information for physicians, nurses, and patients. There are a number of specialized areas within hospital pharmacy, such as nuclear pharmacy, drug and poison information, and intravenous therapy. Hospital pharmacists are seeking to change the pharmacy from a supply department, which is a product-oriented technical function, to a patient-oriented clinical service of drug experts who would be more involved in monitoring and counseling on matters relating to drugs.

The Accreditation Council for Pharmacy Education (formerly the American Council on Pharmaceutical Education) accredits over 100 schools of pharmacy in the United States. In 2006, over 48,000 students were enrolled in first-degree pharmacy programs. Among them, 32.3 percent were minority students and 64.2 percent were women (see Tables 6–5 and 6–6). Of an additional 3,713 students already holding PharmD degrees, 2,773 were enrolled in doctor of philosophy (PhD) programs, and 940 were enrolled in master's degree programs (American Association of Colleges of Pharmacy 2007a).

TABLE 6–5 First Professional Degree Enrollments (Baccalaureate, PharmD1[a])

	1998	1999	2000	2001	2002	2003	2004	2005	2006
Total	33,090	32,537	34,481	35,885	38,902	43,047	43,908	46,527	48,592
By Gender									
Male	11,777	11,411	11,763	12,253	12,815	14,264	14,696	16,069	17,397
Female	21,313	21,126	22,718	23,632	26,087	28,783	29,212	30,458	31,195
Graduate Degree Enrollments									
	1998	1999	2000	2001	2002	2003	2004	2005	2006
Masters	783	753	812	820	770	734	781	796	940
PhD	2,088	2,038	2,167	2,264	2,439	2,597	2,566	2,643	2,773

[a]Beginning in 2005, enrollments include PharmD1 only.

SOURCE: AACP Institutional Research Report Series: Profile of Pharmacy Students, Fall 2006. American Association of Colleges of Pharmacy. VA: Alexandria, April 2007.

TABLE 6-6 First Professional Degrees Conferred

Year	2000–01	2001–02	2002–03	2003–04	2004–05	2005–06
Total	7,000	7,573	7,488	8,158	8,268	9,040
Male	2,484	2,595	2,636	2,721	2,634	2,875
Female	4,516	4,978	4,852	5,437	5,634	6,165
White	4,469	4,648	4,473	4,954	5,031	5,650
Black or African American	0426	575	591	612	720	668
Hispanic or Latino	253	303	310	295	361	377
Asian or Native Hawaiian or Other Pacific Islander	1,456	1,625	1,691	1,857	1,683	1,822
American Indian or Alaska Native	26	47	38	32	53	39
Other/Unknown	194	198	182	190	226	265
Foreign	176	177	203	218	194	219

SOURCE: AACP Institutional Research Report Series: Profile of Pharmacy Students, Fall 2006. American Association of Colleges of Pharmacy. VA: Alexandria, April 2007.

Students are accepted in pharmacy schools after graduation from high school. At least two years of preprofessional study are required prior to four academic years of professional study leading to a PharmD. The BS degree in pharmacy in no longer offered (American Association of Colleges of Pharmacy 2007b).

Pharmacy graduates must pass the North American Pharmacist Licensure Examination (NAPLEX), developed by the National Association of Boards of Pharmacy, before practicing pharmacy in all states. Each state also requires applicants to take a special examination on the legal aspects of pharmacy practice in that state (Multistate Pharmacy Jurisprudence Examination), and some also require the disease state management examinations. License transfer between states is possible for pharmacists under a uniform licensure agreement that all states recognize (National Association of Boards of Pharmacy 2007).

Some professional organizations in pharmacy have urged that training be extended to a one-year residency after graduation. The additional experience would better prepare new pharmacists to function as true members of the health care team. There is no clear consensus on the residency issue and therefore no current requirement for credentialing or licensing (American Society of Health System Pharmacists 2006).

DENTISTS

About 150,000 **dentists** were practicing in the United States in 2004. They diagnose and treat diseases, injuries, and malformations of teeth, gums, and related oral structures. Most (approximately 92 percent) of the nation's dentists are in private practice, and about 85 percent are general practitioners. Of the more than 31,000 dental specialists, most are practicing orthodontics or oral surgery. Approximately 78 percent of private practitioners work in solo practice, although 14 percent work in partnerships (Bureau of Labor Statistics 2006c).

Much like medical school, the first two years of dental school training are focused mainly on academic study, with the last two years devoted to clinical experience. Graduates from dental schools are awarded either a DDS (doctor of dental surgery degree) or a DMD (doctor of dental medicine degree), depending on the school. The American Dental Association's Commission on Dental Accreditation accredits fifty-six U.S. dental schools. There are also a number of postgraduate opportunities in dentistry. Some consist of residencies to qualify for credentialing as a specialist; others consist of advanced study for a combined master's degree or doctorate. In 2005, the first-year class entering dental school was about 44 percent female and about 34 percent minority students. The numbers of female dentists has been slowly growing but the number of minority practicing dentists is similar to what it was in the early 1990s, with the greatest numbers of minority students being Asian and Pacific Islanders (American Dental Education Association 2006).

To be licensed, candidates must pass Parts 1 and 2 of the National Board Dental Exam (the American Dental Licensing Examination—ADLEX) and a clinical examination that the individual states or a regional testing agency administers. Specific requirements may differ among states. The National Exam is scheduled to be restructured in 2007. Forty-six states plus the District of Columbia and Puerto Rico have reciprocal agreements or licensing by credentials for those holding active licenses in other states (American Dental Association 2007a). Credentialing in a specialty requires examination by a chosen specialty board, much like medical board certification (American Dental Association 2007b).

In August 1859, 26 dentists representing various dental societies in the United States founded the American Dental Association (ADA) in Niagara Falls, New York. Today, the ADA has more than 141,000 members, 54 constituent (state or territorial) and 529 component (local) dental societies, and it is the largest and oldest national dental association in the world (American Dental Association 2007c). The ADA's Commission on Dental Accreditation is the accrediting agency for dental educational and dental auxiliary educational programs in the United States. The U.S. Department of Education grants its accrediting authority. The ADA formally recognizes nine specialty areas of dental practice: (1) dental public health, (2) endodontics, (3) oral pathology, (4) oral and maxillofacial surgery, (5) orthodontics, (6) pediatric dentistry, (7) oral and maxillofacial radiology, (8) periodontics, and (9) prosthodontics (American Dental Education Association 2006).

The widespread use of fluorides has dramatically reduced the incidence of tooth decay in children and has changed the nature of dental practice. Since the 1970s, tooth decay in American children has declined, and more time and effort are now spent on other dental problems, such as the management of periodontal (gum) disease and cosmetic dental procedures. Because of the success of preventive dentistry, growing older populations will retain their teeth longer and require regular dental care, contributing to a growing need for dental services. However, the number of graduating dentists is declining, from a high of 5,756 in 1983, to only 4,478 in 2005 (American Dental Education Association 2006). Shortages exist in some rural areas and in some dense urban areas, although an oversupply exists in some of the major suburban areas—much like the distribution of physicians.

OPTOMETRISTS

An **optometrist** is a doctor of optometry (OD—not to be confused with the DO, the degree conferred to a doctor of osteopathy). Optometrist training is quite different from the training of an **ophthalmologist,** who is a medical doctor (MD) with a specialty in medical and surgical treatment of eye diseases.

Optometrists are providers of primary eye care, trained and licensed by the state to examine the external and internal structure of the eyes; diagnose eye diseases and vision conditions; prescribe eyeglasses, contact lenses, and low-vision aids; and provide vision therapy services. In recent years, optometrists have been granted expanded rights to prescribe medication and perform certain surgeries (mainly laser treatments). Optometrists serve as major points of entry into the vision care system and may refer patients to ophthalmologists or other physicians for treatment of more serious ocular and systemic diseases. Optometry differs from ophthalmology in that optometrists provide the vast majority of primary eye care services but are limited in the amount of treatment they may provide. The nature of these limitations sometimes causes tension between the ophthalmology and optometry professions. The differences in treatment privileges are often the results of the lobbying strengths of the professional organizations, and optometry has a very strong lobbying effort (Bureau of Labor Statistics 2006d).

Historically, most optometrists were self-employed, mostly in solo practice. However, optometrists today work in private practices, retail practices, multidisciplinary medical practices, hospitals, teaching institutions, research positions, community health centers, and the ophthalmic industry. Over 32,000 optometrists were active in the United States in 2000. The need for practicing optometrists is expected to grow through 2014, as the need increases for care of the aging baby boomers (Bureau of Labor Statistics 2006d). However, the number of students graduating from schools of optometry in 2006 was 1,220, slightly fewer than the 1,251 graduates in 2005. The total number of optometry students in the 2006-07 academic year was 5,488, 64.2 percent female and 35.8 percent male. In the same year, only 32 percent of optometry students were minorities (Association of Schools and Colleges of Optometry 2007).

Today, optometrists are trained at nineteen schools of optometry in the United States and Canada, which are accredited by the Council on Optometric Education. The four-year postgraduate degree consists of classroom and clinical training, including training in the basic sciences. Unique to the education of optometrists is the advanced study of optics (the science of light and vision) and extensive training in lens design construction, application, and fitting (American Optometric Association 2007).

The curriculum emphasizes a comprehensive, holistic approach to patient care. Most state licensing boards now accept for licensure the results of a national board examination and also require continuing education as a condition for license renewal. However, there is increasing concern in optometry, as in other professions, that participation in continuing education courses is no guarantee of competency in practice and of incorporating the latest developments into daily practice. One way optometrists demonstrate clinical proficiency is by becoming a Fellow of the American Academy of Optometry, which requires careful examination of clinical skills. Following further tests, fellows of the academy can be awarded diplomat status in specialty areas (for example, contact lenses, binocular vision, and perception).

PODIATRISTS

A **podiatrist** is a doctor of podiatric medicine (DPM). Podiatrists are licensed to practice in all fifty states, the District of Columbia, and Puerto Rico. They diagnose and treat diseases of the foot and related or governing structures by medical, surgical, or other means. Most are in private practice, although many podiatrists serve on the staffs of hospitals, nursing homes, medical schools, armed forces, and health departments (American Podiatric Medical Association 2007).

Candidates for admission to colleges of podiatry are expected to complete a baccalaureate degree. About 95 percent of all first-year students entering colleges of podiatry have a bachelor's degree (students with exceptional promise and a minimum of ninety college credit hours are sometimes admitted without the degree); about 10 percent have a master's degree. Training includes four years in one of the nation's seven colleges of podiatry accredited by the Council on Podiatric Medical Education, followed by a hospital residency. The residency must also be accredited by the Council on Podiatric Medical Education. Most states require a state exam in addition to the national board exam. There are over 12,000 active podiatrists in the United States who practice in such areas as surgery, sports medicine, biomechanics, geriatrics, pediatrics, orthopedics, and primary care (ibid.).

CHIROPRACTORS

The word *chiropractic* is derived from Greek words that mean "done by hand." The profession of **chiropractic** evolved in the United States in the late 1800s, and focuses on the treatment of illnesses by manipulation (particularly of the spinal column), physiotherapy (physical therapy), and dietary counseling, without the use of drugs or surgical intervention. Chiropractors use standard procedures and tests to diagnose conditions, and they rely heavily on X-rays of the skeletal system as a diagnostic tool.

Chiropractic education consists of four to five years of study at a chiropractic college after completing a bachelor's degree. The first two years of chiropractic education emphasize the biological sciences and clinical disciplines. The last two years emphasize practical studies, with about half of the time being spent in college clinics. Upon graduating, students are awarded a doctor of chiropractic (DC) degree, but graduates must obtain a license by passing an examination given by state chiropractic boards to practice. The Council on Chiropractic Education accredits fifteen programs and two chiropractic institutions in the United States, and has joint accreditation agreements with colleges in Canada and other international locations (Council on Chiropractic Education 2007). There were over 50,000 chiropractors in the United States in 2004, and the need is projected to grow through the year 2014 (Bureau of Labor Statistics 2006e).

The AMA and American Hospital Association (AHA) previously opposed insurance coverage, hospital-admitting privileges, and physician referrals to chiropractors, maintaining that there was no scientific evidence of chiropractic's curative powers. Policies have changed, and some physicians do refer patients to chiropractors if they are unable to successfully treat certain back problems. Medicare, Medicaid, state workers' compensation programs, and most private health and accident policies authorize reimbursement for chiropractic services. Some managed care organizations have also approved chiropractors as primary care gatekeepers for patients who choose that option. Reimbursement policies and competition for patients continue to feed the tension between chiropractic and medical doctors.

COMPLEMENTARY AND ALTERNATIVE MEDICINE

The following sections describe some of the many forms of medicine that are not considered traditional, but are still used as popular remedies to ailments in the United States.

Acupuncture

Oriental medicine includes a variety of therapies; however, acupuncture is probably the most widely known. "**Acupuncture** describes a family of procedures involving the stimulation of anatomical points on the body using a variety of techniques, the most common being penetration of the skin with thin, solid, metallic needles that are manipulated by the hands or by electrical stimulation" (National Center for Complementary and Alternative Medicine 2008a).

Acupuncture originated in China more than 2,500 years ago, but its entry into U.S. medicine is more recent. Forty-one states and the District of Columbia license, certify, or register acupuncturists; one state allows them to practice under a licensed medical doctor. Acupuncture is largely unregulated in the remaining states.

Currently there are forty-six schools of acupuncture in the United States accredited by the American College of Acupuncture & Oriental Medicine (ACAOM). The National Certification Commission for Acupuncture and Oriental Medicine (NCCOAM) administers licensing exams. Currently, over 22,000 licensed acupuncturists are working in the United States (American Association of Acupuncture and Oriental Medicine 2007a).

According to the American Association of Oriental Medicine, this is how the Oriental system of medicine works:

> It has been scientifically determined that human beings are unique bio-energetic systems. For thousands of years oriental medicine has acknowledged that there is a vital life force that flows through all things which is called "qi" (pronounced "chee"). In Western culture, it is often referred to as "energy." Energy (qi) flows along pathways in the human body, which are related to the organs, the muscular system, and nervous system. When the balance of this energy is disturbed due to trauma, poor diet, medications, stress, hereditary conditions, environmental factors, or excessive emotional issues, then pain or illness results. Oriental medicine focuses on correcting these imbalances, which stimulates the body's natural ability to heal itself. In other words, *Oriental medicine focuses on treating the factors that cause disease.* (American Association of Acupuncture and Oriental Medicine 2007b)

Although acupuncture has long been categorized as "alternative medicine," it is making its way into mainstream medicine. The World Health Organization of the United Nations has issued a provisional list of forty-one diseases amenable to acupuncture treatment. The American Osteopathic Association, the American Chiropractic Association, the American Veterinary Medical Association, former Surgeon General C. Everett Koop, and the National Institutes of Health have in various ways recognized the promise of acupuncture treatment. In April 1996, the U.S. Food and Drug Administration reclassified acupuncture needles from experimental status to a Class II medical device (Food and Drug Administration 1996).

Homeopathy

Homeopathy developed earlier than conventional medicine, at a time when few medical interventions were available to treat illnesses and injuries. The concept of homeopathy is treatment and prevention of disease through the use of "remedies" (substances that might create symptoms, but could relieve symptoms in the right doses). Practitioners of homeopathy also believe in treatment of the whole person, not just the disease. Therefore, lifestyle, nutrition, and emotional and mental states are all considered during treatment (National Center for Complementary and Alternative Medicine 2008b).

In the 1800s, there were many colleges of homeopathy and many homeopathic hospitals in the United States. However, in the late nineteen century and the twentieth century, the colleges and hospitals either closed or were replaced by conventional medical facilities as medical knowledge grew. Many people today still use homeopathic remedies. Although some countries have integrated homeopathy into conventional medicine, most patients in the United States use homeopathy without the help of a medical doctor (National Center for Complementary and Alternative Medicine 2008b).

There are many different types of complementary and alternative medical therapies. Not all can be presented here. Check the National Center for Complementary and Alternative Medicine website (http://nccam.nih.gov) for more information.

THERAPISTS

Therapists are most often linked with rehabilitation or development of skills lost through injury or illness. Many services today are designated as therapies, and it is impossible to include them all in this discussion. However, a few are described here.

Physical Therapists

Physical therapists work mainly with strengthening the joints and muscles. Treatment performed includes therapeutic exercise, cardiovascular endurance training, therapeutic pain relief, and training in activities of daily living. Physical therapists are trained to evaluate patients for treatment needs, and thus they work as part of the health care team for developing a case management approach.

More than 130,000 physical therapists were employed in the United States in 2004 (Bureau of Labor Statistics 2006f). They work in hospitals, private physical therapy offices, sports facilities, nursing homes, home health agencies, and a variety of other settings. Although historically there has been a shortage of physical therapists, a new interest in physical therapy as a career in the 1990s has increased the number of physical therapists in practice. At the same time, new regulations from the CMS have restricted payment for physical therapy services through the Medicare program and decreased salary ranges for many physical therapists. The demand, however, is expected to grow through 2014, as the numbers of elderly increase, and new technologies allow people with serious injuries to survive those injuries and require therapy. The number of new graduates decreased from 2001 through 2004, with a slight increase in 2005 (see Table 6–7).

In 2004, the Commission on Accreditation in Physical Therapy Education accredited 205 colleges and universities. Physical therapy education requires a minimum of a master's degree. In 2004, 94 accredited programs offered the masters degree, and 111 offered a doctoral degree. After graduation, candidates must pass a state-administered national exam to be licensed to practice (American Physical Therapy Association 2007a).

Physical therapy assistants (PTAs) are trained to work under the supervision of a licensed physical therapist to provide direct patient care, transport patients, and prepare and maintain physi-

cal therapy equipment. There were 233 accredited educational programs and thirteen developing programs in 2006, most often in community colleges or junior colleges offering an associate degree. Although the number of graduates increased throughout the 1990s to a high of 5,455 in 1999, the numbers have decreased to only 2,925 in 2005. Over half of the states require PTAs to be licensed, registered, or certified. The major difference in training of PTAs from that of physical therapists is the physical therapist's ability to work independently in providing therapy and in the training to evaluate patients and provide treatment plans. Physical therapy assistants work under the direction of a physical therapist, providing the therapy planned by the therapist (American Physical Therapy Association 2007b).

Occupational Therapists

Occupational therapists work to help people regain and build skills lost to illness or injury, or to develop skills blocked by developmental or psychological impairment. Their primary objective is to help people develop skills for living independent, productive, and satisfying lives and avoiding institutionalization or long-term care. They help clients develop basic motor skills and reasoning abilities and teach them to compensate for loss of function.

More than 80,000 occupational therapists were providing independent hands-on care to patients in the United States in 2004. Since 2007, the minimum educational requirement for occupational therapists is a master's degree. The Accreditation Council for Occupational Therapy Education accredits approximately 150 programs. All fifty states regulate the practice of occupational therapy, and most requiring licensure. Occupational therapists are expected to be in high demand through 2014, in hospitals, rehabilitation facilities, and schools for children with disabilities (Bureau of Labor Statistics 2006g).

In a related profession, occupational therapy assistants complete a two-year associate degree program and work directly with clients, providing therapy under the direction of an occupational therapist according to a developed treatment plan. Candidates for occupational therapy vary greatly: The needs may stem from such impairments as arthritis or other chronic illnesses, head or spinal cord injuries, burns, head trauma, stroke, and developmental disabilities (Bureau of Labor Statistics 2006h).

In 2005, the Accreditation Council for Occupational Therapy Education accredited 135 occupational therapy assistant

TABLE 6-7 Physical Therapist—Degrees Conferred for Selected Years

Year	Master's	Doctorate	Total
2001	5,652	552	6,560
2003	3,646	1,473	5,119
2004	3,014	1,921	4,935
2005	2,431	2,811	5,242

SOURCE: Reprinted from 2005–2006 Fact Sheet, January 2007, with permission of the American Physical Therapy Association. This material is copyrighted, and any further reproduction or distribution is prohibited.

programs. Occupational therapy assistants are regulated in most states, and most take the national certification exam to become certified occupational therapy assistants. Like occupational therapists, therapy assistants are expected to be in high demand through 2014 (Bureau of Labor Statistics 2006h).

Radiation Therapist

Radiation therapists work with cancer patients. As part of a team that includes a radiation oncologist, radiation therapists administer the radiation, monitor patients for any adverse effects, and answer any questions patients may have.

Radiation therapists receive training in either a two-year associate degree program or a four-year bachelor's program. In 2005, there were ninety-four accredited radiation therapy programs in the United States. The formal training is followed by a certification exam. Some states require licensing to practice; however, many of them default to the certification exam for licensing purposes (American Registry of Radiologic Technologists 2006). About 15,000 radiation therapists currently practice, and need in the future is expected to grow. Because of the nature of working with cancer patients, radiation therapists must be psychologically able to be supportive, caring, and have good communication skills (Bureau of Labor Statistics 2006i).

Respiratory Therapist

Respiratory therapists work with patients who have breathing problems and other cardiopulmonary disorders. Like radiation therapists, respiratory therapists work directly with patients, delivering treatment and consulting with a physician to develop and modify individual patient treatment plans (Bureau of Labor Statistics 2006j).

Entry into the field of respiratory therapy requires formal training. Programs are offered at the associate and bachelor's level. In 2005, the Commission on Accreditation of Allied Health Education Programs accredited fifty-one entry-level programs and 329 advanced-level programs in the United States, including in Puerto Rico. All states, except Alaska and Hawaii, require respiratory therapists to be licensed. The need for respiratory therapists is expected to grow through 2014 (ibid.).

ALLIED HEALTH PERSONNEL

The term *allied health* includes a large number of health-related areas of work that assist, facilitate, and complement the work of physicians and other health professionals. The AMA's Committee on Allied Health Education and Accreditation (CAHEA) had worked collaboratively with various specialty societies, allied health organizations, and educational associations to accredit allied health programs, but this responsibility was turned over to an independent, nonprofit agency, the Commission on Accreditation of Allied Health Education Programs (CAAHEP), in 1995. CAAHEP accredits nineteen allied health professions and more than 2,000 programs offered by universities and colleges, academic health centers, junior and community colleges, hospitals, and others (CAAHEP 2007). Among the more familiar allied health professions accredited by CAAHEP are athletic trainers, emergency medical technicians or paramedics, medical assistants, perfusionists, and surgical assistants and technicians (ibid.).

Many other allied health programs are accredited by bodies other than CAAHEP, such as programs in physiotherapy, health education, medical dietetics, dental hygiene, and graduate programs in health administration. In addition, a large number of other allied health occupations have no formal program accrediting process at this time, except that some of them are parts of regionally accredited academic institutions. There is a shortage of many allied health personnel, especially in rural geographic areas and inner-city urban hospitals. Although many new graduates choose the hospital as their first place of employment, many later go into outpatient or other nonhospital settings where the pay is better and the work conditions are more appealing.

HEALTH ADMINISTRATORS AND HEALTH PLANNERS

The health sector is large and complex. It is labor-intensive—requiring a lot of people—and a large amount of money to fuel its operations. Skilled health administrators are much in demand to run hospitals, nursing homes, group medical practices, managed care organizations, health departments, mental health centers and hospitals, home care agencies, and other health care facilities. "To run" means to plan the services and their provision, to assemble or secure the resources, and to manage the use of those resources to fulfill the purposes of the organization. Planning is, of course, an essential part of every administrative job, but the planning function in large organizations is frequently delegated to those whose planning skills are well developed, to allow those people to focus on planning only, and to advise the administrators of what they should adopt as the planned course of action for the organization. In recent years, planning has become known as strategic planning and often includes a strong consideration of marketing because of the complex interrelationships and dependencies between health agencies and government, the competitive nature of health care delivery, and the increased awareness of health care consumers.

Historically, the top administrator in most large health institutions was a physician or a nurse. Few were trained for their administrative roles. Even today, one finds health administrators and health planners who grew or fell into their jobs, whose academic preparation was not geared to either of these roles. In recent years, however, health care organizations have turned increasingly to people who have academic training in health administration or health planning. The necessity for specially trained health-oriented people, and not just any business administration or planning program graduate, stems from the complex nature of the health sector and the historical context within which the organizations and health professions operate. People are needed who understand not only planning and administration, but also the special aspects that apply to the health field—the constraints under which health professionals operate and the culture of health care professionals. In 2004, there were some 248,000 positions for health services managers. The outlook through 2014 is for a growing need for qualified people in medical offices, hospitals, home health agencies, and outpatient centers (Bureau of Labor Statistics 2006k).

The time-honored doctrine of the physician–patient relationship is increasingly experiencing interference from many arenas. An experienced health administrator must know how to orchestrate that intercession without altering the confidentiality of the physician–patient relationship and without affecting the ability of physicians to render the best care for their patients. Well-trained health administrators and health planners are sensitive to these special circumstances and are able to apply their administrative or planning skills in that context to achieve the aims of the organization in terms of seeing that the highest-quality service is delivered.

The academic training of health administrators and health planners traditionally took place in a number of settings. Some were trained and awarded a master's degree by schools of public health, which were geared initially to the training of a variety of public health workers, of which public health administrators were

only one type. Some were trained in schools of health administration, which were geared primarily to the training of hospital administrators. In fact, until about 1970, most of these schools were known as schools of hospital administration. The name change was designed to reflect the recognition by the schools that they were training not only hospital administrators, but also administrators for other kinds of health services organizations. Today, health administration programs are associated with a variety of organizational units of colleges and universities, including schools of public health, business administration, and health and human services, among others. To reinforce the training for more than hospital management, programs have begun to use the term "health services management."

Baccalaureate programs in health administration are certified through the Association of University Programs in Health Administration (AUPHA), on the basis of self-study and peer review. As of 2005, AUPHA certified thirty-five undergraduate programs in health administration. The Accrediting Commission on Education for Health Services Administration (ACEHSA) was organized in 1968, to replace the program that AUPHA conducted for accrediting master's programs. In 2004, ACEHSA changed its name to the Commission on Accreditation of Healthcare Management Education (CAHME) to reflect a need to ensure that health services education was meeting the needs of the changing health services industry. As of April 2005, there were seventy-two accredited graduate programs in health administration in the United States and Canada. Accreditation is a rigorous process of self-study documentation, site visits and reporting by a peer panel, and review by the commission of the program's mission, curriculum, and faculty (Association of University Programs in Health Administration 2005).

Doctorate programs in health administration and/or health planning do not currently have accrediting programs from AUPHA or CAHME, but fall under accreditation processes for the specific colleges or divisions of the universities granting the degrees.

The field of higher education is experiencing a great deal of change that is affecting the training of health administrators (as well as other health care professionals). Particularly at the master's level, new programs are becoming available in growing numbers through distance learning, condensed executive programs, web-based programs, and combined degree programs. Some are accredited and some are not. Prospective students are responsible for determining the quality of such programs by inquiring about accreditation status. Accreditation becomes important for a number of reasons. Postgraduate residencies and fellowships are only offered to students of accredited programs. Scholarships are often limited to students of accredited programs. A strong affiliation exists between accredited programs and the American College of Healthcare Executives, the professional organization that provides opportunities for individual certification and continuing education events.

SUMMARY

The definition of a *profession* is somewhat debatable, and the description of the various health care personnel provided in this chapter is certainly not all-inclusive. Some may even debate the appropriateness of inclusion of some personnel. The goal, however, is not to place the label of professional on some personnel and withhold it from others. The goal is to make readers aware of the various people involved—directly or indirectly—in patient care and to provide a background for understanding the complexity of health care delivery.

By far, nurses make up the largest group of health care professionals. However, it is important to understand the distinction between RNs and LPNs because of the skill sets involved in training. There is a great need for more registered nurses to provide the type and quality of care that is needed now and will be needed in the future. The most difficult issue involved in increasing the number of registered nurses is the shortage of qualified teaching faculty for nurse education.

The nature and scope of health care services available today requires technical skills that go well beyond those physicians and nurses provide. The need for pharmacists is increasing as new pharmaceuticals are developed and the number of patients with chronic conditions grows. Chronic care requires more medical treatment, including pharmaceuticals, rather than invasive treatments such as surgery. As people live longer but not necessarily healthy lives, the need for therapists, alternative medicine professionals, chiropractors, and others grows. As patients seek care, it is important that they understand the various options available to them and are educated as to the appropriateness of each.

Conflicts exist at various levels—government, institutions, and individuals—over what professional might deliver certain levels of care. In a competitive and cost-conscious environment, alternative delivery processes are attractive, yet quality must be the overriding consideration. Education, licensing, accreditation, and certification are only a part of the efforts to ensure quality of care. Other quality assessments will be discussed in later chapters.

ACTIVITY-BASED LEARNING

Many different professions are described in this chapter. Most professionals receive credentialing or they simply affiliate through membership with a national professional organization. General information about education and licensing is available on websites for these organizations but, often, individual state regulations guide the professionals more specifically.

- Interview a health care professional (other than a physician) in your local area to hear the story of the individual's education, licensing, credentialing, and so on, to learn about the differences or challenges that the professional faced in practicing.

A QUESTION OF ETHICS

- Is it the government's role, through licensing and regulation, to ensure the competency of health care professionals? Can licensing and regulation be indicators of quality, or are they simply processes to protect the domain of certain health care providers?

- What is the individual's responsibility when choosing a health care provider, and what information regarding the provider should be made available to individual consumers (patients) to help them determine the provider's competency?

- Is health insurance reimbursement for "alternative medicine" increasing consumer choice or simply a matter of providing less expensive health care treatment?

REFERENCES

1. American Academy of Nurse Practitioners. (2007a). *What is a nurse practitioner?* Retrieved from www.aanp.org

2. American Academy of Nurse Practitioners. (2007b). *Legislation and practice, practice, authorization to practice, issues and updates.* From www.aanp.org

3. American Academy of Physician Assistants. (2007). *Information about PAs and the PA profession: General information.* Retrieved from www.aapa.org/geninfo1.html

4. American Academy of Physician Assistants. (2006). *2006 AAPA physician assistant census report.*

5. American Association of Acupuncture and Oriental Medicine. (2007a) *About AAAOM*. Retrieved from www.aaaomonline.org/default.asp

6. American Association of Acupuncture and Oriental Medicine. (2007b). *Overview: How does the system work*. Retrieved from www.aaaomonline.org/default.asp

7. American Association of Colleges of Nursing, News From. (2007). *Journal of Professional Nursing*, 23(2), March–April, 73.

8. American Association of Colleges of Pharmacy. (2007a). *Institutional data, trends data*. Retrieved from www.aacp.org

9. American Association of Colleges of Pharmacy. (2007b). *Is pharmacy for you? PharmD degree*. Retrieved from www.aacp.org

10. American Association of Nurse Anesthetists. (2007a). *AANA overview, who we are*. Retrieved from. www.aana.com

11. American Association of Nurse Anesthetists. (2007b). *Anesthesiologist distortions concerning quality of care: Summary*. Retrieved from www.aana.com/resources.aspx?ucNavMenu_TSMenuTargetID=51&ucNavMenu_TSMenuTargetType=4&ucNavMenu_TSMenuID=6&id=677

12. American College of Nurse-Midwives. (2005). *Fact sheet, basic facts about midwives*. Retrieved from www.midwife.org/siteFiles/factsheet/Basic_Facts_About_Midwives.pdf?CFID=579144&CFTOKEN=53740566

13. American Dental Association. (2007a). *Dental boards & licensure: Information for the new graduate*. Retrieved from www.ada.org/prof/ed/students/handbook/handbook_newgrad.pdf

14. American Dental Association. (2007b). *Dental specialties: Requirements for recognition*. Retrieved from www.ada.org/prof/ed/specialties/index.asp

15. American Dental Association. (2007c). *ADA timeline*. Retrieved from www.ada.org/ada/about/history/ada_timeline.asp

16. American Dental Education Association (2006) "Trends in Dental Education." Retrieved from http://www.adea.org/publications/trendsindentaleducation/Pages/default.aspx

17. American Dental Education Association (2006). Retrieved from http://www.adea.org.

18. American Nurses Association. (2007a). *What is nursing?* Retrieved from www.nursingworld.org/EspeciallyForYou/StudentNurses/WhatisNursing.aspx

19. American Nurses Association. (2007b). *About ANA*. Retrieved from www.nursingworld.org/FunctionalMenuCategories/AboutANA.aspx

20. American Optometric Association. (2007). *Why choose optometry?* Retrieved from www.aoa.org/x5130.xml

21. American Physical Therapy Association. (2007a). *Education programs: Commission on accreditation in physical therapy education [CAPTE]: PTA program information*. Retrieved from www.apta.org

22. American Physical Therapy Association. (2007b). *Education programs: Commission on accreditation in physical therapy education [CAPTE]: PTA program information*. From www.apta.org

23. American Podiatric Medical Association. (2007). *What is podiatry?* Retrieved from www.apma.org/s_apma/sec.asp?CID=8&DID=2819

24. American Public Health Association. (2007). *Public health nursing overview*. Retrieved from www.apha.org/membergroups/sections/aphasections/phn/

25. American Registry of Radiologic Technologists. (2006). *Licensing versus certification and registration*. Retrieved from www.arrt.org/index.html?content=licensing/certvslic.htm

26. American Society of Health System Pharmacists. (2006). ASHP policy positions, 1982–2006. Retrieved from www.ashp.org/s_ashp/docs/files/About_policypositions.pdf

27. ANCC. (2006). *Accreditation of continuing nursing education providers*. Retrieved from www.nursecredentialing.org/accred/index.html

28. Association of Schools and Colleges of Optometry. (2007). *Student & advisor information*. Retrieved from www.opted.org/info_profile.cfm

29. Association of University Programs in Health Administration. (2005). Healthcare management education: Director of programs 2005–2007. Arlington, VA: AUPHA.

30. Buerhaus, P., Donelan, K., Ulrich, B., Norman, L., & Dittus, R. (2005). Is the shortage of hospital registered nurses getting better or worse? Findings from Two Recent National Surveys of RNs. *Nursing Economics*, 23(2), 61–73.

31. Bureau of Labor Statistics. (2006a). *Licensed practical and licensed vocational nurses.* From www.bls.gov/oco/ocos102 .htm

32. Bureau of Labor Statistics. (2006b). *Bureau of Labor career information: Pharmacists.* Retrieved from www.bls.gov/ k12/print/science02.htm

33. Bureau of Labor Statistics. (2006c). U.S. Department of Labor, *Occupational outlook handbook, 2006–07 edition: Dentists.* Retrieved from http://www.bls.gov/oco/ocos072.htm

34. Bureau of Labor Statistics. (2006d). U.S. Department of Labor, *Occupational outlook handbook, 2006–07 edition: Optometrists.* From www.bls.gov/oco/ocos073.htm

35. Bureau of Labor Statistics. (2006e). U.S. Department of Labor, *Occupational outlook handbook, 2006–07 edition: Chiropractors.* Retrieved from www.bls.gov/ oco/ocos071.htm

36. Bureau of Labor Statistics. (2006f). U.S. Department of Labor, *Occupational outlook handbook, 2006–07 edition: Physical therapists.* Retrieved from www.bls.gov/oco/ocos080.htm

37. Bureau of Labor Statistics. (2006g). U.S. Department of Labor, *Occupational outlook handbook, 2006–07 edition: Occupational therapists.* Retrieved from www.bls. gov/oco/ocos078.htm

38. Bureau of Labor Statistics. (2006h). U.S. Department of Labor, *Occupational outlook handbook, 2006–07 edition: Occupational therapist assistants and aids.* Retrieved from www.bls.gov/oco/ocos166.htm

39. Bureau of Labor Statistics. (2006i). U.S. Department of Labor, *Occupational outlook handbook, 2006–07 edition: Radiation therapists.* Retrieved from www.bls.gov/oco/ocos299.htm

40. Bureau of Labor Statistics. (2006j). U.S. Department of Labor, *Occupational outlook handbook, 2006–07 edition: Respiratory therapists.* Retrieved from www.bls.gov/oco/ocos084.htm

41. Bureau of Labor Statistics. (2006k). U.S. Department of Labor, *Occupational outlook handbook, 2006–07 edition: Medical and health services managers.* Retrieved from www.bls.gov/oco/ocos014.htm

42. CAAHEP. (2007). CAAHEP accredited program search. Retrieved from http://www.caahep.org/Find_An_Accred-ited_Program.aspx

43. Council on Chiropractic Education. (2007). *Directory of chiropractic degree programs and solitary purpose chiropractic institutions holding accredited status.* Retrieved from www. cce-usa.org/CCEPublicationofAccreditedPrograms.pdf

44. Folland, S., Goodman, A., & Stano, M. (2007). *The economics of health and health care* (5th ed.). New Jersey: Pearson Prentice Hall.

45. Food and Drug Administration. (1996). *Center for devices and radiological health, annual report, fiscal year 1996,* p. 7. Retrieved from www.fda.gov/cdrh/ode/ annrp296.pdf

46. Friedman, E. (1991). Nursing: Breaking the bonds? *JAMA, 264*(24), 3117–20; 3122.

47. Friedson, E. (1985). The reorganization of the medical profession. *Medical Care Review, 42*(1), 11–35.

48. Moskowitz, D. (1999). *The 1999 health care almanac & yearbook.* New York: Faulkner & Gray.

49. NACNEP. (2003, November 2003). *Third report to the Secretary of Health and Human Services and the Congress,* Executive Summary. Retrieved from ftp.hrsa.gov/bhpr/nurs-ing/nacreport.pdf

50. National Association of Boards of Pharmacy. (2007). *Examinations.* Retrieved from www.nabp.net

51. National Center for Complementary and Alternative Medi-cine. (2008a). About acupuncture. Retrieved from http:// nccam.nih.gov/health/acupuncture

52. National Center for Complementary and Alternative Medi-cine. (2008b). What is homeopathy? Retrieved from http:// nccam.nih.gov/health/homeopathy/#q1

53. NCSBN. (2007). *What is NCLEX?* From www.ncsbn. org/1200.htm

54. Phelps, C. (2002). *Health economics* (3rd ed.). New Jersey: Pearson Addison Wesley.

55. Rutherford, P., B. Lee, and A. Greiner. (2004). Transforming care at the bedside. IHI's Innovation Series white paper, Institute for Healthcare Improvement, Cambridge, MA.

56. Starr, P. (1982). *The social transformation of American medicine.* New York: Basic Books.

57. Torres, D. (1991). *What, if anything, is professionalism?: Institutions and the problem of change. Research in the Sociology of Organizations, 8,* 42–68.

58. U.S. Department of Health and Human Services, Health Resources and Services Administration, Bureau of Health Professions. (2004). Preliminary Findings: 2004 National Sample Survey of Registered Nurses. Retrieved from bhpr. hrsa.gov/healthworkforce/reports/rnpopulation/preliminary-findings.htm

Chapter 7

Ambulatory Care

CHAPTER OBJECTIVES

After completing this chapter, readers should have an understanding of the following:

- The definition of ambulatory care
- The variety of settings for the delivery of ambulatory care
- The importance of ambulatory care services as a part of the U.S. health care system

INTRODUCTION

Ambulatory care covers a wide range of services for noninstitutionalized patients and, in its most basic description, is simply care that does not require an overnight stay by patients. Office-based physicians provide the majority of ambulatory care. An estimated 910 million visits were made to doctors' offices in 2004, or about 3.2 visits per person. More than 58 percent of those visits were made to primary care specialists (family practice, pediatrics, internal medicine, or obstetrics/gynecology). However, ambulatory care is delivered in a number of other ways, and they are described in this chapter (Hing et al. 2006).

In recent years, the number and type of ambulatory or outpatient facilities have increased to allow more patients to receive treatment outside of the more costly acute care hospitals. Because of advances in technology and technique, many of the procedures formerly done in hospitals can now be performed on an outpatient basis. In fact, since the mid-1980s, payers have designated many procedures as outpatient procedures, meaning

the procedures will not be paid for if performed in an inpatient setting. More familiar ambulatory care facilities, such as hospital outpatient departments and community health centers, have expanded to include surgery centers, diagnostic imaging centers, **cardiac catheterization** laboratories, and other freestanding facilities. Some facilities are for-profit and are operated by chains, either independently owned or affiliated with a hospital. In other cases, nonprofit health care systems with hospitals have expanded their ambulatory facilities as part of an integrated, cost-efficient way to provide care. When addressing health care comprehensively, it is also important to recognize pharmacies, dental care, and "alternative" care such as chiropractic as fitting into what we categorize as ambulatory care. We look now at just a few of the major types of ambulatory care.

MEDICAL PRACTICE

Extraordinary changes are taking place in the practice of medicine in the United States. The sheer number of physicians has more than doubled since 1970. Women, who made up only 9.7 percent of the physician population in 1970, accounted for 27 percent of all physicians in 2005. A larger percentage of female than male physicians (55 percent versus 34.8 percent, respectively) were in primary care specialties in 2005 (American Medical Association 2007).

After decades of "business as usual," physicians are increasingly faced with a decline of professional autonomy, increased competition, and changes in the methods of payment for their services. Although much of this change can be attributed to cost-containment efforts that seek to provide more efficient, effective medical care, and to the alternative delivery systems that have developed, the growing supply of physicians is also a major factor.

In 2005, 718,473 physicians were in patient care[1] in the United States, or 242 physicians for every 100,000 people—more physicians than ever before (American Medical Association 2007). Although the focus in the 1960s was concern over a shortage of physicians, current discussions focus on whether there is an oversupply of physicians (see Table 7–1). In 2005, the majority (62.4 percent) of physicians were in office-based patient care (see Table 7–2). Not everyone agrees that we have an oversupply, but there is general agreement that there is an imbalance in primary care versus specialty care physicians, and a shortage of

physicians practicing in certain geographic areas. Although the sheer numbers of physicians in primary care specialties has been increasing, the overall percentage of physicians in primary care dropped from 36.5 percent in 1980, to 34.6 percent in 1990, and 33.3 percent in 2005 (see Table 7–3) (American Medical Association 2007).

The increase in the U.S. physician-population ratio intensifies competition and is one reason why physicians join large group practices or accept salaried positions with hospitals and managed care organizations. An adequate supply of physicians fosters easy access to care. The level of our knowledge and technology affects the number of physicians needed. New knowledge and new technology permit physicians to do what was previously not possible, and increases the need for more physicians. Determination of need is complex and often elusive. Need is affected by the age characteristics of the population (the elderly having greater needs), by the existing health problems that the population recognizes as problems, by public decisions about which health services insurance or government programs should cover, and by the level of investment that should be made in research and facilities. The need for physicians is also affected by the extent to which physicians are willing to use other health workers, by the population's willingness to accept other practitioners, and

TABLE 7–1 Physician Population and Physician Population Ratios, U.S., for Selected Years

Year	Total Physicians in Patient Care	Physicians Per 100,000 People	Total Population Per Physician
1965	259,418	132	760
1970	278,535	134	747
1980	376,512	163	614
1990	503,870	200	500
2000	647,430	234	427
2003	691,873	238	420
2005	718,473	242	413

SOURCE: American Medical Association. Physician characteristics and distribution in the U.S., 2005 edition, Table 5–16; 2007 Edition, Table 5–16. All rights reserved.

[1] Physicians in patient care exclude those in research, teaching, administration, and other indirect patient care positions.

TABLE 7-2 Physicians by Age, Activity, and Gender, 2005

Physician Activity	Total	Percentage	Male	Percentage	Female	Percentage
Total physicians	902,053		657,140	72.80	244,913	27.20
Office-based practice	563,225	62.40	413,105	45.80	150,120	16.60
Hospital-based practice	155,248	17.20	97,810	0.11	57,438	6.40
Residents	95,391	10.50	55,055	0.06	40,336	4.50
Full-time staff	59,857	6.60	42,755	4.70	17,102	1.90
Other professional activity	43,965		34,664		9,301	
Administration	14,997	1.70	12,294	5.90	2,703	0.29
Medical teaching	10,223	1.10	7,673	0.90	2,550	0.28
Research	14,471	1.60	11,527	1.30	2,944	0.30
Other	4,274	0.50	3,170	0.40	1,104	0.10
Inactive or unknown	139,615		111,561		28,054	

SOURCE: American Medical Association. 2007. Physician characteristics and distribution in the U.S., 2007 edition, Table 1–1. Chicago, IL. All rights reserved.

by the expectations of the population regarding health care services delivery. Thus, there is no more consensus on the correct number of physicians than there is consensus on the amount of money to spend on health care.

In 2005, about 40 percent of physicians were in the primary care areas of internal medicine (17.1 percent), family and general practice (10.3 percent), and pediatrics (8 percent). The majority of U.S. physicians are under 54 years old. Just over 27 percent of practicing physicians are women, about 21 percent of physicians are international (foreign) medical graduates, and 56 percent of all physicians are board-certified in their specialty. Another 3 percent of physicians are certified by their specialty board and others (dual certification), and 10 percent are certified by boards other than their own specialty. About 30 percent of physicians are not board-certified. The average annual income for physicians is difficult to provide because of the range of specialties and range of practice settings. The averages can range from $170,000 to $180,000 for family practice and internal medicine to more than $400,000 for orthopedic surgery or neurological surgery (American Medical Group Association 2006). Although over 62 percent of all physicians provide office-based patient care, an increasing number of physicians are hospital-based or engaged in other professional activities, such as research, teaching, and administration (see Table 7–2) (American Medical Association 2007).

The Development of Medical Practice

The practice of medicine brought neither financial wealth nor social prestige in early America. Medicine was practiced by a wide array of individuals, from those who had studied medicine in Europe to people with little or no medical training. Most families cared for themselves. Many medical practitioners found it difficult to support themselves solely from medical practice and were forced to resort to a second occupation. Most patients who were treated by physicians remained at home, and their physicians spent many hours traveling to visit them with a horse and buggy for transportation. The hours spent traveling severely limited the number of patients a physician could attend. As transportation and roads improved, physicians were able to travel between patients more quickly; patients were also more able to visit the doctors' offices.

Most physicians essentially practiced alone and had little need for hospitals. Medical societies were few and tended to draw only the most elite members of the profession—that is, the ones who had more formal training and who were seeking to upgrade the educational process and the overall quality of medical practice.

The practice of medicine began to change significantly as hospital use increased. In the late nineteenth century and early

TABLE 7-3   Primary Care Physicians by Self-Designated Specialty for Selected Years

	1980	Percentage	1990	Percentage	2000	Percentage	2003	Percentage	2005	Percentage
Total physicians	467,679	100	615,421	100	813,770	100	871,535	100	902,053	100
Active physicians	435,545	93.1	559,988	91.0	737,504	90.6	786,658	90.3	801,742	88.9
Primary care	170,705	36.5	213,514	34.7	274,653	33.8	293,701	33.7	300,022	33.3
Family medicine	27,530	5.9	47,639	7.7	71,102	8.7	78,375	9.0	80,809	9.0
General practice	32,519	7.0	22,841	3.7	15,210	1.9	13,170	1.5	11,049	1.2
Internal medicine	58,462	12.5	76,295	12.4	101,353	12.5	109,317	12.5	112,934	12.5
Obstetrics/ gynecology	24,612	5.3	30,220	4.9	35,922	4.4	37,725	4.3	38,285	4.2
Pediatrics	27,582	5.9	36,519	5.9	51,066	6.3	55,114	6.3	56,945	6.3
Primary care subspecialties	16,642	3.6	30,911	5.0	52,294	6.4	60,589	7.0	65,420	7.3
FM subspecialties	0				483	0.1	691	0.1	835	0.1
IM subspecialties	13,069	2.8	22,054	3.6	34,831	4.3	40,598	4.7	43,552	4.8
OBG subspecialties	1,693	0.4	3,477	0.6	4,319	0.5	4,191	0.5	4,315	0.5
PD subspecialties	1,880	0.4	5,380	0.9	12,661	1.6	15,109	1.7	16,718	1.9
All other specialties	227,569	48.7	302,885	49.2	365,421	44.9	381,921	43.8	396,996	44.0
Inactive/ unknown	52,763		68,111		121,402		135,324		139,615	

SOURCE: American Medical Association. 2007. Physician characteristics and distribution in the U.S., 2007 edition, Table 4–1. Chicago, IL. All rights reserved.

1900s, the number of hospitals grew rapidly as hospital sanitation improved, hospital infections decreased, and antiseptic surgery was introduced. Urban life that accompanied industrialization (working away from home and having smaller living accommodations) also contributed to the increased use of hospitals, although well-to-do families still preferred treatment in their homes. Around this time and as a result of these developments, "hospitals moved from the periphery to the center of medical practice as well as medical education" (Starr 1982).

As hospitals became a necessary part of medical practice, medical practitioners increasingly sought access to them, to admit their patients and to continue treatment. Physicians did not become employees of the hospitals, but rather used the hospitals as one of the tools necessary for patient care. Sometimes they established their own hospitals, particularly when they encountered resistance to joining the staffs of existing institutions, which the professional elite frequently dominated. Hospitals had no control over patients' treatment. This was solely the responsibility of individual physicians.

Solo Practice

Historically, most physicians were in the **solo practice** of medicine; that is, they practiced alone. In 2004, however, more than half (64.2 percent) of all physicians worked in **group practices**, compared to 35.8 percent who were in solo practice (Hing and Burt 2007). The advantages of solo practice, however, are hard to dispute from an individual standpoint. They include (1) greater autonomy for the physician, (2) a more personal patient–physician relationship, and (3) little bureaucracy for both the patient and the physician.

Risks, however, are great for solo practitioners. Among them are the following:

- Financial risks
  - Investing in facilities and equipment
  - Attracting a sufficient patient base
- Administrative responsibilities (hiring staff, contracting insurance, and so on)
- Long hours
  - Providing scheduled care convenient to patients, usually including evening and weekend hours
  - Covering for emergency care
- Limited access to capital
- Difficulty in contracting with payers in a market-driven environment.

Group Practice

A rapidly growing number of physicians are in group practice—either in a group made up of physicians of the same specialty or in a multispecialty group. Group practice is normally defined as consisting of three or more physicians who have organized to practice together, typically sharing offices, personnel, equipment, and other expenses (two physicians are usually referred to as a partnership). Groups can, however, be much larger, even numbering in the hundreds (see Figures 7–1 and 7–2). How they are paid varies from fee for service, to salary, to share of the group's income. The income of group practice physicians tends to be a little higher than that of solo practitioners because of economies the group achieves by sharing support personnel and other resources. Financial risk is also shared, such as raising capital and investing in facilities and equipment. Group practice appeals for reasons other than economic advantages, including the following:

- More peer interaction (ease of consultation and intellectual stimulation)
- More flexible time (shared emergency coverage, vacation coverage, administrative responsibilities)
- Availability of a professional manager (appropriate staffing allows physicians to relinquish direct concern for the financial aspects of patient care)

Group practice, however, is not without its disadvantages. In making the decision to share risks, costs, and administrative responsibilities, physicians also lose some individual autonomy. Group decisions are made regarding office hours, office locations, staffing, and capital investments. Although sharing financial risk has advantages, group practice places an additional risk on physicians—legal and ethical risks. The peer group is expected to be aware of each physician's medical practice habits and decision-making capabilities, and act as bearers of standards for each member of the practice. If a member of the group is sued for malpractice, other members of the group may be held liable if there is any indication that the group was aware of the shortcomings of the physician accused of malpractice.

Another difficulty often shared in group practice situations results from the financial structure of the organization. Particularly in multispecialty practices, formulating an income distribution policy that satisfies all parties is often difficult. Fee structures, capitation rates, and operational expenses vary greatly with the specialty of the physician. Some specialties require a high use of technology and years of intensive training. Other specialties

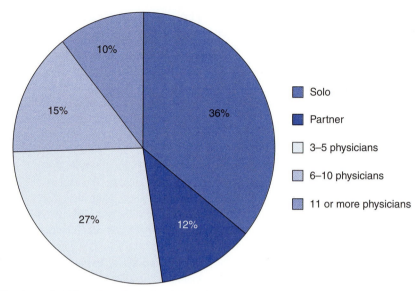

Solo — 36%
Partner — 12%
3–5 physicians — 27%
6–10 physicians — 15%
11 or more physicians — 10%

Figure 7–1 Distribution of Office-Based Medical Practice, 2003–04

SOURCE: Hing, E., and Burt, C. (2007). *Advance data from vital and health statistics, office-based medical practices: Methods and estimates from the National Ambulatory Medical Care Survey, Table 1.*

rely more on cognitive skills, greater time spent with patients, and less use of technology. Various models have been developed to address income disbursement.

Historically, group practices consisted of independent physician-owners (often called "partners") sharing office space and personnel, but each tracking their own income and expenses.

This model was somewhat easy to follow in the atmosphere of fee-for-service medicine. As groups became larger, some practices went to a combination of physician-owners and employed physicians. Physician-owners act as the board of directors and hire additional physicians as the need arises. Hired physicians may be offered a share in ownership after

Medical Group Practice	Number of Physicians
Saint Barnabas Health Care System	4,620
Permanente Medical Group	3,600
Mayo Health System	2,808
Johns Hopkins University School of Medicine	1,808
Barnes-Jewish Hospital	1,724
University of Washington School of Medicine	1,637
Mercy Health Partners of Southwest Ohio	1,524
Cleveland Clinic	1,100
Dartmouth Hitchcock Medical Center	900
Henry Ford Health System	900

Figure 7–2 Sample of Some of the Largest U.S. Group Practices from Medical Group Management Association Membership, 2003

SOURCE: Used with permission of Modern Healthcare Copyright 2009. All rights reserved. (ModernHealthcare.com. 2003, July 21. By the numbers, p. 33)

an initial period of employment or may stay on as employees indefinitely. As managed care and capitated payment structures have become more prominent, so too has the employed physician model.

Why would a physician choose to be an employee of a practice rather than a partner or owner? The advantages are many. Employed physicians do not need to invest in the organization, and thus they carry limited financial risk. They have more defined working hours, few if any administrative responsibilities, and little legal risk for actions of other physicians, yet they have access to greater resources of equipment, facilities, and peer interaction. The disadvantages, however, include limited income potential, an atmosphere of greater regulation and review, and limited input into management decisions. The security of an employed position often outweighs the limitations for many new physicians entering practice in today's uncertain health care environment.

Some larger group practices follow scheduling patterns that make it difficult for physicians to build continuing relationships with their patients. However, most group practices do try to have a specific physician, particularly in primary care specialties, follow each patient. So, although there is some risk of loss of the physician–patient relationship, a group practice setting often provides many advantages to patients. Patients can receive a wider range of care—a type of one-stop shopping—from one medical practice. Medical records are available to all of the patients' physicians without duplicating the information. Patients benefit from improved emergency coverage and, often, a better-informed staff to aid patients in understanding their diagnoses and treatments, as well as the costs, insurance benefits, and financial responsibilities surrounding their care.

EXHIBIT 7–1

Mayo Clinic

Drs. Will and Charlie Mayo shared a single bank account throughout their lives. Every penny the brothers earned was deposited into it, and each withdrew the money needed for his family's expenses without consulting the other. At the end of the year they divided what was left.

Henry Plummer, MD, was one of the Mayo brothers' first partners. In 1914, he designed a structure for the clinic that would enable the group's physicians to practice the kind of medicine they believed in.

"As we grow in learning," declared Will Mayo, "we more justly appreciate our dependence upon each other. The sum total of medical knowledge is now so great and wide-spreading that it would be futile for one man to attempt to acquire, or for any one man to assume that he has, even a good working knowledge of any large part of the whole. The very necessities of the case are driving practitioners into cooperation. The best interest of the patient is the only interest to be considered...."

Plummer's design brought the Mayo Clinic's medical departments, laboratories, workshops, editorial services and business office together within the same four walls in Rochester, Minnesota.

Patient files—individually numbered dossiers he'd devised to replace the cumbersome traditional medical ledger system, soon universally adopted—were shuttled by conveyor belt to every floor as requested.

Physician calls were transmitted over an internal telegraph ticker. Doctors could speak directly to each other, to the operator or to a patient or consultant outside by telephone—a capability Plummer had been told by engineers was impossible until he convinced them otherwise.

Cleveland Clinic

George Crile, MD, learned the value of teamwork on the battlefield in France during World War I. With two other former Army surgeons and an internist, he set up a group practice after the war that would introduce the same combinative style of medical care to Cleveland.

Its informal motto, he recalled in his journal, was "To Act as a Unit."

Ochsner Clinic

Alton Ochsner, MD, was a celebrated surgeon at Tulane University when he and four partners talked of starting a clinic in New

(continues)

EXHIBIT 7-1 (Continued)

Orleans that would redefine health care delivery in the region and make the city a medical mecca for Latin America.

The banker husband of a patient advanced them the start-up funds on the strength of Ochsner's reputation alone.

In 1952, on the tenth anniversary of the opening of the clinic his partners had insisted on naming after him, Ochsner reminded his colleagues: "While working for the 'benefit of humanity,' let us not forget that our work is also for the 'benefit of the patients,' the individual men and women who seek us out in their hours of trial and who need compassion and understanding as well as scientific care."

Not just platitudes

Lofty ideals, inspiring words, exemplary actions—these were the common currency of the founders of what have become the nation's best known, most respected and most successful physician-led medical organizations.

The preeminence of the individual patient's needs ... the transcendent responsibilities of the physician ... collegiality ... trust ... openness ... synergy ... consummate skill (a prerequisite) ... imagination and invention (a hallmark) ... the

motivating principles these founders voiced might be dismissed by cynics as echoes from a less complicated age.

But talk to the doctors who lead and practice in these remarkable groups today and one hears the same phrases, the same unembarrassed invocations.

SOURCE: Weber, D. O. 2007. Leaders of the pack: A look at some of the top group practices in the country, and how they achieved success. *Physician Executive* 33(2, March-April), 6(7). Retrieved May 25, 2008 from *Academic OneFile*. Gale. University of Memphis.

Discussion Questions

This particular article tells of the culture of successful group practice. The following section of this chapter, however, tells us that introduction of the group practice was not without controversy.

1. What are the advantages and disadvantages of group physician practices compared with solo physician practices?

2. In today's complex healthcare environment, will solo practitioners be able to survive?

The Controversy over Contract Practices

Although contract (employed) and group practices are today commonplace, growing, and accepted by organized medicine as appropriate and ethical ways to deliver medical care, many individual practitioners initially resisted what they perceive to be an unwise trend. These trends are represented today by salaried group practices and health maintenance organizations (HMOs). When they first appeared, they were seen as a threat to other practitioners. The cry of unethical practice was heard, and the organizations that represented the aggrieved physicians—the state and local medical societies and the AMA—went to battle. The controversies seem at first to be economic—that is, a threat to the incomes of protesting physicians—but some very real issues lie behind the protests. To understand the resistance to salaried physician groups, it is important to define contract practice and group practice, and then look at the storms that surrounded their development.

Certain industries (for example, railroads, mining, lumbering, steel) traditionally employed company doctors to do preemployment health examinations, treat occupational injuries, and, in some instances, to develop employee medical programs. These physicians were mostly salaried—that is, under contract. Medical societies opposed this type of practice (except when physicians were under contract to serve the military), which they regarded as exploitative because doctors bid against each other for the contracts, thus reducing the price of their services. Over time, the opposition of the medical profession discouraged employers from expanding medical services, except in remote areas where physicians were generally unavailable.

The medical societies were also concerned about contract doctors undercutting them economically, doing work for less than they would normally charge on a fee-for-service basis. The AMA, which was as interested in upgrading the medical profession and preserving the independence of doctors as it was in improving medical education, also objected to contract practice. As Starr (1982) notes, the AMA could see "no economic excuse or justification" for this type of practice in 1907, and it objected "to the unlimited service for limited pay and the 'ruinous competition' it 'invariably' introduced" (p. 208). This type of contract practice declined over time as the supply of physicians decreased and there were enough patients for a physician to earn a living without resorting to contracting. However, it began to rise again with the development of HMOs posing a threat to the traditional form of fee-for-service solo practice, which many physicians still feel serves the best interests of patients and physicians.

Group practice has been a part of the American scene for a long time. The founding of the Mayo Clinic in Rochester, Minnesota, at the end of the nineteenth century, is generally cited as the beginning of organized group practice as we know it today, although there were some antecedents. Mayo was followed by other groups, among them the famous Ross-Loos Clinic in Los Angeles, which served the city water department employees and others under contract. Some group practices operated on a loose fee-for-service basis as in solo practice; however, as the groups became organized, many paid their member physicians a salary, and sometimes also a percentage of the net business income or a bonus. MacColl (1966) notes that the quality of care in many of the early groups "was reasonably good, but there were others which did not reflect much credit on either the organizers or the physicians involved" (p. 12).

During the early period of group practice development, the AMA was somewhat ambivalent about it. Where groups existed, physicians outside the groups often expressed concern about the quality of care the groups provided, as well as concern about the competition from lower fees the groups sometimes charged. Then, in 1932, the Committee on the Costs of Medical Care, a national committee, issued a report titled Medical Care for the American People.

The committee recommended, albeit with some medical and dental member dissent, that medical care should be provided by organized group practices and that "the costs of medical care [should] be placed on a group payment basis, through the use of insurance, through the use of taxation, or through the use of both these methods. This is not meant to preclude the continuation of medical services provided on an individual fee basis for those who prefer the present method" (U.S. Department of Health, Education, and Welfare 1970, 120). As noted, the report was published in 1932, and it galvanized the opposition of the AMA to both group and salaried practice.

"In 1933, the AMA declared that groups of physicians in salaried practice were considered unethical when there is solicitation of patients either directly or indirectly..., when there is competition and underbidding to secure the contract..., when compensation is inadequate to secure good medical practice..., when there is interference with reasonable competition in a community..., when free choice of physicians is prevented." (U.S. Department of Health, Education, and Welfare 1970).

This change on the part of the AMA reflected widespread concern within the profession. The concern was professional as well as economic, although critics all too frequently focus on the economic component, ignoring the professional objections.

The AMA became directly involved in a local issue in the late 1930s and was found guilty of restraint of trade in 1941. The case involved the AMA and the Medical Society of the District Columbia (MSDC) in their actions relating to the Group Health Association (GHA) of Washington. Opposition to the GHA by the MSDC arose almost immediately after the GHA was organized in 1937. The MSDC notified "all the physicians in the area that the plan was unethical. The GHA's salaried physicians were expelled from the society, and a list of 'reputable physicians' was circulated to all the hospitals for their guidance" (MacColl 1966, 140). The MSDC and the AMA were subsequently indicted, found guilty, and fined for having conspired to **monopolize** medical practice. The GHA physicians were later admitted to the society and had no subsequent difficulty over hospital privileges. In other parts of the country, specifically Seattle and San Diego, the local medical societies (not the AMA) were the defendants in similar cases, and lost in their efforts to block development of group health plans in each case the medical societies. After the AMA fine in the GHA case, the AMA disengaged from "further legal entanglement." Local societies were left to interpret or misinterpret the code of ethics (MacColl 1966).

At times, the objections to group practice took on rather nasty characteristics. In metropolitan New York, for example, the Health Insurance Plan (HIP) was established in the mid-1940s, as a demonstration project for national health insurance. HIP, the fiscal agent, contracted with medical groups, paying each group so much for each person on its list (today referred to as capitation). How the group divided the money was up to the group. In return for the capitation payment, the group was responsible for providing comprehensive physician services, prevention, and treatment. For hospital care, Blue Cross covered most HIP subscribers at that time. Though the local medical societies might not have been able to keep HIP physicians from joining, they could ostracize them socially. As late as the 1960s, HIP physicians were denied hospital privileges.

The intensity of feelings on the local level did not need fuel from the AMA. At its inception, HIP had proclaimed itself a demonstration project for a national system, and many New York physicians were accustomed to government systems before coming to the United States. In addition, the economic pressures on physicians in New York City were considerable because many believed that New York City had an oversupply of medical practitioners in the 1950s. At every turn, non-HIP physicians challenged HIP physicians. Blue Shield, which was sponsored by the medical profession, used paid salesmen and advertising; when HIP did this, "the charge of unethical conduct was raised. Ben E. Landis, one of the HIP physicians, took the matter to the AMA's Council on Ethical and Judicial Affairs, which ruled in his favor, finding that HIP was a legally organized plan and had as much right to advertise as did Blue Shield so long as the personal qualifications of the physicians were not promoted" (MacColl 1966, 139). By the late 1970s in New York, all wounds were healed, and HIP physicians were fully accepted by medical societies and hospitals. The AMA's Council on Ethical and Judicial Affairs also reversed, on appeal, the earlier expulsion of the developers of the Ross-Loos Medical Group from the Los Angeles County Medical Society (in addition to the Landis case).

Opposition to contract practice, group practice, and salaried practice has all but disappeared. Organized medicine no longer opposes them, and each of these forms of practice is growing. The change came about partly as a result of effective legal challenges against organized medicine. Perhaps more importantly, the change came as a direct result of a recognized physician shortage in the 1950s that would ensure fee-for-service, solo practice physicians an ample number of patients to maintain a good income, regardless of the presence of contract and group practice. By this time, group practice had also evolved; advocates now saw it as a way to regularize their hours, obtain easy consultation, and afford ownership of expensive technology that they could not economically justify by themselves but could justify on a shared basis. All forms of medical practice could thus live together in harmony.

Group practices are expanding in size, and they increasingly compete for patients with one another, with solo practitioners, and with hospital-based physicians. Many groups now contract with managed care plans. Even though they compete with hospital ambulatory clinics, these groups can have considerable influence on hospitals because they control the admission of a significant number of patients to any particular hospital. In the 1990s, groups affiliated with hospitals to form integrated systems of care to survive in a much more competitive environment. The balance of influence is much harder to identify in a dynamic health care system, in which hospitals, physicians, and insurance plans all operate under the same umbrella organizations.

Medical Practice Costs and Financing

The costs to maintain a medical practice, which in many ways must function as any other business or organization, are considerable. As in most service organizations, the greatest expenses are wages and benefits, including those of physicians, clinical personnel, and office personnel. Additional expenses are incurred for facilities (rent, lease, or real estate), office and medical supplies, medical equipment, liability insurance, and other expenses. Depending on the specialty of the medical practice, malpractice insurance can be one of the largest expenses incurred. Increasingly, physicians' offices are investing in computer systems (see Table 7–4), not only for the business function of the practice, but to maintain clinical records.

At one time, medicine was the highest-paid profession in the United States. Given the state of the health care environment and the growth in computerization, telecommunications, and Internet industries, medicine may no longer be as attractive a career as it once was. The average physician's income varies by specialty and practice design. Specialists with the highest average earnings were cardiac and thoracic surgeons, radiologists, neurosurgeons, orthopedic surgeons, and surgical sports medicine physicians. Lowest average earnings were found among psychiatrists, general or family practitioners, and pediatricians (American Medical Group Association 2006).

In a fee-for-service atmosphere, concern over increased health care costs centered on the possibility of overservice. A number of U.S. and Canadian economists advance what is called the target income hypothesis. This hypothesis contends that physicians set their sights on a given income level, and that they adjust their fees to reach it. When the demand for services is down and threatens attainment of the desired income, physicians raise fees. When fees are decreased (as in the cost-containment environment), physicians provide more services, which could be for the purpose of augmenting income rather than for more comprehensive and appropriate medical care. Supporters of this hypothesis point to the rise in physician incomes despite increased competition for patients and reduced third-party payments per

TABLE 7-4 Trends in Distribution of Patient Care Physicians by Metropolitan/Nonmetropolitan Status

Year	Total Physicians	Metropolitan		Nonmetropolitan	
		Number	Percentage	Number	Percentage
1980	363,915	312,687	86.4	49,228	13.6
1990	487,796	429,396	88.0	58,400	12.0
2000	631,431	553,208	87.6	78,169	12.4
2003	691,873	587,286	84.9	104,453	15.1
2005	718,473	567,201	78.9	151,129	21.0

SOURCE: American Medical Association. Physician characteristics and distribution in the U.S., 2002–2003 Edition, Table 5–14; 2005 Edition, Table 5–14; 2007 Edition, Table 5–14. All rights reserved.

patient encounter. Surgery is often cited in this regard, particularly accusations of unnecessary surgery being performed simply to compensate for decreased fees per procedure.

Others argue that more critical factors in rising physician incomes may be (1) increased demand and productivity that result from providing additional, appropriate diagnostic and therapeutic services made possible by new knowledge and technology; (2) fear of possible malpractice suits (the practice of **defensive medicine**); (3) a more educated population seeking medical care with higher expectations for improved outcomes; and (4) a rapidly aging population with correspondingly increased morbidity. Managed care has tried to curb overservice through capitated payment mechanisms; however, charges have been made of an overcorrection and fears that some patients might actually be underserved because of the costs involved in providing needed services (see more on the costs and financing of health care in Chapters 2 and 3).

Malpractice and Professional Liability

Medical professional liability (medical malpractice liability) continues to be an important issue. Questions arise regarding whether physicians have overused tests as a defense against possible malpractice charges and whether patients have used charges of malpractice to demand perfection rather than prevent negligence or incompetence. Malpractice insurance is a significant expense to medical practitioners. Premium rates are highest for obstetrician gynecologists and surgeons, which is a direct reflection of claims filed.

As a defense to malpractice claims, physicians have become more careful. They are keeping better records so that they can defend themselves in court. They are improving their communication skills to enhance the physician–patient relationship and to help patients to better understand the risks involved in procedures because there are fewer lawsuits when the physician–patient relationship is good. Physicians may try to reduce the risk of lawsuits by practicing "defensive medicine," ordering more diagnostic tests than may be necessary to confirm a patient's diagnosis but also adding to the rising costs of medical care.

The adoption of standards of care by some specialty groups and medical societies may reduce the number of malpractice actions. For example, in 1990, the American Society of Anesthesiologists adopted a standard that requires its members to use certain devices to measure the oxygen level in the blood, which it estimates could have prevented serious injury or death in almost one-third of the cases in which anesthesiologists have been accused of malpractice. The federal legislature has attempted to pass medical liability reform, but has failed to do so. As of 2005, thirty-five states adopted law changes, but the content of the reform varies. Some have targeted total monetary awards, others payment for "pain and suffering," whereas still others limit attorney fees. Some states set new statutes of limitations and provisions for penalties for frivolous lawsuits. A recent study indicates that there is some effect of state tort reforms on malpractice payments, but there remains an inconsistency as to which reforms are most effective (Waters et al. 2007).

Both hospitals and the government are increasing efforts to identify doctors with a history of malpractice. In 1990, the federal government established a **National Practitioner Data Bank (NPDB)** to keep track of doctors who have been successfully sued for malpractice, who have been disciplined for incompetence, and/or who have had hospital privileges revoked. Hospitals are required to access the data bank prior to granting hospital privileges to physicians. Unfortunately, this information is not available to patients when they are choosing a doctor.

About half of the states limit the amount or type of damages that can be recovered in malpractice suits. Still, the average annual malpractice premium for physicians was $15,000 in 2007. Premiums for primary care physicians are about $1,000 less. Since 1990, premiums have been somewhat consistent and have dropped in some states. More than half of all doctors in private practice are insured by risk retention groups, physician-owned companies set up to assume the risk of their members. Twelve of these companies were set up in 2006 alone. Part of the rate increases in the past was caused by insurers leaving the malpractice market. However, this trend is reversing, and new insurers are now entering the market (Insurance Information Institute 2007).

PRIMARY CARE PHYSICIANS

In 1975, the Coordinating Council on Medical Education (CCME) defined primary care physicians as those who provide an individual or family with continuing health surveillance, along with the needed acute and chronic care they are qualified to provide and referral service to specialists as appropriate. General practitioners and family practitioners fall within this category, as do pediatricians, internal medicine physicians, and obstetrician gynecologists, although not everyone would agree about these last three.

Pediatricians typically limit their clientele to children and adolescents; internal medicine physicians typically do not handle some things that family practitioners might handle, such as obstetrics and pediatric problems. Obstetrics and gynecology has more recently evolved as a primary care specialty for categorical care for women, including obstetric and/or gynecological problems, with female patients going directly to ob–gyn practitioners without referral.

The definition of primary care specialties that the CCME developed leaves much to be desired. Other specialties handle a considerable amount of routine primary care that a family practitioner or other health professionals might handle in other settings. Prior to the growth of managed care and the gatekeeper concept, many people had the tendency to self-diagnose and self-refer to a specialist—psychiatrist, surgeon, dermatologist, orthopedist—when, in fact, the family physician or other primary care practitioner might well handle many of the problems. For example, some patients frequently used ophthalmologists and orthopedic surgeons when optometrists and podiatrists might well have sufficed. Part of the recent emphasis on primary care physicians is economic. The rising costs of health care make principal payers want a mechanism to control costs. They believe that one way to control costs is to decrease the use of specialists by encouraging primary care physicians to treat mild illnesses rather than refer patients to expensive specialists. When specialists and primary care physicians treat patients with comparable illnesses, specialists hospitalize patients more often, write more prescriptions, and order more diagnostic tests (Greenfield et al. 1992). Of course, when an illness is complicated or severe, treatment by specialists is appropriate. Primary care medicine provides the majority of preventive services, such as counseling about healthy lifestyle changes, immunizations, and regularly screening for detection of illnesses before they become serious, all of which are becoming more important in maintaining good health.

Managed care organizations use primary care physicians as "gatekeepers" to prevent the unnecessary use of specialists. Medical students are being encouraged to enter primary care fields by the increased payment for their services by Medicare and some insurance companies using the resource-based relative value scale (see Chapter 3 for more details).

Before the American College of Surgeons (ACS) was established and for many years after, general practitioners did everything, including general surgery. In some communities in the United States, particularly in the more remote areas, family practitioners still provide a wide range of services because of the limited availability of specialists.

With managed care organizations placing emphasis on ambulatory care and particularly on care a primary care physician delivers, the percentage of surgical procedures, particularly minor surgery that practitioners other than surgeons perform is difficult to determine. The American College of Surgeons has long sought to curb surgery by those not specializing in surgery. However, the content of family practice residencies requires some training in a variety of other specialty areas, including surgery.

THE APPEAL OF SPECIALIZATION

Physicians specialize for many reasons. People in general have always held specialists in high regard—as physicians who could do things that general physicians could not do and whose special skills warranted a higher fee. Often, the medical school faculty physicians were considered the best of these specialists. There has always been a certain aura that surrounded physicians—a mystique that was even more pronounced for specialists, who had knowledge and skills that saved lives, eased pain, and improved functioning.

Medical students must choose an area of medicine they will practice. Many factors may enter this decision process, but, because most members of the faculty are specialists, the pressure to respond to one of those specialty role models is ever present. Specialization has a certain intellectual appeal, which enables individuals who are curious to know more about the problems that afflict humans. Because the problems are complex, individuals who are curious specialize to understand them.

Other factors may enter. A person's own medical history or that of the family frequently channels a physician's interest. For some specialties, very high incomes are ensured; for others, more orderly personal lives are possible because of fewer emergencies and more regular hours.

Most of the factors that affect the location of a primary care physician also influence the specialist's choice of practice location. Hospital access, however, may be even more critical for specialists, in terms of the supportive services they may need for the effective practice of their specialty. Studies have also shown that specialists tend to locate in areas close to where they did their residency because new specialists are familiar with the area clinicians and tend to know and be comfortable with other specialists for referrals. At the same time, because many of the local physicians know the new specialist, a new specialist can anticipate some helpful referrals. Notwithstanding the pull to practice in urban settings, the overall increase in the supply of specialists, the spread of technology, and the disadvantages of urban life have influenced the movement of new specialists to outlying areas during the past decade.

MEDICAL SOCIETY MEMBERSHIPS

Most physicians find it valuable to belong to a county or city medical society in the area in which they practice and to their state medical society. Not all physicians elect to join the AMA, for a variety of reasons. Many disagree with the AMA's policies (although the association probably truly represents the views of its members), others are more interested in a specialty society, and still others are concerned about the rising costs of membership, particularly in view of the many other memberships physicians feels they must maintain.

Membership in local and state societies is more vital for practicing physicians. These organizations enable physicians to meet their colleagues, to learn about the skills and abilities of other physicians for the purpose of referring patients to them, and to facilitate an intellectual interchange among physicians, which has always been a key element in the continued learning process. Medical societies provide an organizational focus for representation of medical viewpoints about matters affecting the health of the population and about other matters of interest or concern to them. In addition, if any government, industry, or other body wishes to communicate something to the medical community, the medical society is perhaps the most effective vehicle. Finally, membership often enables physicians to receive such financial benefits as group life, health, and malpractice insurance.

Physicians often belong to other medical societies, depending on their interests and specialties. Among the many other societies is the National Medical Association (NMA), an association representing the special interests of African American physicians (see www.nmanet.org).

RURAL AND INNER-CITY MEDICAL PRACTICE

However one chooses to define primary care physicians, rural areas and inner cities have had considerable difficulty in recruiting and retaining them. The lack of appeal of rural practice stems from fear of professional isolation: lack of professional interactions, inaccessibility of hospitals, absence of consultation and continuing medical education opportunities, lack of career opportunities for a spouse, and cultural deprivation (no theater, concerts, or lectures, limited adult education activities, and so on). Physicians today and their spouses are urbanites by virtue of their long periods of education and training in urban professional settings, and the adjustment to rural living, though sometimes inviting in moments of idyllic dreaming, has not been successful in most cases. There seems to be a greater chance of retention if a physician is originally from a rural area, but no one yet has devised a generally valid formula for the successful establishment of rural practices. Professional as well as personal isolation are factors that are very real. Government-sponsored health plans have adjusted payments to rural physicians and facilities to increase the attractiveness of rural practices. Medical schools and residency programs have established training centers in rural outreach clinics, and student loan programs have offered loan reductions for services to rural areas. Still, rural areas struggle to maintain health services for what is often a deprived socioeconomic population.

There is some ambiguity in the word *rural.* One federal agency set the definition of rural as an area with a population of 35,000 or 50,000. Other agencies have used other, usually lower, figures. For those rural regions of 35,000 to 50,000 that have recruited physicians, the reasons for their successes are several: (1) There are more physicians available, and the supply-and-demand factor operates to secure a more even distribution; (2) the large urban settings are congested and are plagued by high costs and high crime rates; (3) the assets of urban life are not as remote as road networks improve; and (4) the small communities have sought to make their areas attractive to primary care and other physicians by developing the best hospital facilities their communities can support, and sometimes more than they can support. These small communities, however, do not face the levels of sparse population scattered across a large geographic area that are problematic in truly rural areas.

Inner-city problems are somewhat different. In large cities, individuals who are poor have not always used private doctors. Hospital outpatient departments and emergency rooms have served as primary sources of care. As people moved to the suburbs, physicians followed their paying patients. The out-migration of physicians and lack of interest from new physicians are a result of the high cost of office and parking spaces, transportation hassles, and crime. In addition, the cities are far more litigiously inclined, and malpractice insurance rates are generally higher. The movement of physicians out of cities has become a matter of concern because individuals who are poor under Medicaid are entitled to private physician care, but the availability of private physicians is limited. Managed care programs for Medicaid recipients are attempting to provide more comprehensive and continuous care to underserved populations, but the insufficient number of physicians practicing in areas where the Medicaid population resides continues to be a problem (see Table 7–4).

HOSPITAL OUTPATIENT DEPARTMENTS

Hospitals offer ambulatory care services in clinics where people with nonurgent medical problems can receive treatment. Clinics are separate from emergency department services, but an emergency department often handles nonurgent patients during hours when clinics are not open. Clinics may be general or specialized (for example, in diabetes, oncology, women's health). Historically, only hospitals with teaching programs or those in areas (usually urban) where patients could not or would not go to doctors' offices had clinics, and they served mostly those with low incomes. The situation has changed because competition among hospitals has increased and inpatient reimbursement has decreased. Hospitals have established and expanded clinics, some of them in a community away from the hospital (freestanding). These clinics also attempt to attract people with middle incomes to provide the hospital with additional income and to "feed" patients to their hospitals for admission. The emphasis on outpatient services that hospitals provide is a result of medical advances that allow new treatment modalities that do not require an overnight stay, and changes in hospital reimbursement that have pushed hospitals into new service areas to supplement income from outpatient services.

COMMUNITY HEALTH CENTERS

Community neighborhood health centers began to develop in the late 1960s, with funding initially from the Office of Economic Opportunity and later from the U.S. Department of Health, Education, and Welfare (HEW). These centers provided primarily comprehensive ambulatory services for a defined population of people who are poor. These people had always received large amounts of care from health departments and in hospitals. The larger hospitals, and particularly medical school hospitals, had long histories of caring for individuals who are poor on both inpatient and outpatient bases. However, outpatient care was often demeaning, with impersonal, crowded surroundings, and long waits on hard benches. Neighborhood health centers were designed to overcome these demeaning features by providing a broad range of primary and secondary ambulatory care services by salaried physicians and other health professionals, by emphasizing prevention, having available a wide range of supporting nonmedical services, and providing these services in the neighborhoods in which the people lived. Important, too, was the concept that the people who were served, the consumers, should be involved in the control of their centers.

When possible, Medicare, Medicaid, and other vendor payments and government grants financed the centers on a fee-for-service basis. As with so many other government programs, priorities shifted and funding tapered off. In addition to decreased funding, community health centers faced other problems. The demand for services far exceeded their availability because these centers were the only source of medical care for individuals who were poor in many rural areas and in many inner-city neighborhoods. Many of these centers provide prenatal and obstetric care for women with low incomes who are considered high risk and who might otherwise not have access to care.

Much of the focus of community health centers has turned to primary health care. The centers provide a more limited range of services and refer patients to clinics and hospital centers for more specialized care. Many of these centers have developed with support from one of several federal programs: the National Health Service Corps, the Rural Health Initiative, Health Underserved Rural Areas Program, and the Appalachian Regional Commission. Such support augmented local organizational efforts and local building of facilities. Although the original concept of the typical federally supported center often had two family practitioners and one dentist, many centers are now staffed by nurse practitioners and physician assistants who provide primary care.

The supporting services vary from center to center. Some in very remote areas have implemented telemedicine. Telemedicine, a fairly new concept made possible by advances in technology, links primary care providers with specialists who are able to "examine" patients and provide consultation without physically being in the remote site. Health care providers in remote areas who use **telemedicine** are equipped with monitors that transmit medical information to a "home base" (emergency room, hospital specialty department, and so on) where consulting physicians receive vital diagnostic information regarding patients. In some cases, a consultant is able to see a patient on a TV monitor. The consultant is therefore able to assist in or direct the patient's care. Studies are under way to determine the effectiveness of possible applications of telemedicine in a variety of settings.

The long-term survival of community health centers depends on attaining financial resources from grants and cooperative ventures with larger medical centers, and on finding ways to attract and retain quality professional personnel and implement new technologies within limited funding opportunities.

AMBULATORY SURGERY CENTERS

Technology and reimbursement patterns have increased the amount of surgery performed on an ambulatory basis. Hospitals all over the country are experiencing a rise in the number of surgical patients who come into the hospital and go home on the same day, cases that previously required at least an overnight stay in the hospital, if not a two- or three-day stay. In many cases, ambulatory surgery is not optional; third-party payers require that many procedures be done on an outpatient basis. The move to outpatient treatment can significantly affect a hospital's use of beds and its overall organization.

Many surgeons, however, have been accustomed to performing a limited amount of ambulatory surgery in their offices, depending on their facilities, support services, and self-imposed limits. One of the major limits was anesthesia. Surgeons typically provided only surgery requiring a local anesthetic, not a general anesthetic, because anesthesiologists or nurse anesthetists administer general anesthesia. Advances in technology make it possible to perform an increasing number of surgical procedures on an outpatient basis and with general anesthesia. During the 1970s, a number of freestanding—that is, not hospital-based—surgical centers began to develop in several parts of the country.

After the American College of Surgeons began to approve freestanding ambulatory surgical centers (ASCs) in 1981, the number of facilities increased rapidly throughout the country. In 1999, there were just over 2,700 Medicare-certified, freestanding outpatient surgery centers; in 2006, there were approximately 4,700 such centers. Some 10 million surgical procedures were performed at such centers that same year, up from 4.3 million in 1996 (Ferreter 2000; American Association of Ambulatory Surgical Centers 2006; MedPac 2007). The most common procedures performed at these ASCs are in ophthalmology, gynecology, otolaryngology, orthopedics, and plastic surgery. Demand for procedures at ASCs is expected to grow by between 12 percent and 20 percent through 2010, depending on the specialty. The rapid growth of ambulatory surgery has been due to a demand by insurance companies and government to provide surgery at lower costs. ASCs are able to function at lower costs because they incur lower overhead costs than hospitals. With the increase of freestanding centers, hospitals perform some 53 percent of all outpatient surgery, freestanding surgical centers perform about 23 percent, and doctors in their offices perform about 24 percent (Haugh 2006).

ASCs are able to compete effectively with hospitals because Medicare covers many procedures on an outpatient basis only. Surgery centers also affiliate with HMOs and preferred provider organizations (PPOs), thereby competing with hospitals for a certain flow of patients. Hospitals have responded to the growth of ASCs by establishing their own freestanding centers, by affiliating or going into partnership with some of the freestanding centers, and by aggressively marketing and expanding their own hospital-based outpatient surgical services.

ASCs may be independently owned, some by surgeons who are competing with the very hospitals in which they perform their more complicated surgical procedures. Some independently owned facilities are small, single-specialty centers with fewer physicians than those owned by hospitals and corporate chains (see Figure 7–3). The development of ASCs in an area depends on such factors as state regulations, certificate-of-need requirements, competition, and reimbursement policies. Most states require ASCs be licensed and undergo inspection and reporting. All ASCs serving Medicare patients must be Medicare-certified. Many also choose to be certified by the Joint Commission, the Accreditation Association for Ambulatory Health Care, the American Association for Accreditation of Ambulatory Surgery Facilities, or the American Osteopathic Association. ASCs are limited by the federal government as to what procedures they may perform, limitations that do not apply to hospital outpatient departments. However, Medicare is due to expand that list for 2008 (Haugh 2006).

EMERGENCY CARE

When considering emergency treatment, most people still think of the hospital emergency room. However, changes have taken place even in this area of health care delivery on the basis of costs, competition, and quality of care. Many communities have tried to provide care to individuals without insurance in more suitable settings, recognizing that emergency rooms are overburdened with treatment requests that could be better served in a primary care setting. Managed care companies try to address this issue by requiring that primary care providers (gatekeepers) be the initial contact even in emergent cases, mandating that primary care physicians provide twenty-four–hour contact options for their patients. The emergency care described in the following sections is just a sampling of the care that is available, and it may vary greatly in local communities.

Hospital Emergency Departments

The emergency room (ER) or emergency department (ED) is still the most familiar setting for emergency care and is the most appropriate for acute and all life-threatening medical situations. Hospital ERs have at their disposal all of the hospitals' resources of equipment and specialty care. They also have the referral mechanisms in place for care not available in house. Although each hospital may have its own method for staffing the ER, most hospitals today either directly employ physicians trained and certified in emergency medicine or contract with emergency medical groups for continuous coverage. In 2005, over 29,000 physicians specialized in emergency medicine. In

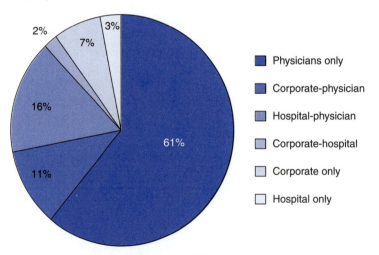

Figure 7–3 Ownership Structure of Ambulatory Surgery Centers

SOURCE: American Association of Ambulatory Surgery Centers. 2006. *Ambulatory surgery centers: A positive trend in health care* (p. 2).

very specialized areas of care, area physicians may be on call to provide care rather than such care being available in house.

Although most hospitals do have emergency rooms or emergency departments, there is no general mandate to have an ER. However, if a hospital does have an emergency department, it must treat all patients who present for care, regardless of ability to pay. The mandate to treat is defined as a requirement to stabilize a patient. A 1986 federal "antidumping law" states that hospitals cannot inquire about patients' insurance status before providing emergency care (California Health Line 1999). The statute often places ERs in a difficult situation because many managed care organizations refuse to pay for emergency care without prior authorization. An ER also places stress on the hospital's financial status because most acute trauma cases are very expensive to treat and many patients requiring such treatment are uninsured or underinsured and unable to pay for this very expensive care. ERs also face financial stress in that patients who have no regular source of care and/or no or very inadequate insurance often use them as primary sources of care.

Emergency rooms are considered outpatient services of hospitals. Patients most often are provided care and return home on the same day. Those requiring additional care are either admitted to an inpatient service of the facility or referred to another appropriate facility.

Freestanding Emergency Centers

Freestanding emergency centers (urgi-care centers) provide episodic emergency care twenty-four hours a day for problems that are not life-threatening. It is estimated that there are over 5,000 such centers in the nation. They provide primary care on a "walk-in" or appointment basis, as well as more acute care. Sometimes they are storefront operations located in large shopping malls, but more often they are fully equipped clinics that provide a wide range of care for situations that are not life-threatening. Like ambulatory surgical centers, they provide the opportunity for physicians and for-profit organizations to compete with hospitals and office-based physicians for patients. They provide treatment options to the use of hospital emergency departments and other practitioners whose location or appointment systems are inconvenient for patients. Unlike medical clinics that hospital outreach programs provide, urgi-care centers are often cash-and-carry operations. They require payment at the time of service (cash, check, or credit card) and do not bill insurance. Patients are given proper documentation to submit to any insurance plans they may have for reimbursement after paying the center.

Other forms of freestanding emergency centers might be referred to as "minor medical centers." These provide the same type of care as for-profit urgi-centers but are owned by hospitals as outreach clinics into the community. They are open during extended hours to care for patients who have emergent conditions that are not life-threatening or who either cannot get to or do not have a regular source of care. Minor medical centers are intended to relieve the pressure on hospital emergency rooms. They accept insurances from those who have coverage.

AMBULANCE SERVICES

A variety of agencies provide ambulance services. Depending on the community, services may be provided by police and fire departments, hospitals, volunteer groups, and private ambulance companies. Considerable effort has been made in recent years to train ambulance crews in dealing with the kinds of emergencies they are likely to encounter, and in connecting ambulance services via sophisticated communications equipment to emergency facilities to provide care swiftly to patients at the point of contact. As part of their ambulance services, many communities have paramedic teams and emergency medical technicians (EMTs) who are able, in communication with the hospital emergency room staff, to provide treatment prior to a patient's arrival in the emergency room.

On the other hand, ambulance services can also provide routine transport for patients being transferred from a hospital to more appropriate sites of care, such as a rehabilitation center, nursing home, or home care. Transport can also be arranged for a bed-bound patient from home to physician visits or other ambulatory care. Costs and reimbursement policies for ambulance services vary by insurance company and the reason for transport, and can be a financial burden to patients required to pay out of pocket. Some voluntary community ambulance companies provide free services to individuals who become annual "members" of the ambulance service by making an annual contribution to the ambulance corps.

FAMILY PLANNING CENTERS

Family planning centers were first established in 1970, when Congress passed Title X of the Public Health Service Act, which provided federal funding for establishing family planning services on the local level. Depending on the state and geographic area, local health departments, hospital agencies, or voluntary agencies established the centers, which typically provided gynecological examinations, breast or cervical cancer screening, contraceptive information and supplies, and other services related to reproductive health care. Many centers have expanded their services to include genetic screening; routine child health screening; and sexually transmitted disease diagnosis, treatment, and follow-up. During the early 1980s, federal funding became less available as the Reagan administration cut back on many health and social services, so funding now comes from a combination of federal and state funds, private donations, fund-raising, and sliding-scale client fees.

Planned Parenthood is probably the most familiar family planning organization in the United States, with over 860 health centers nationwide. They are a private nonprofit organization funded through clinic revenues, government grants, and private contributions. The core services of Planned Parenthood are contraception, education, sexually transmitted disease (STD) testing and treatment, cancer screening, women's health services, and abortion services (which are only 3 percent of their services). Clients include both males and females. The Planned Parenthood Action Network is a separate organization that advocates at the state and federal level to advance comprehensive reproductive health services (Planned Parenthood 2007).

CLINICAL LABORATORIES

Physicians may require a variety of laboratory analyses to facilitate diagnosis and treatment of their patients. Some physicians do their own tests or have their own technicians carry out whatever tests are desired. However, some tests are very complicated and require rather costly equipment. For these tests, as well as some of the simpler tests, physicians may have an arrangement with a nearby hospital or may use a freestanding clinical laboratory run by a pathologist or by a registered medical technologist. Sometimes physicians send patients to a lab; sometimes physicians send specimens to the lab. In rural settings, physicians may have to mail a specimen to a lab, or the lab may arrange for periodic pickup of specimens.

Although there is state licensing of clinical laboratories and federal monitoring of those labs that work across state lines, there has been concern about the quality of laboratory analyses over the years. Periodically, studies are completed that call into question the accuracy of clinical lab results. This is, of course, a serious matter because physicians treat patients on the basis of lab reports.

The Clinical Laboratory Improvement Amendments of 1988 (CLIA-88)—changes to the Clinical Laboratory Improvement Act of 1967—brought much-needed regulation to laboratories to ensure the quality of test results. CLIA-88 brought standards to freestanding and office-based laboratories similar to those imposed on hospitals and reference laboratories by CLIA-67. Laboratories must be registered, must be open to periodic inspection, must perform proficiency testing, and must follow staffing guidelines to receive payment from government programs for their services. These requirements have helped to improve the quality of laboratory findings, which ultimately lead to higher-quality treatment planning. There have been many CLIA updates since 1988, each an effort to improve quality in laboratory testing. In 2007, over 200,000 laboratories were registered with the Division of Laboratory Services at the Centers for Medicare and Medicaid Services (CMS). Certification of laboratories is also carried out by the Joint Commission, Commission on Office Laboratory Accreditation (COLA), the College of American Pathologists, and others (CMS 2007).

VOLUNTARY HEALTH AGENCIES

Many national health agencies operate state and sometimes local chapters. These agencies are typically oriented toward special disease and are financed largely by charitable contributions. Some of the more prominent agencies include the American Heart Association, American Cancer Society, the Arthritis Foundation, American Diabetes Association, and National Mental Health Association. Some of these agencies provide direct service (for example, diagnostic services, clinical consultation), some support research, some help finance needed services, and most conduct some health education activities to educate the population about a health problem of their concern.

SUMMARY

The move from inpatient to outpatient care has become more predominant since changes in reimbursement in the Medicare system in the early to mid-1980s. However, it is important to note that several types of care have always been found in outpatient settings. Key among those services is physician services, but dentistry, pharmacy, and visiting nurse services have also historically been ambulatory services.

As new technology develops, we will continue to see new forms of care in all settings. Although hospitals have been the focal point of health care delivery in the past and continue to consume a large portion of health care expenditures, the hospital is no longer synonymous with the health care system. The system is more diverse and more complex than ever before and, at least for the near future, continues to change in its functions, size, and scope of services.

Ambulatory surgery centers house much of the outpatient surgical procedures once considered inpatient procedures. These centers may operate in competition with the hospital or may actually be the service of a hospital. Outpatient surgical departments of hospitals also house many outpatient surgeries. There is no "one" business model for the provision of outpatient surgery.

Emergency rooms have always been major providers of outpatient care, although they are not often thought of as outpatient facilities because they are housed in hospitals. To relieve hospitals of some emergency treatment cost, various freestanding emergency facilities now provide care for emergencies that are not considered life-threatening.

Various clinics and hospital outpatient departments also provide primary or chronic care to patients who do not have a regular physician or live in areas where access to a private physician may be difficult. Oftentimes, clinics fill gaps to provide care to individuals who are poor and uninsured, and the greatest challenge to these facilities is to find funding to provide the amount and the quality of care patients need.

ACTIVITY-BASED LEARNING

- Identify a group medical practice in or near your community and determine its characteristics: number of physicians, single or multispecialty practice, and history of its development and growth. Do the physicians own the practice, or does a corporate entity employ physicians?

- Identify an ambulatory surgery center in your community and determine its ownership and/or affiliation. Research the year it first opened, procedures most commonly performed, number of operating rooms, and number of physicians performing procedures in the facility.

A QUESTION OF ETHICS

- It has been said that an increased number of physicians is related to an increase in the utilization of health care services—a concept known as physician-induced demand. In your opinion, is the utilization of health care related to greater access to care for those who previously could not get care, or do physicians provide unnecessary care to maintain their income in a competitive environment?

- The move from inpatient to outpatient care is driven by cost containment, as well as by new technologies. Are there risks to care provided in the ambulatory setting?

- Many freestanding ambulatory care facilities came into being as an opportunity to capture payments diverted from inpatient services. Does the ownership structure or profit motive of an ambulatory care facility have any bearing on the quality of its services?

REFERENCES

1. American Association of Ambulatory Surgical Centers. (2006). Ambulatory surgery centers: A positive trend in health care. Retrieved from www.aaasc.org/features/documents/ASCTrendReport118061.pdf

2. American Medical Association. (2007). Physician characteristics and distribution in the U.S., 2007 Edition. Chicago, IL: AMA.

3. American Medical Group Association. (2006). AMGA physician compensation survey. Retrieved from www.cejkasearch.com/compensation/amga_physician_compensation_survey.htm

4. CMS. (2007). CLIA statistical table/graphs. Retrieved from www.cms.hhs.gov/CLIA/17_CLIA_Statistical_Tables_Graphs.asp

5. Ferreter, M. (2000). Taking their cut. *Modern Physician, 4*(1), 40.

6. Greenfield, S., Nelson, E., Zubkoff, M., Manning, W., & Ware, J. (1992, March 25). Variations in resource utilization among medical specialties and systems of care. *JAMA, 269*(12), 1624–1630.

7. Haugh, R. (2006). Competition keeps getting hotter for ambulatory surgery. *Hospitals & Health Networks, 80*(10), 68.

8. Hing, E., & Burt, C. (2007). Advance data from vital and health statistics, office-based medical practices: Methods and estimates from the National Ambulatory Medical Care Survey. Retrieved from www.cdc.gov/nchs/data/ad/ad383.pdf

9. Hing, E., Cherry, D.K., & Woodwell, D.A. (2006). National ambulatory medical care survey: 2004 summary. Advance data from vital and health statistics; no. 374. Hyattsville, MD: National Center for Health Statistics.

10. Insurance Information Institute. (2007). Medical malpractice: The topic. September 2007. Retrieved from www.iii.org/media/hottopics/insurance/medicalmal/

11. MacColl, W. A. (1966). *Group practice and prepayment of medical care.* Washington, DC: Public Affairs Press.

12. MedPac. (2007) A data book: Healthcare spending and the Medicare program. Retrieved June 2007 from www.medpac.gov

13. California Health Line. (1999, February 19). Patient dumping: Hospitals caught between feds, HMOs. Retrieved from http://www.californiahealthline.org/Articles/1999/2/19/PATIENT-DUMPING—Hospitals-Caught-Between-Feds-HMOs.aspx

14. Planned Parenthood. (2007). Planned Parenthood services. Retrieved from www.plannedparenthood.org/about-us/who-we-are-4648.htm

15. Starr, P. (1982). *The social transformation of American medicine.* New York: Basic Books.

16. U.S. Department of Health, Education, and Welfare. (1970). Medical care for the American people: Final report of the Committee on the Costs of Medical Care. Chicago: University of Chicago Press.

17. Waters, T., Budetti, P., Claxton, G., & Lundy, J. (2007). Impact of state tort reforms on physician malpractice payments. *Health Affairs, 26*(2), 500.

Chapter 8

Hospitals

CHAPTER OBJECTIVES

After completing this chapter, readers should have an understanding of the following:

- The historic development of hospitals
- Characteristics and functions of hospitals
- Developments in the health care environment that have imposed changes on hospital functions
- The response of hospitals to environmental changes
- Competitive and regulatory influences on hospitals

INTRODUCTION

Although hospitals in their very early history were considered places to die, advances in medical knowledge transformed hospitals into centers for medical care and cure. The hospital became the focus of medicine for acute patient care, and the center for medical education. Physicians provided the bulk of their services in hospitals, laboratories were located in hospitals, nurses were employed by hospitals, and research was conducted in hospitals. Because the hospital was the focus of care, it naturally follows that hospitals have also experienced the greatest amount of change over many decades. Technology, developments in drug therapy, cost-containment efforts focusing on efficiency and efficacy, and a competitive environment have all changed the structure and function of hospitals as we see them today. The history and transition of hospitals are the focus of this chapter.

HISTORY OF HOSPITALS

Seventeenth-Century Hospitals

Religions and wars had a great deal of influence on the development of hospitals, particularly because the earliest conception of a hospital was as a facility for care of people who were poor and infirm. One of the earliest hospitals in what was to become the continental United States was established in 1658, in New Amsterdam, now New York City. It consisted of several houses and accepted soldiers and slaves; civilians were not accepted until 1791. **Voluntary hospitals** were the first hospitals in the continental United States built specifically to care for people in the general population who were sick . They were based on the British voluntary hospitals that flourished in the provincial centers outside of London in the eighteenth century. They differed from the earlier royal hospitals in Britain in that voluntary contributions maintained them, and consulting physicians served without pay, whereas both municipal governments and voluntary contributions maintained royal hospitals, and their physicians were salaried.

The initiative in founding voluntary hospitals came largely from laypeople and depended on gifts and subscriptions from donors who, for religious or humanitarian reasons, felt some responsibility for those less fortunate. The wealthy and social elite governed the hospitals. The success of these hospitals depended on the willingness of wealthy individuals to help the poor because poor sick people were virtually all of the hospital's patients. It was still preferable to endure illnesses at home, if possible, and the wealthy were better able to do this. Britain's first voluntary hospital was established in 1720; numerous reports of success of this and similar hospitals made their way to the United States and influenced the development and administration of U.S. hospitals.

The First Permanent Hospitals

The Pennsylvania Hospital, in Philadelphia, was the first permanent hospital for civilians in the continental United States; it was also a voluntary hospital. During the nineteenth century, the United States experienced dramatic growth in territory, population, and industry. New York became the largest and most influential city. Municipal and state hospitals were becoming permanent, and the role of hospital leadership passed from Pennsylvania Hospital to hospitals in New York and Boston.

Because Boston was an important seaport, confronted with many sick and injured seamen with no homes or families to care for them, the city opened the Boston Marine Hospital in 1804, to accommodate about thirty patients. This hospital was possible because, in 1778, Congress enacted a law requiring that 20 cents a month be withheld from the wages of each seaman on U.S. ships to support seamen's hospitals in seaports. This was the first compulsory health insurance law in the United States. In addition, Boston, like many other U.S. cities, had an almshouse that functioned mainly to give food and shelter to those who were poor but that also provided a few beds for the poor who were sick. In addition to a lack of facilities for the sick poor, training opportunities for physicians in New England were also lacking. In a period when medicine was beginning to make relatively significant advances, hospitals were important

centers for the dissemination of new knowledge. There, a variety of cases with similar clinical symptoms could be studied. Hospital experience was becoming indispensable for the training of new physicians, but few of them could afford to study in Philadelphia, London, or Paris.

These facts were very much on the minds of a number of the distinguished Bostonians who, in 1810, met to consider the establishment of a general hospital for those who were sick, poor, pregnant, and insane.[1] People who could afford it still preferred to be cared for at home. Supporters of the hospital petitioned the General Court (the Massachusetts legislature) for a hospital charter. The problems of those who were poor and insane were described, but the concluding paragraphs emphasized the need for medical students in New England to have hospital training. They cited the advantages that physicians from Philadelphia or New York had because hospital training was available to them.

The hospital was incorporated as the Massachusetts General Hospital in 1811. This voluntary hospital was a corporation composed of contributors with twelve trustees, four of whom were to be appointed by a board composed of the governor, lieutenant governor, president of the senate, speaker of the house, and the chaplains of both houses. Thus, the state had a share of control from the beginning. As an endowment, the legislation also granted the Province House (an unproductive estate that was initially considered and then rejected as a possible temporary hospital), on the condition that the corporation raise an additional $100,000 in private subscriptions—the concept of matching funds for establishing a hospital. The legal owner of the hospital was the corporation, which met once a year, but the trustees managed the institution. Government regulation or interference was not a problem because the trustees were all Federalists with many friends at the state capitol.

The hospital design included kitchens, laundry, a small sickroom for dying patients, morgue, storerooms, large wards to care for those who were sick, smaller rooms, water closets (lavatories), and accommodations for nurses and physicians. The water closets made the Massachusetts General Hospital the first U.S. hospital to have interior plumbing. The hospital, noted for its imposing structure and utility of interior design, was completed and ready for patients in 1821. At this time, the

---

[1] Although the term *insane* is today politically incorrect, the term was used widely during the times described here. Its use is not in any way meant to be disparaging to those with mental illness.

structure of the American hospitals was superior to that of their European counterparts, mainly because American architects were able to design new buildings rather than remodel old ones.

Finances were a major problem for the Massachusetts General Hospital. The operating expenses exceeded the income from endowments; thus, although only half of the hospital beds were occupied, many deserving people were turned away because of a lack of operating funds. In 1825, the Boston trustees proposed a successful method of increasing operating funds, called the free bed subscription. People who contributed $100 would support one patient in the hospital free of expense during the following year. People and organizations responded well to the idea, and the drive for free bed subscriptions became an annual event. Because of these subscriptions, the hospital was able to give free care to about 40 percent of its patients, which was comparable to the percentage of free beds at the Pennsylvania Hospital during the same period.

During the early 1800s, an important source of money for the hospital was the Massachusetts Hospital Life Insurance Company, which, by an 1824 agreement, gave the hospital one-third of all its profits over 6 percent and frequently lent money to the hospital. In addition, as the reputation of the hospital increased, many citizens remembered it generously in their wills.

The hospital's board of trustees met monthly to deal with matters that ranged from ratifying the decisions of the superintendent concerning wages for attendants, building repairs, and purchase of supplies to selecting personnel and investing the corporation's capital. The hospital's admission policy followed the precedent the Pennsylvania and New York hospitals set in forbidding the admission of patients who were incurable. The reasoning was that the institution was intended to cure disease; if they admitted or kept patients who were incurable, in free beds, they would soon have no room for treating and curing diseases.

One very persuasive reason for establishing a hospital was to provide care for individuals with mental illness. The care of those considered insane had been studied in Pennsylvania and New York. In contrast to the Pennsylvania Hospital, the Massachusetts General Hospital housed its patients considered insane in a separate building from the beginning. One of the first activities of the board was to purchase an estate overlooking the Charles River, which was designated for the insane and named the McLean Asylum. The patients came from towns and villages throughout New England. The asylum was under the

direction of the hospital trustees, but the financial accounting was separate. By this time, bleeding and purging were no longer used in the treatment of those considered insane, and there was an emphasis on keeping patients usefully occupied in a strict routine. The asylum had both a resident and an attending physician.

The Massachusetts General Hospital, like the Pennsylvania and New York hospitals, was a teaching hospital. It provided practical clinical instruction for the students of the Harvard Medical School. Lectures in surgery and medicine at the medical school were supplemented with classes at the hospital. In time, the hospital also became the leading New England center for medical research, largely because it had an adequate number of patients to study.

Hospitals moved westward with the population. They appeared along the Mississippi River as navigation increased. In New Orleans, St. John's Hospital (later known as Charity Hospital) was founded in 1736, from an endowment left by a French sailor. It began serving about twenty-four people, but grew over time to over 2,500 beds. Charity Hospital became part of the Medical Center of Louisiana at New Orleans in the 1990s. The hospital, like many others, incurred extensive damage during Hurricane Katrina in 2005, and remains closed.

The first hospital west of the Mississippi River was established because of the efforts of the Catholic bishop of St. Louis. John Mullanphy, an Irish American trader and merchant in St. Louis, donated some land on which to build a three-room log cabin. Four Sisters of Charity journeyed from Emmitsburg, Maryland, to St. Louis to run the hospital. The hospital opened on November 28, 1828, and the cabin was used for four years. By 1832, John Mullanphy and other citizens had provided a two-story brick building, which later became the City Hospital of St. Louis. In 1845, St. Louis built a new hospital that became the official City Hospital, and the old St. Louis Hospital operated by the Sisters of Charity was renamed the Mullanphy Hospital.

Mullanphy Hospital was the first private institution in the West to establish a regular nursing school, and the first hospital in the United States to establish a maternity hospital and **foundling asylum**. Mullanphy Hospital was also a teaching hospital for the Washington University School of Medicine. After a tornado virtually destroyed the hospital in 1927, a larger institution was built at a new site and was named De Paul Hospital to honor St. Vincent de Paul, who was instrumental in establishing the Daughters of Charity of St. Vincent de Paul.

The design and management of hospitals was largely influenced by Florence Nightingale, although she is more widely known for her reforms in the nursing profession. In the 1850s, the relationship between filth and disease was recognized, and sanitary measures for preventing disease were accepted. At that time, the prevalent theory of disease was that a vaporous emanation from humans could "enter into the putrefactive condition," causing disease. The germ theory of disease was yet to come.

In Nightingale's design, the dangerous emanations were quickly and continually removed by proper ventilation. The dominating theme of the Nightingale ward was pure air. To deprive those who were sick of pure air "is nothing but manslaughter under the garb of benevolence," according to Nightingale. Her ideal ward, described in *Notes on Hospitals,* was oblong with windows on each side extending from two feet from the floor to one foot from the ceiling. Windows would make up one-third of wall space, and there would be one window for every two beds. The wards would be 111 feet to 128 feet long, 30 feet wide, and 16 feet to 17 feet high. These dimensions were all calculated to provide the optimal flow of air. There would be thirty to thirty-two patients in a ward, each bed with 8 feet by 12 feet of "territory to itself." The water closets, lavatory, and baths, independently ventilated, would be located at the far end of a ward. The head nurse's room would be at the entrance to the ward with a window onto the ward so that she could see all the patients. Behind the nurse's room, Nightingale called for a room for cleaning and storing dishes, washing vegetables, and the like. Fireplaces in the center of the ward would serve for both heating and further ventilation. Each ward would open onto a long corridor. Wards designed on these principles were used in the United States and Britain (Nightingale 1863).

Scientific Advances Influencing Hospital Care

Advances in science and medicine during the mid-nineteenth century revolutionized medicine and had a great impact on hospitals. Hospitals became important centers for disseminating new knowledge and places where all classes of society could benefit from treatment.

Surgery was radically changed with improved ways to deaden pain during operations. Until the mid-1800s, operations were limited mainly to amputating, repairing wounds, setting fractures, reducing dislocations, suturing muscles and tendons, and removing kidney stones and some tumors. Pain was somewhat lessened by administering large doses of brandy, wine, opium, or henbane (a plant extract resembling belladonna), by constricting the limb above the portion to be amputated, and by hypnotism. Morphine was not introduced into general practice until 1844. In 1846, ether was first used for an operation at the Massachusetts General Hospital. From that date forward, operations could be performed on the inner cavities of the body without pain, but most patients died nonetheless from subsequent infection.

EXHIBIT 8-1

Surgical Amphitheatre

Pennsylvania Hospital is home to the oldest existing surgical amphitheatre in the United States. It was constructed in 1804 and is located in the center portion of the Pine Building. The initial portion of the hospital, the East Wing, had been completed earlier in 1755 but had no provision for surgical operations; all available space was designated for housing patients and staff of the hospital. Forty-nine years after the initial construction project, when all other parts of the hospital were finished, a large circular amphitheatre opened on the third floor.

The amphitheatre is approximately 30 feet high and 28 feet in diameter. The upper gallery has rows of wooden benches that hold approximately 130 students and observers, but it was often overcrowded when an unusual operation or particularly popular lecturer was scheduled. Since the skylight was initially the only source of lighting, operations were scheduled for midday and preferably during clear weather. Procedures were performed in an unsterile environment, since the sterile technique was not mandatory in American hospitals until the turn of the century (1900). In addition, until about 1840, operations were performed without the benefit of anesthesia; patients were given a choice of opium, liquor, or a knock on the head with a mallet to render them unconscious.

The surgical amphitheatre helped to inaugurate American clinical teaching by bringing the patient into the lecture room with the students. Dr. Benjamin Coates initiated

(continues)

EXHIBIT 8-1 (Continued)

the practice of demonstrating with patients in 1834. This approach followed the earlier example of Dr. Thomas Bond's bedside clinical teaching, which had been carried on in the wards since the earliest days of the hospital. Several other distinguished physicians made use of the amphitheatre over the years, such as Dr. Philip Syng Physick, Dr. George W. Norris, Dr. Joseph Pancoast, Dr. D. Hayes Agnew and Dr. Thomas G. Morton.

In the early nineteenth century, Philadelphia became known as the "Athens of America." The city had begun to attract students seeking medical education and clinical instruction not available anywhere else in the United States. The opening of the amphitheatre marked the establishment of surgery as a recognized discipline. Prior to its inception, what little surgery had been taught was done so as a practical aspect of anatomy classes. The amphitheatre filled a long-held desire of the University of Pennsylvania's faculty for a place in which a large class of students could receive formal lectures as well as witness surgical operations.

The surgical amphitheatre has been continually used for a variety of purposes since it ceased to function as a clinical amphitheatre in 1868. Immediately after a larger amphitheatre opened in another wing, the room served as a dining room for nurses and patients. It later served as a lounge for the house staff. In 1976, funds were raised to renovate the space, and the amphitheatre was returned to its original state; visitors are now welcome to visit this "time capsule of surgery."

Information for portions of this essay was gleaned from Alfred R. Henderson, Note on the 'Circular Room' of the Pennsylvania Hospital, *Journal of the History of Medicine* and *Allied Sciences*, 1964, Volume XIX, Number 2.

Discussion Questions

1. Describe some specific ways that medical education at Pennsylvania Hospital still influences medical education today.
2. In what ways has technology evolved to widen the scope of medical education.

In 1865, an English surgeon, Joseph Lister, dramatically reduced surgical infections by using carbolic acid sprays during surgery. Lister postulated that microorganisms in the air caused infection. He later realized that the organisms were also present on hands and instruments and insisted on the use of antiseptics on hands, instruments, and dressings. His introduction of antiseptic procedures was based on the work of the French chemist Louis Pasteur, who, in opposing the theory of spontaneous generation, showed that organisms found in putrefying materials originated from the organisms found in the air. The introduction of antiseptics so revolutionized surgery that the history of surgery can be divided into two periods: pre-Listerian and post-Listerian.

Robert Koch, a German physician, firmly established the germ theory of disease, in 1876. Since the sixteenth century, it had been thought that a person who was sick could transmit something and make a person who was well to become sick. After microorganisms were discovered, it was generally believed that they caused disease, but there was no proof. Koch studied anthrax, a disease of cattle that occasionally occurs in humans. He established that anthrax bacteria were always present in the blood of animals with the disease, and that if blood from an infected animal were injected into a well animal, the well animal would develop anthrax. Koch also grew the bacteria in nutrients outside the animal's body and found that, when those cultured

bacteria were injected into a well animal, that animal also developed anthrax. On the basis of this and other experiments, Koch proved that specific bacteria produce specific diseases.

Using Koch's methods, investigators isolated and identified bacteria that caused a wide variety of contagious diseases. Once the causative agents were identified, cures were possible either by immunization with killed bacteria or blood serum from recovered animals, or by other methods.

Koch used the microscope to identify disease-causing bacteria, and Rudolph Virchow used it to study diseased body tissue. In 1893, the first real hospital laboratory was set up in Paris, and laboratories soon became an integral part of every hospital. In the first part of the nineteenth century, other instruments, such as the stethoscope, clinical thermometer, and sphygmomanometer (blood pressure monitor), were introduced to aid in the diagnosis and treatment of disease. Toward the end of the century, Wilhelm Röntgen's discovery of the X-ray had an important impact on medical care.

The Johns Hopkins Hospital

The Johns Hopkins Hospital in Baltimore became world-renowned because it incorporated many of the advances in hospital design and function, medical education, and medical care. In 1867, a Baltimore businessman, Johns Hopkins, endowed the city with $7 million to be divided equally for the funding of a university and a hospital. The university and the hospital were to form two separate corporations with separate boards of trustees, but there was some liaison between the two because several men sat on both boards. Johns Hopkins purchased the thirteen-acre site for the hospital and pledged $100,000 a year toward construction costs while he lived. He died within a year, but the income from the $2 million that he also willed the hospital amounted to approximately $120,000 a year. The construction was to be financed only from the income; after the hospital was completed, the income was to be used for maintenance.

This was to be no ordinary hospital. Hopkins stipulated that the hospital's staff should be surgeons and physicians of the highest character and greatest skill. Hopkins also requested that the facility be used as a teaching hospital for the university's medical school and should provide care free of charge to those in the city and state who were **indigent** and sick, without regard to sex, age, or color. He specified that there be space for a limited number of paying patients, and the income from their care should be applied to the care of those who were poor. Although the administration of the hospital was to be nonsectarian, Hopkins wanted a religious spirit to be apparent. In addition, he wanted a training school for female nurses to be established. The hospital trustees interpreted Hopkins's mandates as meaning they should build the best hospital in the world. The hospital was opened for patients in 1889.

An important function of the hospital was its integration with the medical school's curriculum. The clinical methods established at the hospital enhanced research and promoted improved teaching of future physicians. The nurse training school introduced a two-year course of systematized instruction at the hospital rather than the usual practice of placing nursing students with private families during the second year. A very generous endowment, international consultation, early recruitment of leading clinicians, and careful planning resulted in a hospital with a worldwide reputation for excellence to which others would look for the latest and best in medical care and training for many decades.

Increased knowledge, new technology, and societal pressures caused hospitals to modify and develop as the decades advanced. Hospitals changed in many ways. For example, the type of patient changed when the principles of the germ theory of disease were understood and **aseptic techniques** were practiced, and as a result hospital infections began to decrease. It became advantageous for who were ill, regardless of their financial status, to be treated in hospitals. The number of separate wards for paying patients and

expensive private rooms increased; this change, in turn, altered the way in which hospitals were financed. In addition, as the number of paying patients increased, there was an increasing patient demand for privacy, which led to the replacement of the large wards for paying patients with semiprivate rooms accommodating two to four patients. This development forced changes in the nursing supervision of patients and also increased construction and operating costs. Infection control also affected hospital planning. No longer were separate buildings or separate floors necessary for certain conditions. With the introduction of iron and steel for construction, along with the development of elevators, hospitals could be built with multiple stories and occupy less ground space, a most fortunate development as city populations grew and land prices rose.

Changes in U.S. hospitals have been dramatic. "Nevertheless, the modern hospital's basic shape had been established by 1920. It had become central to medical education and was well integrated into the career patterns of regular physicians; in urban areas it had already replaced the family as the site for treating serious illness and managing death. Perhaps most important, it had already been clothed with a legitimizing aura of science and almost boundless social expectation" (Rosenberg 1987).

Hospitals are still evolving in response to technological developments, societal needs, pressure from special interest groups, payment policies, and a competitive environment.

MODERN HOSPITALS

The environment in which hospitals function is changing dramatically, forcing them to significantly change how they are organized and operated. Following World War II, the federal government encouraged the construction, expansion, and renovation of hospitals by providing grants under the Hill-Burton Act (Hospital Survey and Construction Act of 1946). The legislation provided federal aid to states under the Public Health Service Act for surveying hospitals, planning construction, and authorizing grants for the construction. Grants were designed under a formula, taking into account greater need for hospitals in the states with the poorest population. Those who received grants were required to provide matching funds. Once in operation, the institution was required, for twenty years after receiving the funds, to provide uncompensated services to those who could not pay. The results were impressive: New hospitals were built, and existing institutions were expanded and upgraded. However, the "planning" portion of the legislation fell short, and some areas of the country remained without hospitals whereas other areas became "over bedded" (Stevens 1989). In 1975, the act was amended to require grant recipients to provide uncompensated services in perpetuity (Health Resources and Services Administration 2007).

Simultaneously, the rapid growth of health insurance, followed by the introduction of Medicare and Medicaid, increased the demand for health care. Government also facilitated growth by allowing nonprofit hospitals to issue tax-exempt bonds for construction and acquisition of capital-intensive new technologies. These developments were in large measure dictated by the development of antibiotics and other new drugs, anesthetics, instrumentation, and knowledge that permitted physicians to treat what was previously untreatable, as well as to treat other patients more effectively.

By the late 1960s and early 1970s, concern began to mount over the rapidly rising cost of health care. Many states passed certificate of need (CON) legislation to prohibit the construction or expansion of hospitals unless they could prove that more beds were needed. As health care costs continued to climb dramatically, government and others encouraged shorter hospital stays and more outpatient services. Seeking to contain costs their employees incurred, corporations began to require second opinions about the necessity for surgery before insurance would cover the surgery, and they modified their health insurance policies by requiring higher co-payments and deductibles. They began to review the length of and necessity for inpatient hospital stays, and they encouraged their employees to join cost-effective health maintenance organizations (HMOs) and other alternative delivery systems. A number of state governments started to control the rates that hospitals charged. Then, in 1983, the federal government tried to slow the cost spiral by implementing prospective payment to hospitals for patients eligible for Medicare. These patients accounted for about 40 percent of hospital revenues.

As government and businesses moved to control health costs, hospitals were transformed from expanding institutions with little regard for costs (because they were largely reimbursed for them) into institutions with a declining number of patients, in an environment that had become very competitive and in which the payers were questioning the efficiency and quality of their services. To understand this shift in emphasis, it is important to understand the basic structure of the hospital field as it developed in the second half of the twentieth century, which will be the focus of the remainder of this chapter.

HOSPITAL CHARACTERISTICS

A **community hospital** is the type of hospital with which we are most familiar. Community hospitals are defined as nonfederal,

short-term (average length of stay less than thirty days), general and specialty care providers whose facilities and services are available to the public. They provide a variety of diagnostic and therapeutic services for both medical and surgical cases. Excluded from the definition of community hospitals are those hospitals not available to the general public, such as prison hospitals or college infirmaries (American Hospital Association 2006). At their most advanced development, community hospitals handle almost every kind of case; they are truly general hospitals. However, there are and always have been compromises of this ideal. In the early part of the twentieth century, it was easier for hospitals to approach the ideal because the limits of our knowledge and technology did not suggest or permit the sophisticated differentiation that we now find.

Patients with mental health issues and tuberculosis were separated, and if one goes back far enough, one finds patients with other contagious diseases isolated in special hospitals. In some communities, obstetric and gynecological cases were reserved for special women's hospitals; eye, ear, nose, and throat (EENT) cases went to EENT hospitals; and children requiring special services for severe cardiac and orthopedic problems were in separate hospitals. Many of these private hospitals later evolved into larger for-profit or nonprofit community hospitals.

Today, technology and cost largely dictate the differentiation from, and compromises on, the ideal model of a general hospital. Some medical care requires highly trained clinicians whose skills cannot be maintained unless those clinicians are employed in a large hospital with a high volume of cases. Open-heart surgery is one example. Cardiac surgeons cannot maintain their skills working solely in rural general hospitals with twenty-five beds. Cost is another issue, and a related one, for highly specialized services typically require extensive support from other hospital services. An open-heart surgery team requires, among other things, skilled technicians, diagnostic imaging, and sophisticated laboratory support. None of these could be justified clinically or economically in small general hospitals. Thus, general hospitals today are almost always compromises on the ideal, with the smaller hospitals tending to compromise more than the larger ones.

Differentiation in hospital services and structures is even more difficult to describe since the 1980s. Competition and restructuring has led to unprecedented partnering among hospitals, so much so that describing the "average" hospital or even categorizing hospitals is difficult. We therefore simply present some of the characteristics of hospitals today.

Hospital Ownership

Hospital ownership can be described in broad terms as falling into three major categories: nonprofit, for-profit, or government. These broad categories may be somewhat less definitive when we consider integrated systems with umbrella for-profit organizations owning hospitals that are nonprofit. Whatever the ownership configuration, understanding the major categories is still a worthwhile endeavor.

In 2004, there were 4,919 community hospitals, down from 5,194 in 1995, and continuing a downward trend since 1980. Of those, 2,967 were nonprofit, 835 were for-profit, and 1,117 were government hospitals (see Table 8–1). The downward trend in the number of hospitals is largest in the number of government hospitals, with slower decreases in the number of nonprofit hospitals and a somewhat consistent number of for-profit hospitals (National Center for Health Statistics 2006, Table 112).

Nonprofit Hospitals

Nonprofit (voluntary) does not mean that the hospital cannot make a profit; rather, it means that there are restrictions on what can be done with the profit. Profits must be turned back into the hospital's operation rather than distributed to shareholders. **Nonprofit hospitals** do not have shareholders; rather they have boards of trustees who serve on a voluntary basis, receiving no pay, to guide and govern the hospital. Nonprofit organizations are exempt from paying taxes, but they must follow certain criteria to qualify and remain nonprofit. Tax-exempt status must be granted on each of the government levels separately.

The federal statutes (501[C][3]) require that hospitals serve those unable to pay for services and be nonrestrictive toward physicians; that is, the facilities cannot limit participation to a particular group of physicians to the exclusion of other qualified physicians. Nonprofit hospitals' earnings also cannot be used for the benefit of any individual. Earnings must be turned back to the hospitals' operations or used for the benefit of the community. State requirements are similar to federal requirements, but each state may have specific definitions of charitable activities or of the use of revenues. Local tax-exempt status usually means property tax exemptions, and qualifications again may differ from locality to locality. All levels of tax exemption, however, do require some level of charity care or community service on the part of the hospitals.

The reliance on community business, industrial, and professional leaders to serve on hospital boards has long-standing historical roots. These people were the very ones who could provide leadership in raising funds to support the hospitals, and they underwrote hospital deficits with personal checks in a great many cases. Though the latter practice has declined sharply, community leaders still tend to dominate hospital boards (1) because of their ability to exercise influence on behalf of the hospitals, (2) because of the valued entrepreneurial skills that they apply to hospital work without cost to the hospital, and (3) because of their positions, in which they can readily allocate some of their working time to hospital activities.

Church-affiliated hospitals are often the most readily recognized nonprofit hospitals. They are different only in that they are owned, or heavily influenced by, the churches or church groups

TABLE 8-1 Hospitals, by Ownership, for Selected Years

	1980	1990	2000	2003	2004	2005
All hospitals	6,965	6,649	5,810	5,764	5,759	5,756
Federal	359	337	245	239	239	226
Nonfederal	6,606	6,312	5,565	5,525	5,520	5,530
Community	5,830	5,384	4,915	4,895	4,919	4,936
Nonprofit	3,322	3,191	3,003	2,984	2,967	2,958
For-profit	730	749	749	790	835	868
State-local government	1,778	1,444	1,163	1,121	1,117	1,110

SOURCE: National Center for Health Statistics, Health, United States, 2006, Table 112.

that sponsor them. A large number of Protestant denominations and Catholic orders and dioceses own and operate hospitals. Their roles in this field have deep historical roots. Though rooted in a religious denomination, none is discriminatory in terms of access to care (save the limitation dictated by whether or not one's physician has admitting privileges); a church hospital may, however, be sensitive to the special spiritual or dietary needs of the denomination that sponsors it.

Churches are tending to lessen the extent of their control on their hospitals. This trend is reflected in the makeup of their boards, on which nonchurch members and fewer church officials and ministers serve. This may be a reflection of the increased secularization in U.S. society, as well as recognition of the need for many other talents for the successful direction of hospitals. On the other hand, it may also be a necessity, given the decreased numbers of people joining religious orders and able to directly carry out the work of the orders.

For-Profit Hospitals

Unlike nonprofit hospitals, **for-profit hospitals** do operate with the goal of making a profit to distribute to their shareholders. The shareholders elect a board of directors to govern the hospital. Board members may or may not be compensated for their services. Responsibilities are somewhat the same as the nonprofit's board of trustees. For-profit organizations do not qualify for tax exemption, although they may provide some charity care. Because of the responsibility to shareholders and owners and the burden of paying taxes, for-profit organizations often operate more efficiently, with an eye to cost-effectiveness. For this reason, for-profit health care organizations are often criticized for paying more attention to the bottom line than to quality of care. Competitive pressures and reduced reimbursement rates, however, have made both for-profit and nonprofit hospitals more aware of the bottom line. Studies bring mixed results as to the quality of care provided by each. Accreditation, outcomes research, and a more watchful consumer eye make it difficult for any hospital to remain in operation if not providing quality care.

Among the investor-owned hospitals, corporately owned hospitals are perhaps the most visible and controversial. A number of corporations have developed that build, own, and/or operate general and specialty hospitals all over the United States. Most of the firms are small, but some are quite large. Hospital Corporation of America (HCA), for example, which is based in Nashville, Tennessee, owns 167 hospitals in the United

States (Hospital Corporation of America 2008). HealthSouth, a network of rehabilitation hospitals, owns over 150 facilities (HealthSouth 2007), and Tenet Healthcare Corporation owns 56 hospitals in 12 states (Tenet Healthcare Corporation 2008). Most of the investor-owned hospitals are members of the American Hospital Association (AHA) and are accredited by the Joint Commission (formerly the Joint Commission on Accreditation of Healthcare Organizations [JCAHO]). Some are community general hospitals; some are specialized institutions—psychiatric, drug dependency, rehabilitation, and so on. The controversy, again, is focused on the emphasis on profits versus the emphasis on quality health care delivery.

Hospital Boards

In recent years, court decisions and federal regulations caused hospital boards of trustees to become more active in their oversight role. Both for-profit and nonprofit boards are responsible for the following:

- Establishing a hospital's mission and vision
- Hiring and evaluating the performance of the hospital administrator (often called the chief executive officer or CEO)
- Appointing physicians to the medical staff
- Ensuring the quality of care delivered
- Approving long-range plans and budgets
- Monitoring performance against plans and budgets

Where for-profit and nonprofit boards differ is in their ability to sell assets or discontinue operation of the hospital. Boards of for-profit hospitals may sell assets or discontinue the operation of the business and disperse the proceeds to owners. Boards of nonprofit hospitals must follow specific regulations regarding selling or transferring assets. Any proceeds from sales must go into a nonprofit foundation and continue to be used for charitable purposes or community needs (Griffith and White 2002).

Government Hospitals

The federal government owns and operates general hospitals for clientele for whom it is responsible. Specifically, the federal government, through the Department of Defense, has over 200 total facilities, forty-seven of which are hospitals in 2008. Though some of these hospitals specialize, most are general hospitals. The Veterans Administration (VA) also has about 150 hospitals throughout the country, to care for veterans with service-connected disabilities, as well disabilities not connected to service for which the veteran cannot afford private care. Some of its hospitals are psychiatric, but most are general, with strong rehabilitation medicine services.

The Indian Health Service in the U.S. Public Health Service has forty-eight hospitals located on various Native American reservations. The government administers thirty-three and American Indian tribes and Alaskan native corporations administer the other fifteen. The U.S. Department of Justice also provides general hospital services for inmates of federal prisons.

County and city hospitals exist in many parts of the country. In large urban areas, these tend to be safety net hospitals (serving those who are poor and/or uninsured), although these hospitals now also serve private patients since the advent of Medicare and Medicaid and the growth of private health insurance. The governance of these hospitals by local government varies from the highly political to the highly professional, depending on the style or pattern of political practice in that area. In larger cities, these are frequently teaching hospitals and hospitals with strong ties to medical school. Some famous hospitals are in this group, including New York's Bellevue Hospital Center (with 912 beds), Chicago's Cook County Hospital (with 460 beds), and Los Angeles's Los Angeles County-University of Southern California Medical Center (with 984 beds) (American Hospital Directory 2008).

State governments and, in some instances, local governments have been primarily responsible for establishing facilities for the care of those with mental illness. See Chapter 10 for more information on mental health and the providers of mental health services.

HOSPITAL SIZE AND SERVICES

Hospitals may be large or small, teaching or nonteaching. The size of a hospital, typically indicated by the number of beds, depends on the size of the population served, the range of services provided, and whether it is used as a referral hospital. A small community may be able to justify only a small general hospital, just large enough to support the general run of cases (see Table 8–2). Smaller communities must also limit the range of services provided because the volume of patients may be so small in a specialized area of medicine that not enough patients would use the service to justify the expense

of developing and maintaining it. Similarly, in such cases, specialists would not have enough cases to maintain their skills. In these instances, patients would be referred to another facility that has been able to put together and maintain that service. Generally speaking, however, the larger the community served, the larger the hospital, in terms of number of beds, range of specialists, and range of supporting equipment and services (see Table 8–3).

A community hospital may also be a **teaching hospital**. Teaching hospitals are hospitals that have an approved residency program. The presence of nursing or other health professional programs in a hospital does not define it as a teaching hospital. On the other hand, a teaching hospital need not be a university hospital, but merely affiliated with a medical school accredited for medical education. Historically, most teaching hospitals were either public general hospitals for the poor, or other types of general hospitals with a large number of patients considered indigent. These patients were those on whom medical students, interns, and residents learned. The patients, in a sense, paid for their care by allowing their bodies to be used for medical training purposes. Patients who are poor frequently resented this form of payment, and they often looked upon the hospital as the place where "they" experimented on patients. In part, this perception by those who were poor contributed to the development of Medicaid, under which all people are entitled to private care. However, by that time (1966), the practice of teaching hospitals had changed, and all patients, paying as well as indigent, were patients on which students learned. Teaching hospitals became known for their advanced technology and expert practitioners and, as a result, became the centers of choice for many patients.

Hospitals can also be described as allopathic or osteopathic institutions. Although the allopathic-oriented institutions predominate in this country, the same types of hospital standards also apply to hospitals that were established to serve osteopaths (DOs). The separation has historical roots that go back to the time when neither would relate to the other school of medicine. However, times have changed, and now osteopaths serve on the staffs of allopathic institutions, and MDs serve on the staffs of osteopathic hospitals. In some communities, these institutions have merged.

Children's hospitals are community hospitals dealing specifically with chronic, congenital, and/or acute childhood diseases. Whether needed surgical care is performed in these hospitals or in other institutions varies. Advances in technology and

TABLE 8-2 Number of Hospitals, Beds, and Occupancy Rates by Ownership, Bed Size, and Occupancy Rates, 2004

Hospitals by Bed Size	Number of Hospitals	Number of Beds	Occupancy Rate
Community	4,919	808,127	67.0%
Nonprofit	2,967	567,863	68.3%
For-profit	835	112,693	60.5%
State-local government	1,117	127,571	66.4%
6–24 beds	352	6,030	33.8%
25–49 beds	988	33,206	45.8%
50–99 beds	1,028	73,606	58.0%
100–199 beds	1,141	162,914	63.5%
200–299 beds	621	151,197	67.2%
300–399 beds	351	120,509	69.7%
400–499 beds	185	82,071	70.4%
500 beds or more	253	178,594	75.3%

SOURCE: National Center for Health Statistics, Health, United States, 2006, Table 112.

scientific medicine generally dictate a close affiliation with other hospitals to benefit from the latest instrumentation and essential supporting specialties and services.

Maternity hospitals, women's hospitals, EENT hospitals, and other specialty hospitals still retain a significant presence in health care delivery. Cancer treatment hospitals are perhaps the newest specialty hospitals on the rise.

TABLE 8-3 U.S. Community Hospitals, by Location for Selected Years

Location	1999	2000	2001	2002	2003	2005
Urban Hospitals	2,767	2,740	2,741	2,749	2,729	2,927
Rural Hospitals	2,189	2,175	2,167	2,178	2,166	2,009

SOURCE: American Hospital Association. 2005. AHA hospital statistics, 2005. Chicago, IL: Health Forum; and American Hospital Association. 2007. *TrendWatch Chartbook, 2007: Trends affecting hospitals and health systems.*

MULTIHOSPITAL SYSTEMS

The future of many hospitals (especially small, rural hospitals) may well depend in large part on the concept of regionalization, whereby small hospitals affiliate with larger, more urban hospitals. Under regionalization, each level of hospital (the small rural hospital, the moderate-sized hospital, and the large regional referral center) provides only those services that it is able to provide efficiently and effectively. Thus, small rural hospitals provide basic general care; moderate-sized hospitals provide more specialized care and equipment; and regional hospitals provide the most sophisticated and expensive special types of care. Patients have access to a full range of services and are admitted or transferred to the appropriate level of hospital according to their medical needs. With this type of arrangement, hospitals avoid duplicate expensive services, obtain consultation assistance from medical personnel in larger hospitals, and have the advantages of sharing certain support services, such as human resources departments and purchasing departments. The affiliations range from an informal regional working agreement to a merger of institutions into multihospital or multi-institutional systems with a single, coordinated management structure. Many European countries have regionalized their hospital systems to provide hospital services more efficiently. The occasional hesitancy of small institutions in this country to enter into more formal regional agreements stems from a long-standing desire for local control, coupled with a fear that arrangements will serve the financial and occupancy rate needs of the higher-level institution at the expense of smaller institutions.

Advances in telemedicine make it possible for small rural institutions to bring needed expertise to patients' bedsides without bringing costly services into institutions. Regional affiliations make telemedicine and technology diffusion possible and plausible.

Regionalization is not the only motivation for hospital affiliations. Competition and the pressures of managed care contribute to the affiliation frenzy. Nationwide, the numbers of multihospital systems are changing rapidly, with disassociations occurring almost as rapidly as new affiliations. One needs only to go to nationally recognized newspapers (*The New York Times, The Wall Street Journal, The Washington Post*, and so on) to read about changes in affiliation that occur on an almost daily basis. The cost-effectiveness of such ventures is unknown. Promises of consolidation of services fall into low levels of priority when local needs and cultures are taken into account. The entire process is still in a high degree of uncertainty. In 2004, fifty-nine announced mergers or acquisitions involved over 200 hospitals; in 2005, fifty-one announced mergers or acquisitions involved eighty-eight hospitals (American Hospital Association 2007).

HOSPITAL STATISTICS

The most reliable source for data about hospitals is the American Hospital Association (AHA). Each year, the AHA conducts a survey of "all hospitals—registered and nonregistered, in the U.S. and its associated areas . . . with an average response rate of 85 percent" (American Hospital Association 2005, xxxi). Not all registered hospitals are accredited by the Joint Commission, nor are they required to be members of the AHA. In lieu of accreditation, hospitals do have to be licensed and meet a specific list of criteria published by the AHA, such as maintaining at least six inpatient beds, an organized medical staff, continuous nursing services, a pharmacy service supervised by a registered pharmacist, a governing authority and chief executive, up-to-date and complete medical records on each patient, and so on (American Hospital Association 2005).

The AHA's publication *Hospital Statistics* provides useful current and trend data on hospital utilization, personnel, and finances. Other AHA publications provide information on individual hospitals, networks, and systems, as well as lists of organizations, agencies, and providers.

The National Center for Health Statistics (NCHS) of the Centers for Disease Control and Prevention (CDC), and the Center for Medicare and Medicaid Services (CMS) also provide reports and publications related not only to hospitals but also to other components of the health field.

HOSPITAL ORGANIZATION AND ADMINISTRATION

The governing boards of hospitals not only establish policies for the institutions but also hire administrators. The word *administrator* is used in a generic sense. Some hospitals designate the top administrative person as president, chief executive officer (CEO), or executive director. The training and experience of the administrator may vary greatly by size and location of the hospital. Today, many hospital administrators have a master's degree in health administration (MHA) or business administration (MBA). Some administrators have PhDs, whereas others are MDs or DOs. Whatever the formal education structure, administrators must also possess a wide range of experience in the health care field.

Administrators are responsible for carrying out the strategic plan developed by the board and the day-to-day operation of the facilities. It is important for administrators to align themselves with qualified personnel in finance, human resources management, and other management skills while having the ability to work with the medical staff and other clinical managers. Griffith and White (2002) categorize the responsibilities of administrators into four functional areas: to lead, support, represent, and organize (p. 115). As such, administrators are responsible not only for the internal functioning of the organizations, but for their roles, images, and responsibilities in and to their communities.

The organizational functioning of a hospital is not as clear-cut as it is in business and industry. The lines of authority are not precise (see Figure 8–1). Organizational lines of authority are even more difficult to define in multihospital systems (see Figure 8–2). Boards appoint administrators. Boards also appoint

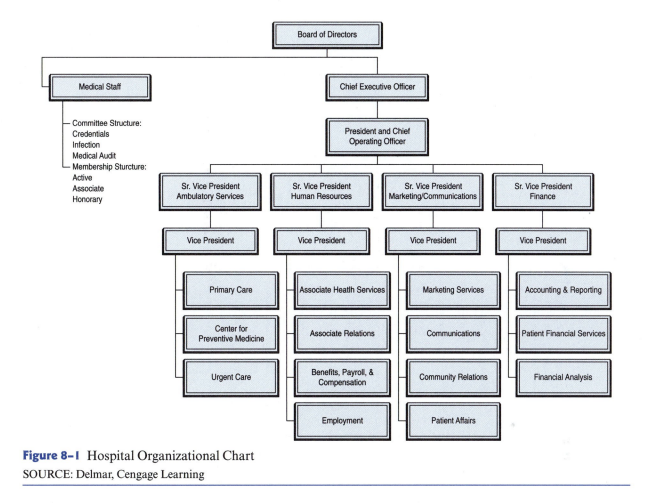

Figure 8–1 Hospital Organizational Chart
SOURCE: Delmar, Cengage Learning

the medical staff. Membership on the medical staff allows physicians to admit patients and continue to treat them and call in specialists as needed. Though the medical staff is technically accountable to the board, it has a daily functional relationship with the administrator. Nursing service is administratively accountable to the administrator but professionally accountable to the medical staff. Other personnel, such as pharmacists, lab and X-ray technicians, and dietitians, are also administratively accountable to the administrator but professionally accountable to the medical staff.

Hospitals are really physicians' workshops, although some argue that they are also centers for meeting all community health needs. However, only physicians can admit patients (except in a few circumscribed areas in which other health professionals hold admitting and treatment privileges), and all others must act

on physicians' orders. However, physicians typically do not hire or fire unless they are employed as members of the hospital's medical staff. Even then, a physician's authority is circumscribed by a certain accountability to the administrator.

Physicians are the driving forces in hospitals. They ask that certain procedures be done for patients and that certain supplies or equipment be purchased. Administrators, the nurses, and others working with the administrators must cooperate to the greatest extent possible with the physicians. Since the 1980s, with additional cost-containment imperatives in place, third-party payers and the utilization review process have added difficulty to the hospital personnel decision-making equation. Conflicts occur: Personality clashes, misunderstandings, and insufficient funds create problems. The various parties try to resolve differences, figure out ways to obtain the needed funds,

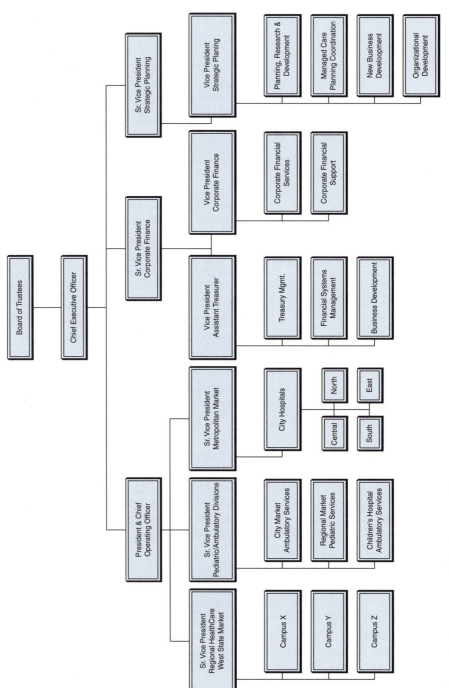

Figure 8-2 Integrated Health Care Delivery System

SOURCE: Delmar, Cengage Learning

and reach agreement on outstanding issues. When the medical staff and administrator cannot resolve differences, the board must enter to decide.

Most hospitals minimize tensions between hospital governing boards and the medical staff by having a physician represent the medical staff as a member of the board. Hospitals depend on physicians to refer patients to them and fill their hospital beds. An individual physician may have admitting privileges at several hospitals. The physician and patient choose the hospital to which the patient will be admitted. Administrators try to make their hospital the most attractive to the physician by making the dealings with the hospital convenient and pleasant. Attempting to meet this objective sometimes means obtaining equipment the physicians want or prefer. At times, physicians and hospitals compete with each other as both develop and expand outpatient services, such as freestanding ambulatory and diagnostic centers, to improve their financial status.

Hospitals are changing their organizational structure to a corporate model and are calling themselves medical centers to create fiscal flexibility at a time when government programs are placing greater constraints upon hospitals. The corporate model permits a hospital to set up profit-making operations, such as a medical office building or a freestanding clinic, with the profits kept completely separate from hospital operations and thus not taken into account by government, insurance companies, and business coalitions as they compare hospital costs and quality. In other words, for-profit operations cannot be counted as an offset against losses in hospital operations, such as in care of those who are poor or who have no insurance or Medicaid protection. The profits are then free for use as the overall governing body sees fit. Corporate restructuring is a rapidly developing phenomenon, although Congress has considered legislation to curtail such profit-making activities by nonprofit organizations, with much opposition from the AHA. To date, such mixed corporate structuring continues to operate. Government is concerned about antitrust issues, but is also concerned about lowering health care costs. The two issues may sometimes collide.

Despite the varieties and complexities of hospital organization, the board delegates to the medical staff retain certain professional responsibilities. These responsibilities are typically described by the medical staff bylaws, which the board approves. More importantly, however, the smooth functioning of the hospital can be attributed to improved quality of administration, which comes with the introduction of sound management practices and appropriately trained administrators.

Medical Staff Privileges

The board also grants admitting and practice privileges to physicians and others, usually on recommendation of the medical staff. Physicians apply to a hospital for **staff privileges**.[2] If the hospital is a closed–group practice hospital, then the only way to become part of the hospital staff is to be accepted by the medical group. Hospital bylaws define how physicians may secure admitting privileges. Typically, in community general hospitals, physicians who seek privileges make applications to the board. The board typically seeks the advice of its credentialing committee (which includes members of the medical staff), which judges the applicant's qualifications and character and makes a recommendation. The decision about appointment to the medical staff is based on a variety of factors, including current state licensure, board certification status, medical school education, residency training, written recommendations, malpractice insurance coverage and history, and the type of privileges sought.

The Health Care Quality Improvement Act of 1986 mandated that hospitals query the National Practitioner Data Bank for information on each new appointment to the medical staff and once every two years for existing medical staff. The data bank legislation requires malpractice insurers to report "all medical malpractice payments they make on behalf of physicians and dentists." It also requires hospitals, state licensure boards, professional societies, and other health care organizations to report adverse actions they take against physicians. The purpose of the data bank is to provide protection to the public from incompetent physicians (Yessian and Greenleaf 1997). Prior to the establishment of a national system, physicians who had lost their licenses could simply move to another state and establish a practice without their previous history becoming known to the community.

The larger and more complex the hospital is, the more precisely defined the admitting privileges are. In some remote rural hospitals, a family practitioner may be doing general medical care, reading electrocardiograms, handling obstetrics, and

---

[2] Hospital privileges may also be dictated by state law, other government regulations, or local custom. Although dentists, podiatrists, chiropractors, midwives, and others may have staff privileges in some hospitals, physicians are those most generally recognized as professionals on the medical staff. References are made to physicians' privileges for the sake of simplicity.

performing a variety of surgical procedures. The same physician in a large urban teaching hospital might be restricted to carefully circumscribed family practice privileges.

Staff privileges fall into several categories. The active medical staff consists of those physicians accorded all rights, privileges, and responsibilities. They provide most of the care, offer leadership in various committees, and may hold a variety of medical staff offices. Associate medical staff members are the more junior physicians, or those who wish to become active staff when vacancies occur. They may have limited access to beds for their patients. Courtesy medical staff is the category for those physicians who seek the privilege of admitting only occasional patients and who do not wish to become part of the active staff, either because the bulk of their admissions are to other hospitals or because they do not have practices that necessitate frequent admission of patients. The consulting medical staff consists of those who serve primarily as specialty consultants to members of the active staff. In some types of cases, for example, the law, or hospital or medical staff bylaws, may require an attending physician to secure consultation, and this staff is available in the event an appropriate consultant is not on the active or associate staff.

The bylaws—rules and regulations—and offices of the medical staff organization vary from hospital to hospital. Typically, however, a chief of staff or medical director is elected by the medical staff for a fixed term and represents the staff's interests to the board and to the hospital administration. This is the formal line for communication, particularly on major issues, but hospitals also have a wide informal mechanism that functions as the rule. Whether a physician is an employee of the hospital varies within organizations. Full-time salaried physicians, other than radiologists, pathologists, anesthesiologists, and emergency department physicians, are usually found in the larger teaching hospitals. When a hospital has divided its staff into clinical departments or services, each clinical area typically has a chief of service, and each chief of service reports to the chief of staff.

Clinical and Supporting Departments

The clinical organization of the general hospital varies depending on its size, the pattern of patient mix among the various specialties, and the extent of specialization of the medical staff. Except in very small hospitals, obstetrics tends to be segregated in a separate wing or on a separate floor of the hospital, along with the newborn nursery. This is done to minimize the risk of infection to newborns and mothers; unfortunately, these units have become locked units to prevent abduction of newborns.

Pediatric cases also tend to be segregated. The assignment of other patients to clinical services or departments varies considerably. If there is any division of patients into separate departments in the smaller hospitals, it tends to be divided into medicine and surgery, with patient assignment as appropriate.

As specialization increases in a hospital and the volume of patients increases within each specialty, departments tend to be established with beds assigned to that specialty. When the volume of patients is sufficient to justify it, the specialty beds may be located in a separate wing or on a separate floor. The establishment of specialty services with assigned beds permits a more effective and efficient concentration of support services peculiar to that specialty (equipment, specially trained nurses, and other personnel) and contributes to the development of the specialty and its scientific work. Assignment of beds to a given specialty has clinical advantages; however, it decreases institutional flexibility in terms of bed use.

In a general hospital, the emergency department (sometimes called emergency room) and the outpatient—or ambulatory services—department have increased importance. Their functions and importance are described in more detail in Chapter 7.

Some of the larger teaching hospitals have departments of family medicine. These departments serve as family physician to a community or to an enrolled group, and they ensure admission to that hospital when necessary. The department of family medicine also serves as a training area for future primary care physicians.

Supporting the patient care services are three medically supervised departments: anesthesiology, radiology, and pathology. In smaller hospitals, part-time specialists staff these services; in larger hospitals, however, the specialists work full-time. They may be paid by salary or fee for service, or the services may be contracted out to independent group practices. Both radiology and pathology are rapidly expanding departments, owing to rapidly developing technology. Anesthesiology services are often staffed by one anesthesiologist supervising a larger number of nurse anesthetists.

All hospitals have a number of other support services. Whether or not they have departmental status depends on the size of the institution and the rationale of those responsible for establishing the organizational arrangements. Some of these services are nursing, pharmacy, health information management (medical records), and dietary. Larger hospitals also have such services as inhalation therapy, physical therapy, occupational therapy, and medical social work.

Increasingly, hospitals are seeking new ways to cope with rising costs. Services shared with other hospitals—such as laundry, purchasing, and computer services—are methods of cost control. Whether a hospital participates in a given shared service or purchases the service from an outside firm depends on whether the hospital's needs can be adequately met and whether it is economically advantageous. Some hospitals find it advantageous to contract to outside firms for services such as food, security, and housekeeping, and even for nurses and other personnel.

HOSPITAL LICENSURE AND ACCREDITATION

Hospitals are licensed to operate by state governments. Each state has its own requirements, but all states' requirements are similar. Originally, the various states focused their attention for licensure on hospital physical plants—for example, fire safety, heating, space allocations, and sanitation. Now, however, states have moved beyond this and are beginning to pay more attention to professional standards, often by defaulting to Joint Commission accreditation (see the following section) as a criterion for licensure.

As noted previously, the American College of Surgeons (ACS) suppressed its 1919 hospital inspection report because the conditions it found were so poor. The ACS and the American Medical Association (AMA), however, have worked consistently for reform of hospitals. Though they were concerned with physical plants, as were the states, these professional bodies were also concerned with matters relating to quality of care. Their efforts at reform culminated in 1952, with the initiation of a hospital accreditation program by the Joint Commission on Accreditation of Hospitals (JCAH).

Joint Commission

The history of the Joint Commission goes back to 1913, when the American College of Surgeons (ACS) was formed. Almost immediately, the ACS embarked upon a hospital standardization program when it found that more than half of the applicants for fellowship in the ACS had to be rejected because the case records they were required to submit were inadequate. ACS developed the minimum standard for approval, and more than half of the hospitals in the United States met the minimum standard by 1950. In 1951, the American College of Physicians, the American Hospital Association, the American Medical Association, and the Canadian Medical Association joined the ACS to form the Joint Commission on Accreditation of Hospitals (JCAH), which offered accreditation to hospitals that applied and complied with its standards. In 1959, the Canadian Medical Association withdrew to participate in its own program, and, in 1979, the American Dental Association became a member of the ACS board of commissioners. In 1966, the Joint Commission, in a major policy decision, changed the standards it used for accreditation from the minimal essential standards for proper patient care to the optimal achievable standards.

As other health organizations developed, the Joint Commission became the accreditation body for them. In 1987, JCAH changed its name to the Joint Commission on the Accreditation of Healthcare Organizations (JCAHO). Now known simply as the "Joint Commission," this "independent, not-for-profit organization sets standards and accredits nearly 15,000 health care organizations in the United States, including hospitals and health care organizations that provide home care, long-term care, behavioral health care, laboratory, and ambulatory care services" (Joint Commission 2007a).

The Joint Commission is governed by a board of commissioners of twenty-nine members composed of nurses, physicians, consumers, medical directors, administrators, providers, employers, labor representatives, health plan leaders, quality experts, ethicists, health insurance administrators, and educators. Among its corporate members are representatives from the American College of Physicians, the American College of Surgeons, the American Dental Association, the American Hospital Association, and the American Medical Association. Seeking accreditation is voluntary; hospitals and other health care organizations apply for accreditation and request an on-site survey. A variety of health care providers are employed by the Joint Commission to conduct the accreditation on-site surveys. The survey team assesses the extent of a hospital's compliance with the Joint Commission's standards by gathering data regarding the organization's activities.

Accreditation is not based simply on the physical environment, such as fire safety, sanitation, and bed space. It is also based on performance in functional areas, such as patients' rights, quality of care, standards for providers, patient-nurse ratios, and outcomes measures. The findings of the survey team are reported to the board of commissioners, which makes the accreditation decision. Site visits take place at least every three years for most organizations and at least every two years for laboratories. Accreditation categories include accredited, provisional accreditation, conditional accreditation, preliminary denial of accreditation, and preliminary accreditation. Those organizations receiving status other than "accreditation" may have certain deficiencies to correct and a specific time period to do so to receive accreditation or qualify for another on-site visit (Joint Commission 2007b).

Accreditation is important for health care organizations, and hospitals in particular, in many ways. Accreditation may fulfill all or part of the state licensing requirements, most health insurance company participation requirements, Medicare and Medicaid certification requirements, and managed care organization contract requirements. In addition, voluntary accreditation enhances consumer and community confidence, medical staff recruitment, quality of care, and staff education. Finally, the accreditation process provides an opportunity for organizations to assess their strong and weak features and make improvements.

The basic question accreditation has answered is: Can this organization provide quality health care? The accreditation process has traditionally focused primarily on organizational structure, processes, and equipment. Now the Joint Commission has moved beyond determining an institution's capability of providing quality care to answer the question: Does this organization provide safe, culturally competent health care? It developed ORYX, a computerized database system, to integrate the use of outcomes and other clinical indicators into the accreditation process.

Although the Joint Commission has contributed much to the improved quality of care in hospitals, many have been critical of its activities, claiming that the organization is not inclined to publicize poor medical care or to strip hospitals of accreditation. The Joint Commission sees its inspections as an educational device for improving performance rather than for removing accreditation. However, Medicare and Medicaid reimbursements depend on accreditation, and the federal government expects certain standards to be fulfilled if hospitals are accredited. In the early 1990s, Health Care Financing Administration (HCFA; now CMS) found that many accredited hospitals did not meet Medicare conditions of participation. Criticisms caused the Joint Commission to create an additional category of "conditional accreditation" and impose stricter timetables for improvement and release of limited information to the federal government about those hospitals that do not meet the standards. The Joint Commission website provides a directory of hospitals and their accreditation status and other general information regarding size, financial status, and the like at www.qualitycheck.org/consumer/searchQCR.aspx.

Other Performance Evaluators

Hospitals have been interested in their efficiency, quality of care, and performance in relation to other hospitals for many years. In 1950, the Kellogg Foundation awarded a grant to the Southwestern Michigan Hospital Council to assist the study of professional activities in hospitals through inter-hospital comparisons of hospital statistical reports. The project was known as the Professional Activity Study (PAS). At the heart of PAS are the medical abstracts of all hospitalized patients in participating hospitals, which permit a hospital to review its performance over a period of time by such factors as the type of service for which the patient was admitted, final diagnosis, length of stay, type of surgery, and name of physician. Reports are prepared for hospitals monthly, semiannually, and annually. The initial PAS studies resulted in establishment of the Commission on Professional and Hospital Activities to assist in evaluating such activities.

Employers, as major purchasers of health care for their employees, compare costs for hospital care but are also interested in the quality of the care provided. Under ERISA (the Employee Retirement Income Security Act; see Chapter 3), many employers self-insure, so evaluating cost and quality becomes even a more direct issue. Many states have begun incentives to help employers, insurers, and others evaluate the performance of hospitals and other health care providers. One of the first such state incentives was the Pennsylvania Health Care Cost Containment Council (PHC4) created in 1986. The purpose of the council is to promote health care cost containment, promote the public interest by encouraging the development of competitive health care services, and ensure that all citizens have reasonable access to quality health care. PHC4 developed a computerized system for the collection, analysis, and dissemination of data. The data reflect the effectiveness of provider quality and services for specific treatment categories. Data collected and analyzed may include such information as the number of cases in the category, severity level at admission, length of stay, discharge condition (mortality), and cost of care, which are compared to expected results (benchmarking). PHC4 issues special reports developed from the data analysis and makes the raw data available to any purchaser requesting it.

Health care purchasers are enthusiastic about having such information available when contracting for care, but hospitals have mixed responses. Although they find the information valuable, they also point out causes of wide variation in results that may not be captured by the data. Other states have followed through with similar outcomes measurements (Sessa 1992). Coalitions of employers in larger communities are asking health care organizations to provide data that will help the coalition to do similar analysis.

HOSPITAL COSTS

We hear a great deal about rising health care costs, and in particular about rising hospital costs—and not without cause. The American Hospital Association provides figures on inpatient expenses, adjusted per inpatient day and adjusted per inpatient stay. In 1980, for example, the average cost of an inpatient day was $245, and the average cost of a hospital stay was $1,851. For 1990, the cost was $687 per day and $4,947 per stay. By 2005, the figures stood at $1,522 per day and $8,535 per stay (see Table 8–4) (National Center for Health Statistics 2007). The increased costs have been a concern of the industry because the phenomenal growth of private health insurance has increasingly been paid as an employee fringe benefit, forcing price increases in industrial products. Since the introduction of Medicare and Medicaid, the government has fretted over cost increases because they force politically unpopular tax increases.

Three factors account for most of the rise in hospital costs and in health costs generally. The first major factor is the increase in population. We simply have a growing population. The population is, moreover, an aging population that requires more, longer, and costlier types of care.

The second major factor is inflation. Everything costs more—drugs, linens, food, fuel, and personnel. More than half of a hospital's budget is consumed by its payroll, and because it is a heavy employer of unskilled labor, hospital labor costs jump accordingly when the federally mandated minimum wage goes up. Similarly, hospital payroll costs overall have risen in recent years as mandated contributions to the Social Security system have risen.

The third major factor in hospital and health care cost increases is new technology and new services. As a result of scientific advances, we are able to do more things to help people than heretofore. However, the price of new technology is high. Not only is the equipment expensive, but the personnel needed to operate it is also costly. A more educated population results in greater demand for health care. This does not necessarily equate to realistic demands. Technology may contribute to a belief that any disease can be cured (resulting in higher costs) rather than a commitment to healthier lifestyles, prevention, and screening (lower costs).

Every few years, there is a new controversy in the health field, a controversy that arises from new technology. The new technology permits more life-saving, more effective clinical management, or better diagnosis. Cardiac care advances, computed tomography (CT), magnetic resonance imaging (MRI), laser therapy, transplantation, and chemotherapy each occupied center stage at one time because of high cost and the alleged desire of all hospitals to develop the new service.

Those who are most concerned about rising health costs often cite the "duplication" of very costly equipment and services, and they are most critical of what they perceive to be competition among hospitals to be the first with the new technology, as well as the desire of other institutions to keep up with the hospital that is first. This rhetoric fails to recognize some very important points and does a disservice to hospitals. What is perceived as duplication may be simple recognition by the hospital that new technology enhances quality patient care and physician efficiency. In some cases, hospitals share costly medical equipment, such as an MRI or CT scanner, by installing it in a mobile van that moves from one hospital to another. This helps hospitals to use it efficiently, to have the technology available locally, and to contain costs.

Even when it is feasible to share facilities and high-tech equipment, a very good case can be made for duplication and the resulting excess capacity. Having technology available in the hospital where the physician practices, rather than having to schedule its use in another hospital, is very convenient and can contribute to excellence in medical care. In a competitive environment, hospitals are inclined to acquire technology to survive. Only the providers of comprehensive services will "win" case management (managed care) contracts. Under such exclusive contracting, some providers will win and some will

TABLE 8-4 Community Hospital Expenses, United States, for Selected Years

Year	1980	1990	2000	2004	2005
Patient expenses per day	$245	$687	$1,149	$1,450	$1,522
Patient expenses per stay	$1,851	$4,947	$6,649	$8,166	$8,535

SOURCE: National Center for Health Statistics, Health, United States, 2007.

lose, but all will attempt to provide a wide range of services rather than default to competitors.

Technology has spread despite the efforts of government and the health-planning agencies. These bodies slowed the process somewhat, but eventually the technology spread basically because the public wanted it, and its acquisition was facilitated historically by cost-based reimbursement to hospitals. It may be fashionable to place the blame for rising costs on physicians, who are accused of providing treatment indiscriminately, and on hospitals, for their overall inefficiencies. Demand from regulators and consumers for quality care and access to all members of the community places technology development and diffusion at odds with cost-control efforts.

Certificate of need (CON) legislation, utilization review, and the shifting of more costs to patients have also been employed to contain costs, but the costs continue to rise. The federal government made the most dramatic attempt to slow the rise in hospital costs when it introduced its prospective payment system (PPS) for hospital patients covered by Medicare, with fixed payments based on assignment of each patient's diagnosis to a diagnosis-related group (DRG). Efforts to control costs are described in the sections that follow.

Peer Review Organizations

Since the advent of Medicare and Medicaid, government has assumed an increasing share of the costs of medical care, and the costs have risen rapidly. The initial legislation for Medicare in 1965 required utilization review; in 1967, this was extended to Medicaid. Peer review, in its initiation, focused on assuring medical necessity. The review process emphasized quantity rather than quality and was accomplished by retrospective review of records by physicians and largely handled within the hospitals themselves. The process was ineffective in controlling costs.

The 1971 amendments to the Social Security Act mandated the development of professional standards review organizations (PSROs), an attempt by HCFA (now CMS) to formalize the review process and give assurance that services paid for under Medicare and Medicaid were medically necessary, of high quality, and delivered at the lowest possible cost. HCFA went on to note that these objectives, though complementary, were sometimes in conflict because the medical profession tended to stress the quality assurance element, whereas Congress seemed more interested in the cost-control element.

More than 185 PSROs developed throughout the country. A major part of their work entailed **preadmission review** and **concurrent review** of hospital admissions: On the basis of physician-established criteria for hospital admission, admissions certified as appropriate were certified for a specific number of days, the number depending on the diagnosis and the norms for that area. The PSROs also reviewed admissions that went beyond the norm. The actual review of cases was largely delegated by the PSROs to the respective hospital utilization review committees.

In addition to preadmission and concurrent review activities, PSROs carried out a variety of retrospective studies on quality of care, utilization, and patterns of care that served in part as a basis for the criteria employed in concurrent review. Because the rising costs of Medicare and Medicaid were a significant problem for both federal and state governments, the emphasis on cost efficiency was increasingly impressed upon the agencies, but the results of PSRO efforts were mixed. In early 1978, the president's Office of Management and Budget (OMB) proposed that PSRO funding be deleted from the budget request to Congress because of a Department of Health, Education, and Welfare (HEW) study showing that PSROs had no significant effect on reducing costs and did not contribute significantly to increased quality of care. OMB's view did not prevail; however, congressional dissatisfaction was evident in that the appropriation for 1979 fiscal funds provided for hospital review activities but not enough for the reviews that Congress had earlier directed for ambulatory and long-term care.

In October 1978, the PSROs came under criticism from the General Accounting Office (GAO). The GAO criticized the salary schedules for PSRO executive directors that HEW had issued. The GAO also felt that there was room for improvement of PSRO efficiency in terms of combining some administrative staffs and functions, given the fact that twenty-one states had more than a single PSRO. In those twenty-one states, there were 164 PSROs. A month later, HCFA released a new evaluation that it felt demonstrated PSRO effectiveness in both cost containment and cost control. However, costs were still going up, and the drive to abolish PSROs continued. In 1981, the funding for some agencies was cut off, and the administration again sought to abolish all PSROs. Congress resisted and came forth with a compromise, agreeing to replace the large number of PSROs with a much smaller number of peer review organizations (PROs) that would be responsible for quality control but would also focus more vigorously on controlling hospital costs of patients covered by Medicare.

PROs were now required to review care of all cases in which a patient covered by Medicare was readmitted to a hospital less than thirty-one days after the most recent discharge, as well as to review all written patient complaints (Lohr and Schroeder 1990). If detected, unnecessary care is classified into severity levels with appropriate sanctions on the attending physician and hospital. The basics of the severity levels are as follows:

- Level I: without potential for significant adverse effects
- Level II: with potential for significant adverse effects (but none occurred)
- Level III: with significant adverse effects on the patient

Sanctions move from notification and education, to withholding of payment, to loss of the right to participate with the Medicare and Medicaid programs.

A PRO is an external organization that successfully bids for a contract with CMS to carry out the required peer review functions; thus, peer review is no longer simply left to the hospital to conduct on its own. Hospitals, however, continue to maintain their own utilization review departments to monitor compliance with rules of CMS and other regulatory bodies. Because Congress has been concerned with quality of care as well as cost, it has continually expanded the duties of PROs. By 1987, PROs were required to review the quality of care in HMOs, nursing homes, ambulatory care settings, and hospitals. New emphasis for review includes preadmission and concurrent review, a focus on variations from the standards, and education to communicate desirable processes and outcomes. As internal utilization review has become stronger, many PROs now spend more time and emphasis on data collection and evaluation to work with organizations to establish quality standards and reduce variation.

Certificate of Need

Another approach to curbing rising health care costs has been to require health facilities to secure from state government a certificate of need (CON) for major capital expenditures and major expansions in services. Rising costs had been tied to duplication of services. The National Health Planning and Resource Development Act of 1974 required that states develop regulations setting a dollar amount (typically in the millions of dollars) above which a facility had to secure a CON for new services, beds, or equipment. The legislation also provided funding for new health systems agencies that were required to develop plans for health resource and health status needs for the population residing within the health services areas (Stevens 1989). CON programs peaked in the 1970s, but their effectiveness was questioned. Organizations learned creative ways to

bypass regulation, such as breaking large projects into smaller components to avoid CON review. Politics entered into the approval process because board members were often members of the community in which the project might be requested. Failure to approve a hospital project might mean loss of hospital administration support for other community projects. Members of the community were also hesitant to block a project that might bring more jobs into their community.

In 1987, Congress repealed the CON requirement but allowed the states to continue CON programs if they wished to use their own criteria. Many states continued CON programs; however, many hospitals opposed them, stating that they should be revised to eliminate bureaucratic red tape and delays so that health care organizations can respond quickly in a climate of increasing competition and eroding profits. In 2007, thirty-six states and the District of Columbia still had CON programs in force (American Health Planning Association 2007). Some health care organizations oppose CON programs as being politicized, poorly managed, costly, and ineffective; advocates believe that some regulation is necessary, especially in areas where the population is growing. Whatever its merits, it is clear that the certificate of need has not been effective in controlling costs.

PAYMENT OF HOSPITAL COSTS

Hospitals have historically been paid by most insurance and government programs on a retrospective cost or near-cost basis; that is, they were paid after the costs were incurred. Some private insurance programs even paid whatever the hospital charged, which could be higher than costs. These methods of payment did not encourage hospitals to operate efficiently or to economize. The very nature of these retrospective systems was an inducement to do more and keep patients in the hospital longer. Though physicians made these clinical decisions, neither they nor the hospital had any reason to take into account the cost of care. As the costs of Medicare continued to rise rapidly, there was serious concern about the solvency of the Medicare program, and the federal government sought new ways to contain costs and increase its control over hospital payments.

In 1984, the federal government instituted a PPS based on DRGs. The primary objective of the PPS was to change the economic incentives of hospitals under the Medicare program by offering strong encouragement to reduce hospital costs. As predicted, the introduction of this system brought about

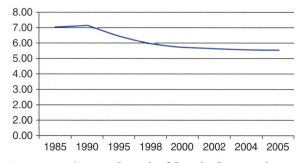

Figure 8–3 Average Length of Stay in Community Hospitals, for Selected Years

SOURCE: American Hospital Association. 2007. *TrendWatch Chartbook, 2007: Trends affecting hospitals and health systems,* Table 3–1.

important changes in hospitals, the medical profession, and the entire health care sector. For the first time in the history of Medicare, there was a decline in the number of discharges (which means that fewer people were hospitalized) and in the length of stay for hospital inpatients (see Figure 8–3).

Occupancy rates in both urban and rural hospitals declined as hospitals worked to discharge patients as early as possible under PPS. The total average occupancy rate for all community hospitals went from 77.3 percent in 1970, to 62.8 percent in 1995 (see Figure 8–4). However, as with hospital admissions, the occupancy rate began to increase slightly and was 67 percent in 2005 (National Center for Health Statistics 2007).

Although it may be true that patients are discharged sicker than prior to PPS, what went along with those early discharges was a greater dependency on discharges to rehabilitation facilities,

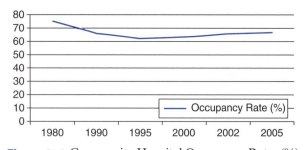

Figure 8–4 Community Hospital Occupancy Rates (%)

SOURCE: National Center for Health Statistics. 2007. *Health United States, 2007, with chartbook on trends in the health of Americans,* Table 113. MD: Hyattsville.

home health care, and other facilities that are less costly than hospitals. Most hospitals have employed discharge planners to facilitate the discharge of patients from acute care hospitals to appropriate post-hospital services. Virtually all hospital discharge planners initially reported difficulties in placing patients in skilled nursing facilities, primarily because of restrictions in Medicare rules and regulations regarding eligibility and coverage, and because of the shortage of such beds (U.S. General Accounting Office 1987). Over 85 percent of the discharge planners surveyed also reported problems with home health care placement because of Medicare rules and regulations. Since the early 1980s, however, the number of nursing homes and home health agencies has increased. In addition, Medicare's payment structures have been modified (see Chapter 10). Thus, as the PPS reduces hospital costs, it exacerbates problems in other health care sectors.

Occupancy rates have also been affected by new technologies. Since the early 1980s, many procedures previously requiring an inpatient stay have been possible on an outpatient basis. Not all of these procedures are done outside of the hospital; however, outpatient care does not factor into occupancy rates. Occupancy rates consider only inpatient admissions, discharges, and beds.

The move from inpatient to outpatient therapy was not optional. Medicare, and other insurers, targeted certain procedures as payable only if done on an outpatient basis. Hospitals were compliant because outpatient payments were higher than inpatient payments and provided the hospital with a new source of revenue. Units with empty beds were consolidated, and space was converted to more profitable outpatient services.

PPS and technology both contributed to a reduction in hospital admissions—from 35,155,000 in 1984, to 30,945,357 in 1995. However, since 1996, the number of inpatient admissions again began to rise and was 35,238,673 in 2005 (see Table 8–5). The number of outpatient visits has continually been increasing from 211,961,000 in 1984, to 584,428,736 in 2005 (American Hospital Association 2007).

The average length of hospital stay has also decreased since the implementation of PPS—a direct cause of the decreased occupancy rates. At 7.7 days in community hospitals in 1975, the average stay was 5.6 days in 2005 (see Figure 8–3). The decreased length of stay was a direct result of PPS and its incentives for hospitals to operate efficiently (ibid.).

Patients are no longer brought into a hospital for preadmission testing as inpatients. All preparatory care is done on an

TABLE 8–5 Hospital Outpatient Utilization for Selected Years

	1984	1985	1990	1995	1996	2000	2004	2005
Total inpatient admissions	35,155,462	33,448,631	31,181,046	30,945,357	31,098,959	33,089,467	35,086,061	35,238,673
Inpatient surgeries	14,378,580	13,161,996	10,844,916	9,700,613	9,545,612	9,729,336	10,050,346	10,097,271
Total outpatient visits	211,941,487	218,694,236	300,514,516	413,748,403	439,863,107	521,404,976	571,569,334	584,428,736
Outpatient surgeries	5,529,661	6,951,359	11,069,952	13,462,304	14,023,651	16,383,374	17,351,490	17,445,587

SOURCE: American Hospital Association. 2007. *TrendWatch Chartbook, 2007: Trends affecting hospitals and health systems.*

outpatient basis. Inpatient services are scheduled on a timelier basis, avoiding lags in time that provide no benefit to patients but increase the total inpatient stays. Technology has also played an important role in decreasing length of stay. New surgical techniques, less-invasive therapies, and laser technology have shortened recovery and response times.

Most hospitals continued to earn profits during the first years of PPS. However, subsequent profits have been dwindling. The profits, we need to be reminded, are necessary to cover losses in other areas—for example, the losses incurred from care of those without insurance and from low Medicaid payments, as well as the purchases a hospital may need to improve the quality of care. As profits decline, hospitals are improving their utilization review departments to minimize unnecessary procedures and practices without affecting the quality of care, but the tensions over providing care and staying financially viable grow.

Government oversight grows following concern that hospitals are increasing their income by manipulating diagnosis codes that are used to describe a patient's condition and treatment and assigning cases to DRGs for which the payment is higher (a practice sometimes referred to as DRG creep or upcoding). According to the Department of Health and Human Services Inspector General's report, the coding mistakes averaged 20 percent, but most of the errors favored hospitals, creating the suspicion that some hospitals are deliberately manipulating DRGs to increase their income. Whether or not this is the case, the errors cost the Medicare program millions of dollars in overpayments to hospitals. Efforts have been made to help curtail deliberate overbilling through federal fraud and abuse legislation such as the False Claims Act, anti-kickback statutes, the Ethics in Patient Referrals Act, and most recently the Health Insurance Portability and Accountability Act of 1996 (Kalb 1999).

PPS has slowed the increase in hospital costs for patients covered by Medicare, and it has also affected other payers for inpatient hospital services. Some state Medicaid programs are using Medicare's PPS as a model for controlling their hospital costs. Blue Cross and other private payers of hospital care are also implementing DRG-based payment systems to control their costs.

Hospitals turn to other services, particularly outpatient procedures, to bring in additional income, but that soon may not be the ultimate answer to increased income. Congress established ambulatory payment groups similar to DRGs that pay a fixed rate according to the group (outpatient payment groups [OPGs]). Fixed payments save the federal government millions of dollars, but hospitals will have to find other ways to recover losses from increasingly less profitable inpatient care and from treating patients who are uninsured or underinsured.

HOSPITAL COMPETITION

A competitive market in health care developed as a result of PPS. A shorter length of stay meant lower occupancy rates. Only a greater flow of patients could counteract the short stay. In some areas, a high penetration of managed care contracting resulted in "exclusive providers," leaving those providers outside the contract to deal with an increasingly smaller patient base. Managed care also changed the emphasis of treatment from inpatient and specialty care to medical management, case management, and prevention—again decreasing the demand for inpatient care. Some areas saw an oversupply of physicians and hospital beds. Under these conditions, a buyers' market developed in the health services sector. Health services payers (insurers and employers) were increasingly able to set the prices and conditions under which they would pay hospitals. A third operative factor in this changing environment was an administration in Washington that wanted to deregulate the health sector, to let market forces prevail to a greater extent than before, and to shift responsibilities from the federal government to the states and the private sector. These factors became even stronger after the failure of the Clinton health plan and other health care reform efforts in the mid-1990s. The Bush administration emphasized market forces in any discussion of reform. In 2009, President Barack Obama proposed health care reform legislation, emphasizing mandates for employer-sponsored health insurance and methods to help those without insurance pay for health insurance. At the time of publication, it was not known if Obama's proposals came to fruition.

In this environment, hospitals are forced to compete for patients with their decreased occupancy rates. They now promote amenities such as homelike patient rooms, improved meal service, and other "customer service" features. Strategic planning involves identifying medical services that are popular with the public (and reimbursed primarily by private insurance). Hospitals advertise on radio, television, and billboards. They affiliate with other hospitals (horizontal integration) to achieve economies of scale in supplies and services, and they contract with large purchasers of health care to provide services at a discount rate to secure a dependable flow of patients.

As profits from inpatient care decreased, hospitals expanded more profitable outpatient services into such areas as primary care, surgery, extended care, rehabilitation, home care, and occupational medicine (vertical integration). Although expanding services was necessary to survive and to provide competitive prices to purchasers of health care, it also frequently put hospitals in the position of competing for patients with physicians on their medical staffs, and with other health professionals and community health agencies. This situation has changed the traditional physician-hospital relationship and the hospital–community health agency relationship. In some cases, when physicians threatened to offer services on their own that would compete with those offered by the hospital outpatient department—such as in surgery and radiology, the hospitals went into a business partnership with those specialists in their freestanding enterprises. Some of the most successful diversification strategies have been freestanding outpatient surgical units, freestanding diagnostic centers, cardiac rehabilitation services, substance abuse programs, inpatient rehabilitation units, occupational medicine clinics, sports medicine programs, home health services, and women's health centers.

their physicians, but most medical staffs still consist primarily of independently practicing physicians.

Over the past few decades, hospitals have changed from expanding institutions with little regard for cost to institutions with reduced occupancy and a great interest in cost containment. They are now more businesslike institutions that stress efficiency, and they compete for patients. The changes were caused by the efforts of government and other large health care purchasers to slow the dramatic increases in health care spending. Medicare changed its method of paying for inpatient services to a prospective payment system based on DRGs, which encourage cost savings. Admissions and lengths of hospital stays decreased, as did the number of hospitals and hospital beds. Quality of care is increasingly important as data collection methods have enabled hospitals and health care purchasers to compare hospital performance records. Hospitals continue to search for ways to maintain or improve their efficiency and effectiveness in a climate of increased competition and cost constraints.

SUMMARY

Hospitals have undergone dramatic changes from their inception as places for poor, sick individuals to spend their final days before death. They have moved from being defined as places to die to being defined as places to be cured. However, in the last twenty years, hospitals have changed in both form and function—so much so that the term *hospital* has even become an inappropriate label in some cases. *Medical centers, health systems, networks,* and *alliances* are terms used to describe the new face of hospital care.

Community hospitals, with which most of us are familiar, continue to serve many communities with short-term acute care. Chances are high, however, that community hospitals are in some way affiliated with an umbrella corporation or large chain of other hospitals.

Nonprofit institutions, governed by a board of trustees, are still the largest group of "hospital" facilities; however, many of them may have affiliations with a for-profit organization or separate business functions that operate on a for-profit basis.

Although teaching hospitals affiliated with universities and providing high-tech tertiary care still tend to provide the bulk of medical education, physician training takes place in a wider variety of health care settings, including community hospitals, primary care clinics, rural health care settings, and public health clinics. A growing number of hospitals directly employ some of

ACTIVITY-BASED LEARNING

- Visit the American Hospital Directory website at www. ahd.com. Choose a city, and find the number of hospitals within that city. Compare the hospitals for size, services offered, and financial statement summary. Are you surprised by the differences? Choose another city that is different in size from your first choice, and compare the two. What are some of the interesting facts you have discovered?

- Visit the Joint Commission website at www.qualitycheck.org/consumer/searchQCR.aspx, and view the accreditation status of the hospitals you found in the previous exercise.

- Do any of the hospitals about which you have inquired have their own websites? Can you determine the members of the hospital board, if the hospital is for-profit or nonprofit, the bed size, and other characteristics from visiting the website, or from other available literature about the hospital?

A QUESTION OF ETHICS

- Hospitals today are faced with many financial challenges. One method of cost containment has been to reduce the length of stay for most patients, transferring them to other locations for some of their care, such as nursing homes, rehabilitation centers, and home health agencies. Is this appropriate utilization of services, or simply a method of "patient dumping"?

- People who are ill and have no regular source of care and no money to pay for care often go to the hospital emergency department to receive care that may not fit the strict sense of "emergency." The hospital is obligated to care for patients without any payment for that service. Should this be the responsibility of the emergency department? If not, what is the answer to caring for people who have no medical insurance and cannot afford to pay?

REFERENCES

1. American Health Planning Association. (2007). *Certificate of need*. Retrieved from www.ahpanet.org/copn.html

2. American Hospital Association. (2007). TrendWatch *chartbook 2007, trends affecting hospitals and health systems*. Retrieved from www.aha.org/aha/research-and-trends/chartbook/2007chartbook.html

3. American Hospital Association. (2006). *Fast facts on U.S. hospitals*. Retrieved from www.aha.org/aha/resource-center/Statistics-and-Studies/fast-facts.html

4. American Hospital Association. (2005). *AHA hospital statistics, 2005*. Chicago, IL: Health Forum.

5. American Hospital Directory. (2008). *Free hospital information*. Retrieved from www.ahd.com/freesearch.php3

6. Griffith, J. R., & White, K. R. (2002). *The well-managed healthcare organization* (5th ed.). Chicago: Health Administration Press.

7. Health Resources and Services Administration. (2007). *Hill-Burton facilities compliance and recovery: About Hill-Burton free care program, Titles VI & XVI*. Retrieved from www.hrsa.gov/hillburton/compliance-recovery.htm

8. Hospital Corporation of America. (2008). Online Press Kit. Retrieved from www.hcahealthcare.com/CustomPage.asp?guidCustomContentID=89AAC3E7-7E84-4E62-9BF0-C33927FBFBC9

9. Joint Commission. (2007a). *About us: About the Joint Commission*. Retrieved from www.jointcommission.org/AboutUs/joint_commission_facts.htm

10. Joint Commission. (2007b). *General public: Fact about the 2007 accreditation decisions*. Retrieved from www.jointcommission.org/GeneralPublic/Decisions.htm

11. Kalb, P. (1999). Health care fraud and abuse. *JAMA*, *282*(12), 1163–1168.

12. Lohr, K., & Schroeder, S. (1990). A strategy for quality assurance in Medicare. *New England Journal of Medicine*, *322*(10), 707–712.

13. National Center for Health Statistics. (2007). *Health United States, 2007, with chartbook on trends in the health of Americans*. Hyattsville, MD.

14. National Center for Health Statistics. (2006). *Health United States, 2006, with chartbook on trends in the health of Americans*. Hyattsville, MD.

15. Nightingale, F. (1863). *Notes on hospitals* (3rd ed.). London.

16. Rosenberg, C. E. (1987). *The care of strangers—The rise of America's hospital system*. New York: Basic Books.

17. Sessa, E. (1992, January). Information is power: The Pennsylvania experiment. *Journal of Health Care Benefits* (44–48).

18. Tenet Healthcare Corporation. (2008). Introduction. Retrieved from www.tenethealth.com/NR/rdonlyres/0599B87D-14E2-4258-B979-5E4A242860CB/149778/IntroductionSept2009.pdf

19. Stevens, R. (1989). *In sickness and in wealth: American hospitals in the twentieth century*. New York: Basic Books.

20. U.S. General Accounting Office. (1987). *Posthospital care*, GAO Report 132066. Retrieved from archive.gao.gov/f0102/132066.pdf

21. Yessian, M. R., & Greenleaf, J. M. (1997). The ebb and flow of federal initiatives to regulate healthcare professionals. In T. S. Jost (Ed.), *Regulation of the healthcare professions* (169–198). Chicago: Health Administration Press.

Chapter 9

Mental Health Services

CHAPTER OBJECTIVES

After completing this chapter, readers should have an understanding of the following:

- The range of services encompassing the mental health system
- The history of the development of mental health services
- The difficulties the mental health sector of health care faces

INTRODUCTION

The mental health system encompasses a large variety of services and service providers. As with medical care, the modern focus is on prevention and early treatment—a move away from the historical focus on isolation and control of those with mental illness. However, many difficulties still arise in the treatment of mental illness, from lack of resources to lack of understanding. Mental illness is described in many ways:

- Carrying normal fears, thoughts, emotions, and beliefs to an extreme
- Behavior dangerous to oneself or others
- Mental function resulting in unproductive activities, unfulfilling relationships with other people, and the inability to adapt to change and to cope with adversity

All of these descriptions are somewhat left to interpretation, and here lies some of the difficulty. Behavior is steeped in culture and values. Diagnosis and treatment must also be culturally based. New understandings of mental health and mental illness must be made available to communities so that those seeking care can come forward and receive effective treatment without stigma and fear.

Mental illness may affect the way a person thinks (**cognitive disorders**), behaves (**behavioral disorders**), or interacts with others (**emotional disorders**). It encompasses a number of psychiatric disorders, including depression, anxiety disorders, schizophrenia and other psychotic disorders, substance abuse disorders, dementia, eating disorders, learning disorders, and personality disorders—a variety of mental illnesses. These are described and categorized in an official code book, *Diagnostic and Statistical Manual of Mental Disorders*, now in its fourth edition (*DSM-IV*), and separate from the diagnosis codes used for physical illnesses.

According to the surgeon general's report:

Mental disorders (collectively) account for more than 15 percent of the burden of disease from all causes. (U.S. Department of Health and Human Services 1999, 3)

Approximately one in five children and adolescents experiences the signs and symptoms of a DSM-IV disorder during the course of a year, but only about 5 percent of all children experience what professionals term extreme functional impairment. A range of treatments exists for many mental disorders in children, including attention-deficit/hyperactivity disorder, depression, and disruptive disorders. (pp. 17–18)

Anxiety, depression, and schizophrenia particularly present special problems in the adult stage of life. Anxiety and depression contribute to the high rates of suicide in this population. Schizophrenia is the most persistently disabling condition for young adults (U.S. Department of Health and Human Services 1999, 18). Substance abuse is a major co-occurring problem for adults with mental disorders (p. 18).

The National Institute of Mental Health (2007) estimates that 26.2 percent of adult Americans suffer from mental disorders in any given year; 6 percent suffer serious mental illness. Normal aging is not characterized by mental or cognitive disorders. Mental or substance use disorders that present alone or co-occur among older adults should be recognized and treated as illnesses (U.S. Department of Health and Human Services 1999, 19).

Remarkable advances have been made in the understanding of mental health and mental disorders, the function of the brain, and the relationship between mental and physical functioning of the body. However, much remains to be done in converting this understanding into care and treatment of those in need. The 2000 supplement to the surgeon general's 1999 report on mental illness indicates that the majority of people with diagnosable disorders do not receive treatment. This fact crosses race and ethnicity (U.S. Department of Health and Human Services 2001).

The large number of homeless people who are mentally ill and seen in the streets, subways, and parks of larger cities forcefully bring the shortcomings of mental health services in the United States to our attention. An estimated one-third of individuals who are homeless suffer from serious mental illness (Pardes 1991). Less obvious is the amount of mental illness that could be prevented or controlled, but is not for fear of the stigma attached to mental illness. The American Psychological Association (1999) points out the following:

> It is a myth that mental illness is a weakness or defect in character and that sufferers can get better simply by "pulling themselves up by their bootstraps." Mental illnesses are real illnesses—as real as heart disease and cancer—and they require and respond well to treatment. (p. 1)

A fragmented system of financing and responsibility has resulted in an inadequate amount of care or care not targeted toward many in need. Sufficient medical care, social support, and help with basic living needs for a prolonged period of time are not available. How this situation came about and what is being done to remedy it is the focus of this chapter.

HISTORY OF MENTAL HEALTH SERVICES

Before the 1800s, families provided the majority of care to people with mental illness; those with mental illness became a public concern only if they had no family support, were unable to care for themselves, or were violent. In the latter cases, local officials assumed responsibility for the welfare of such people by boarding them with families, placing them in public almshouses, or housing them in public jails.

As the population grew and urbanization increased, there was a growing awareness of social and medical problems. Some psychiatric hospitals were established (in that era, these institutions were often referred to as "mental hospitals" or "asylums"). About this time, Dorothea Dix became very interested in the condition of almshouses and jails in her native state of Massachusetts and found, among other problems, that people suffering from insanity (often referred to as lunatics) were held in unheated jails. She convinced the state legislature to assume direct responsibility for the care of people with mental illness. Dix also campaigned for improved conditions for people with mental illness in many other states. Her reforms led to the establishment of large state institutions in almost every state; thus, an era of "moral treatment" began, in which patients were nourished and cared for until they became well again.

The prevailing view at that time was that mental illness was the result of improper behavioral patterns that were associated with an unsatisfactory environment. It was thought that psychiatric institutions could provide a more appropriate environment, where patients could be improved physically, be treated with narcotics to calm violent behavior, and be provided with kind, individual care. Most patients were institutionalized for brief periods of time.

There were relatively few long-term or chronic cases in institutions during the nineteenth century, partly because a large proportion of people with mental illness were still kept at home or in municipal almshouses and partly because the funding of these institutions was divided between state and local governments. States provided funding to build and renovate psychiatric institutions, but local communities paid for the care and treatment of the patients admitted if their family or friends did not assume the cost. Sometimes local officials kept indigent people with mental illness in almshouses, where the costs were less. Other times, local officials pressured psychiatric hospitals to discharge patients prematurely if localities were paying for their care (Grob 1991).

As the number of patients with chronic mental illness increased, the conflicts that occurred because of the divided responsibility resulted in states assuming full responsibility for cases of mental illness. Local officials then redefined **senility** as mental illness and transferred patients who were poor, senile, and elderly from almshouses to state mental institutions to save even more money. As a result, state psychiatric institutions that had high turnover rates saw those rates decline with the rapid increase of patients needing long-term care. They became institutions largely for custodial care for the aged, as well as for patients with chronic mental illness (ibid.).

After 1945, psychiatrists who were associated with institutional care began to leave psychiatric hospitals and move into community and private practice. They were frequently replaced by international medical graduates with little or no training in psychiatry, and psychiatric hospitals deteriorated. Most psychiatrists in the community treated large numbers of patients with psychological problems and had little contact with the institutionalized people with mental illness. As the links between psychiatric hospitals and psychiatrists weakened, there was a movement to strengthen outpatient care and community clinics. By the mid-1950s, there were over 1,000 outpatient psychiatric clinics, most of which were state-supported or state-aided (Grob 1991).

THE MOVE TO DEINSTITUTIONALIZATION

The support for community-based care and treatment grew steadily, on the assumption that early treatment could prevent inpatient care and that patients did better with home and family as support. At the same time, a growing number of private psychiatric hospitals and psychiatric beds in community hospitals became available for short-term treatment and emergencies. The concept of community care and treatment prevailed, supported by

those who did not believe in the concept of mental illness, civil rights advocates who identified people with mental illness as a group deprived of their civil liberties, and social advocates who emphasized that psychiatric hospitals are inherently repressive and dehumanizing (Grob 1991). The Community Mental Health Act of 1963 strengthened community facilities and weakened the central role psychiatric hospitals played in the treatment of patients with mental illness.

After 1965, a number of factors contributed to the rapid decline in the number of patients in psychiatric hospitals. The introduction of **psychotropic drugs** enabled patients rendered dysfunctional by illness to control symptoms and function well within the community. The introduction of Medicaid, which paid the cost of nursing home care for the elderly poor, enabled their transfer from psychiatric hospitals to nursing homes. The transfer of the elderly to nursing homes was encouraged because the federal government partly funded Medicaid, and this reduced the cost of elder care for state and local government.

According to Grob (1991), "Prior to 1940, public policy had been focused almost exclusively on the severely and chronically mentally ill. This policy was based on the assumption that society had an obligation to provide such unfortunate persons with both care and treatment in public mental hospitals. The policies adopted during and after the 1960s rested on quite different assumptions." These later policies created a decentralized system of services that separated care and treatment, and often focused on mild mental illness to the detriment of patients who suffered from severe mental illness more difficult to treat.

In 1964, federal legislation provided construction money for community mental health centers to serve people who were deinstitutionalized and others who could be treated on an outpatient basis. It was hoped that 2,000 centers would be established to meet the need throughout the nation, but the maximum number never exceeded 700. Very little money was obtained from other sources to staff and operate the centers. The federal government provided matching funds for operational costs for eight years; after that, the funds decreased and the community was to assume the financial responsibility for operational costs. That didn't happen. States were forced to provide funds, but it was not enough. Services were reduced, and some centers closed. The separation of care and treatment often resulted in a lack of social services to ensure that patients had their basic living needs covered while they underwent treatment. With decreased funding for community care over time, communities had difficulty providing the volume of care required by the outpatient sector.

Many people with mental illness who lacked sufficient resources and family support experienced what came to be known as the "revolving door" concept. Patients would seek treatment in short-term inpatient facilities. Through the use of psychotropic drugs and intense counseling, patients would be stabilized and discharged, perfectly capable of functioning in the community. However, psychotropic drugs often have significant side effects. After time, as the patients feel better, the side effects of drug treatment become a real burden. Without continued counseling, patients would discontinue drug therapy as community centers became overburdened with many patients, not enough staff, and significant waiting lists for treatment. Predictably, the symptoms would recur (psychotropic drugs help control, not cure, mental illness), and patients would experience an acute episode requiring hospitalization once again. A cyclical pattern would develop—thus the revolving door.

Even with drug therapy, outpatient therapy recognizes that patients will experience difficult periods when more intense care is necessary. Patients can be encouraged to continue drug therapy even when symptoms are minimal (a sign the drug is effective) and side effects continue; however, every patient has the right to refuse treatment (drug therapy), and, although not desirable, it is understandable why patients may not want to continue with a drug when symptoms go away.

Although the current state of treatment for mental illness is still largely focused on outpatient care, inpatient facilities remain available in some state institutions, private psychiatric hospitals, and specialized facilities (substance abuse facilities, children's psychiatric centers, and so on). The majority of short-term inpatient care is available through specific units in general hospitals.

Another level of care for mental disorders is partial hospitalization (or intensive outpatient care). Under this framework, patients receive treatment (medications, individual and group therapy, vocational training, and so on) on an intensive basis for some four to eight hours per day, but they otherwise remain in their own homes. This approach is an alternative to residential care, but it is more treatment-oriented than regular outpatient care.

Like other areas of the health care sector, the mental health delivery system is undergoing a great deal of change. Managed care, Medicare and Medicaid, and government mandates for health insurance coverage for mental health services have affected the delivery of care—in both positive and negative ways.

CHALLENGES TO MENTAL HEALTH SERVICES DELIVERY TODAY

Mental illness is difficult enough to define; identifying a large segment of the population with mental illness—those with chronic mental illness—is even more difficult. The 1999 surgeon general's report reminds us of the following:

> The fact that many, if not most, people have experienced mental health problems that mimic or even match some of the symptoms of a diagnosable mental disorder tends, ironically, to prompt many people to underestimate the painful, disabling nature of severe mental illness. . . . Yet relatively few mental illnesses have an unremitting course marked by the most acute manifestations of illness; rather, for reasons that are not yet understood, the symptoms associated with mental illness tend to wax and wane. These patterns pose special challenges to the implementation of treatment plans and the design of service systems that are optimally responsive to an individual's needs during every phase of illness. (U.S. Department of Health and Human Services 1999, 1)

An estimated one in five American adults has experienced mental illness of some type. About one in five children and adolescents experience diagnosable disorders in the course of a year, but only about 5 percent of all children experience "extreme functional impairment." According to the Agency for Healthcare Research and Quality, national expenditures for treatment of mental illness were $46.4 billion in 1990, and increased to $100.3 billion in 2003 (*National Center for Health Statistics 2007*). The number of people in the United States with expenses for mental disorders increased from 20.1 million in 1997, to 31.2 million in 2002. Treatment in community hospitals and psychiatric hospitals accounted for the largest share of expenditures, $10.2 billion in 2004 (AHRQ 2004). However, most people receiving treatment live in the community.

Community hospitals with separate psychiatric services, private psychiatric hospitals, state and county psychiatric hospitals, and Veterans Administration (VA) medical centers provide inpatient treatment services today. There were 476 specialty

TABLE 9-1 Treatment for MHSA* in Community Hospitals and Specialty Psychiatric Hospitals, 2004

	Community Hospitals: All Adult Stays	Community Hospitals with MHSA*: Adult Stays	Specialty Psychiatric Facilities: All Stays
Number of hospitals	4,919	4,821 (98%)	476
Number of inpatient stays	31,929,000	7,592,000 (23.8%)	807,000
Number of inpatient days	154,786,000	44,295,000 (28.6%)	26,698,000
Mean length of stay, in days	4.8	5.8	33.0

*Mental health/substance abuse.

SOURCE: AHRQ. 2004. *Fact book #10: Care of adults with mental health and substance abuse disorders in U.S. community hospitals* (p. 5).

psychiatric hospitals in the United States in 2004. However, community hospitals provided the majority of patient care days for mental health and substance abuse disorders, as seen in Table 9-1 (AHRQ 2004). Nursing homes and related care are also a major resource for residential care of people with mental illness. Nearly half of the total population of those in nursing homes has been diagnosed with Alzheimer's disease or other forms of dementia.

Few communities have a truly integrated system of treatment and social support for people with mental illness. Managed care's entry into the mental health services market has helped with coordinating medical services but has done little to enhance the types of social services needed by many people who suffer from mental illness. The Substance Abuse and Mental Health Services Administration (SAMHSA) reports that some 700,000 people are homeless in the United States at any given time during a year. An estimated one-half has substance abuse problems, and one-fourth has serious mental illness. However, since 1990, the Center for Mental Health Services has distributed formula matching grants to states to design programs to meet the needs of their homeless population. They also provide grants to public and private community-based nonprofit organizations to provide treatment services for homeless patients with mental health disorders and to link with other social services for individuals who are homeless (*Substance Abuse and Mental Health Services Administration* 2004).

MENTAL HEALTH SERVICES PROVIDERS

A number of different professionals provide mental health services in a variety of settings.

Psychiatrists are medical doctors. Like other physicians, they attend four years of medical school after receiving a bachelor's degree, complete one year of a general residency, and then complete a specialty residency in psychiatry. They are licensed by the state and become certified through the American Board of Psychiatry and Neurology, which issues three types of specialty certification and a number of subspecialty areas such as child and adolescent psychiatry, addiction psychiatry, and forensic psychiatry; they must be recertified every ten years (American Board of Psychiatry and Neurology 2007). Psychiatrists prescribe medications and perform medical procedures with emphasis on clinical work, counseling, and research. In 2005, over 27.6 thousand psychiatrists were in active practice (see Figure 9-1), up from 23,000 in 1995 (National Center for Health Statistics 2007).

Psychologists are licensed by the states to practice after receiving an academic doctoral degree and completing a minimum of two years of supervised experience in direct clinical service. Licensure is required in all fifty states, and board certification is becoming more important. More than 170,000 psychologists provided clinical care, counseling, and research in the United States in 2004 (Bureau of Labor Statistics 2004a). In some states,

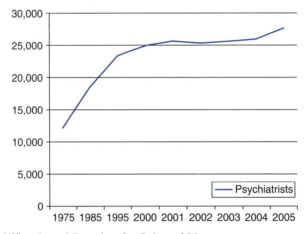

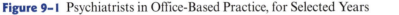

Figure 9–1 Psychiatrists in Office-Based Practice, for Selected Years

SOURCE: National Center for Health Statistics. 2007. *Health United States, 2007, with chartbook on trends in the health of Americans*, Table 107. MD: Hyattsville, MD.

psychologists have lobbied for the right to prescribe medications, pointing to the new advances in drug therapy for such conditions as depression, anxiety, and addictions, as well as the frequency with which psychologists work with patients dealing with such conditions. Psychologists also cite the shortage of psychiatrists to whom they can refer patients for medication consults. However, a very small number of states have enacted legislation to allow psychologists prescribing privileges (Office of Diversion Control 2007). Such lobbying efforts may contribute to tensions between psychiatrists and psychologists as they compete for comparable treatment privileges (Moran 1998).

Psychiatric nurses are trained beyond RNs in caring for the special needs of patients with mental illness. The range of responsibilities of psychiatric nurses varies with the organization in which the nurses practice and the state in which the organization resides. Some psychiatric nurses conduct independent therapy sessions, whereas others simply provide nursing services in a psychiatric setting.

Support services are also provided by social workers and counselors. Social workers have a bachelor or master's degree and work with mental health facilities, providers, and patients to find housing, employment, medical care, and other support services for those in need. Clinical social workers with a master's degree also provide individual and/or group counseling. All fifty states require licensing, certification, or registration to practice (Bureau of Labor Statistics 2004b). Counselors often have "life experience" in a given area of counseling (for example, drug

abuse, alcohol abuse, battered spouse syndrome, and so on). Counselors are not licensed by the states, but many are certified in their field. It is up to the people seeking services to inquire about the credentials of counselors because few states exercise any control. Lack of state control is not an automatic indication of the lack of quality or efficacy of a program.

The twelve-step program, a foundation of Alcoholics Anonymous, has long been recognized as an effective way of dealing with addiction. It is a self-help approach to healing based on support among addicts facing the same or similar problems and does not rely on leadership or facilitation by mental health professionals. Many well-known programs, such as the Betty Ford Center, are based on the foundation of the twelve-step program (although the inpatient portion of the program includes other therapies). Other addiction treatment programs (for example, for drug abuse, codependency, and so on) rely heavily on the principles of the twelve-step approach. Both licensed and unlicensed mental health service providers use the twelve-step approach, and again, consumers are responsible for determining the credibility of the service.

It is important to remember that mental health services are also provided by the general medical or primary care sector of the health care community. Many family physicians provide counseling and medication to their patients with mental health problems, referring the patients to other professionals if and when necessary (U.S. Department of Health and Human Services 1999). Community hospitals provide care in specialized units, scattered beds throughout the hospital, emergency rooms, and outpatient clinics.

EMERGING MENTAL HEALTH CONCERNS

Suicide was the cause of death for some 30,000 people in the United States in 2004. Men are more likely to die of suicide, but women are three times as likely to attempt suicide. Some 179,000 hospital stays are a result of a suicide attempt, and nearly two-thirds of those attempts are by poisoning. Risk factors for suicide are a history of mental disorders (mainly depression) and drug and alcohol abuse (AHRQ 2004).

Depression is a feeling of helplessness and sadness and a loss of interest in things that were once important. Everyone feels depressed occasionally, especially after experiencing a loss or deep disappointment. A diagnosis of depression, however, happens when symptoms continue for a long period of time and interfere with normal functioning. Major depressive disorder is the leading cause of disability in the United States for people aged between 15 and 44 years. It affects approximately 14.8 million American adults, or about 6.7 percent of the adult population and is more prevalent in women than in men (National Institute of Mental Health 2007).

Depression can successfully be treated with therapy and antidepressant medications. The use of antidepressants by the noninstitutionalized U.S. population has grown—from 271.3 million people in 1997, to 288.2 million people in 2002, or from 5.6 percent to 8.5 percent (AHRQ 2005). Antidepressant use increased in both the elderly and nonelderly populations, among men and women, across racial categories, and across income levels (see Figure 9–2). Antidepressants work mainly to control a chemical imbalance in the brain; however, there are many different types of antidepressants, and a physician must determine the best fit for the patient with input from the patient (American Academy of Family Physicians 2005).

EXHIBIT 9–1

From The National Survey on Drug Use and Health (The NSDUH Report), October 11, 2007:

Depression Among Adults Employed Full-Time, by Occupational Category

Depression can seriously impact a person's ability to perform routine activities at work. It negatively affects U.S. industry through lost productivity, employee absenteeism, and low morale. U.S. companies lose an estimated $30 billion to $44 billion per year because of employee depression. Research shows that the rate of depression varies by occupation and industry. . . .

- Combined data from 2004 to 2006 indicate that an annual average of 7 percent of full-time workers aged 18 to 64 experienced a major depressive episode (MDE) in the past year.

- The highest rates of past-year MDE among full-time workers aged 18 to 64 were found in the personal care and service occupations (10.8 percent) and the food preparation and serving related occupations (10.3 percent).

- The highest rates of past-year MDE among female full-time workers aged 18 to 64 were found in the food preparation and serving related occupations (14.8 percent), and the highest rates among male full-time workers aged 18 to 64 were found in the arts, design, entertainment, sports, and media occupations (6.7 percent).

The NSDUH Report is published periodically by the Office of Applied Studies, Substance Abuse and Mental Health Services Administration (SAMHSA). The full report is available online at http://www.oas.samhsa.gov.

Discussion Questions

The number of people suffering from depression is on the increase. Depression strikes men and women of all ages and backgrounds. Consider the number of new drugs developed to treat depression.

1. There are a number of different drugs available to treat depression, but even with those drugs available, what are the barriers against people with depression getting effective treatment?

2. How does the stigma of mental illness effect the treatment of depression?

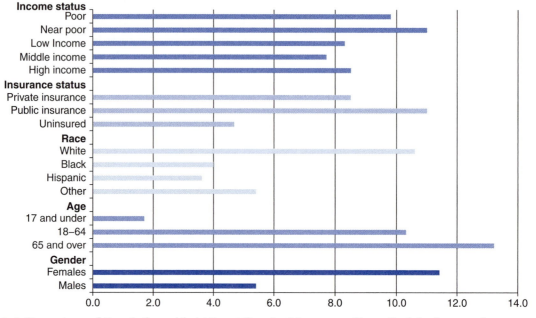

Figure 9–2 Percentage of Population with At Least One Antidepressant Prescribed, by Income, Insurance, Race, Age, and Gender, 2002

SOURCE: AHRQ. (2005b). *Medical expenditure panel survey, statistical brief #76.*

Bipolar disorder, also known as manic-depressive disorder, is a brain disorder that causes wild mood swings. Untreated, it can cause a severe inability to function and can even lead to suicide. Fortunately, bipolar disorder can be treated with medication, and those with the disorder can go on to live normal lives as long as they stay on the medication (National Institute of Mental Health 2007).

FUNDING AND EXPENDITURES FOR MENTAL ILLNESS

The government paid for 58.1 percent of the care of patients with mental illness in 2003, including payments through Medicare, Medicaid, the Department of Veterans Affairs, and the Department of Defense, as well as other federal, state, and local government payments. Insurance and patient payments account for the remainder.

A large portion of treatment for drug abuse takes place in special substance abuse centers, whereas the majority of alcohol abuse treatment takes place in the general service sector, such as community hospitals. Private-sector payments ($4.4 billion in 2003) include private insurance, out-of-pocket, and other private payments. Although out-of-pocket expenses decreased from $1.8 billion in 1986, to $1.6 billion in 2003, the decrease was not accompanied by an increase in private insurance payments, which stayed relatively stable over the same period. It is primarily an increase in public funding that is reducing the percentage of out-of-pocket expenses (National Center for Health Statistics 2007).

In 1995, almost $6 billion dollars were spent on retail pharmaceuticals for mental health and substance abuse treatment separate from facility expenditures. By 2003, the amount spent on psychotropic drugs rose to $23.2 billion. This increase in psychotropic drug spending is greater than the growth in overall drug spending. The largest portion of psychotropic drug use is for antipsychotic medications and antidepressants. Medicaid and the U. S. Department of Veterans Affairs are large purchasers of psychotropic drugs. Now that the Medicare Modernization Act is in force, these expenditures may shift to the federal government (Frank et al. 2005).

Private health insurance has historically been much more restrictive in benefits for mental health services than for medical services. Many people have no coverage at all for mental health services within their health insurance plan. Those that do have coverage experience higher co-pays and deductibles and lower maximum annual and lifetime payments. Some experience limitations on numbers of visits or numbers of days of treatment. The Mental Health Parity Act of 1996 sought to remedy the disparity in coverage. However, after a great deal of compromise over proposed legislation, the final product made only small inroads toward parity. The act mandates that health plans offering mental health services may not impose lifetime or annual limits on those services different from limits for medical services. However, any plan that can show that its premiums have increased by at least 1 percent because of the requirements can apply for a waiver (Newbould 1998). In addition, the act does not require employers or health plans to cover or maintain coverage for treatment of mental illness, and benefits for treatment of substance abuse are excluded from the requirements (American Psychological Association 1999). Additional legislation, at both the state and federal levels, has been introduced to expand parity and close loopholes. The legislation includes a call for elimination in differences in the number of inpatient days, number of outpatient visits, co-payments, deductibles, and other limitations between medical and mental health benefits (American Psychiatric Association 2007; Sullivan 1997).

The growth of managed care in the medical insurance arena has also been felt in mental health services. Managed care's approach to mental health or mental illness is the case management approach. People seeking treatment contact their managed care provider; they are first screened for signs and symptoms and then are given a referral to a professional for further screening. The screening process assures treatment at the appropriate level and for a specific term of treatment. Patients pay only a co-payment for each visit when receiving care from a professional in the network of providers. The approach has been instrumental in containing the costs of mental health treatment. It has, however, created tension among both consumers and providers because of the amount of paperwork required to gain approval for initial and continuing care, and because of the limitations on the number of visits allowed.

The surgeon general indicated that "[m]ental illness is a real health condition" and "mental health is fundamental to [overall] health" (U.S. Department of Health and Human Services 2001, 2). Although adding more resources to treatment of mental health will increase the overall expenditures toward health care, it may decrease health care costs in the long run. Good mental health leads to increased productivity, decreased employee absenteeism among the working population, and fewer early departures from work (Wang et al. 2007). Mental health plays an important part in any consideration of health care reform.

SUMMARY

Mental health care has undergone changes in terms of organization, financing, and services to cope with current realities. The large number of people who are homeless with untreated mental illness continues to remind us of the serious shortage of mental health services at the outpatient community level. A major problem in gaining support for the care and treatment of people with mental illness is that the diagnosis, treatment, and cure are not as precise, certain, and assured as other types of illness—for example, a broken hip, heart disease, or cancer—that can be precisely diagnosed and definitively treated to yield a cure or an alleviation of symptoms or pain. Treatment of mental illness consists of helping patients live with their condition and cannot promise a cure.

The demand for mental health services far exceeds their availability. Too few centers have been built and too few services have been provided to support the community care movement begun in the 1960s. Managed care has provided access to services formerly unavailable to some. However, many in need still have no access to care. The lack of financial commitment to mental health services by government and private insurance places pressure on mental health providers.

ACTIVITY-BASED LEARNING

The trend in mental health services is outpatient treatment. What types of services are available in your community for mental health treatment? For drug addiction? For alcohol addiction?

A QUESTION OF ETHICS

- Review your own health insurance plan. Does it provide mental health benefits? How do the benefits compare to those for medical services? In your opinion, should there be a difference in medical benefits versus mental health benefits? Does it matter to you?

- Community-based mental health services assume a level of patient support from family and friends. Yet many people do not have a personal support system. They cannot or do not adhere to medication regimens, have difficulty maintaining therapy and/or counseling, and so on. Should inpatient, residential care be mandated for those who are unable to maintain outpatient treatment?

REFERENCES

1. AHRQ. (2005). *Medical expenditure panel survey, statistical brief #76.* Retrieved from www.ahrq.gov/data/hcup/factbk76/factbk76.pdf

2. AHRQ. (2004). *Fact book #10: Care of adults with mental health and substance abuse disorders in U.S. community hospitals, 2004.* Retrieved from www.ahrq.gov/data/hcup/factbk10/factbk10.pdf

3. American Academy of Family Physicians. (2005). Antidepressants: Medicine for Depression. Retrieved from familydoctor.org/online/famdocen/home/common/mentalhealth/treatment/012.html

4. American Board of Psychiatry and Neurology. (2007). *Initial certification.* Retrieved from www.abpn.com

5. American Psychiatric Association. (2007). *APA applauds passage of Bill on Equal Mental Health Coverage.* Retrieved from www.psych.org/search.aspx?SearchPhrase=apa+applauds+passage+of+bill+on+equal+mental+health+coverage

6. American Psychological Association. (1999). APA supports full mental health parity bill. Retrieved from www.apa.org/practice/pf/apr99/parity.html

7. Bureau of Labor Statistics. (2004a). *Occupational outlook handbook: Psychologists.* Retrieved from www.bls.gov/oco/ocos056.htm

8. Bureau of Labor Statistics. (2004b). *Occupational outlook handbook: Social workers.* www.bls.gov/oco/ocos060.htm

9. Frank, R., Conti, R., & Goldman, H. (2005). Mental health policy and psychotropic drugs. *The Milbank Quarterly, 83*(2), 271.

10. Grob, G. (1991). *The chronically mentally ill in America.* In V. Fransen (Ed.), *Mental health services in the United States and England: Struggling for change.* Princeton, NJ: Robert Wood Johnson Foundation.

11. Moran, M. (1998, February 9). New twist in push for prescribing: Ballot initiative. *American Medical News* (pp. 7–8).

12. National Center for Health Statistics. (2007). *Health, United States, 2007 with chartbook on trends in the health of Americans.* Hyattsville, MD. Retrieved from www.cdc.gov/nchs/data/hus/hus07.pdf

13. National Institute of Mental Health. (2007). *The numbers count: Mental disorders in America.* Retrieved from http://www.nimh.nih.gov/health/publications/the-numbers-count-mental-disorders-in-america/index.shtml

14. Newbould, P. (1998, February). Federal parity law takes effect. American Psychological Association. Retrieved from http://www.apa.org/practice/pf/feb98/parity.html

15. Office of Diversion Control. (2007). Mid-level practitioners authorization by state. U.S. Department of Justice, Drug Enforcement Administration, Retrieved from www.deadiversion.usdoj.gov/drugreg/practioners/index.html#1-3

16. Pardes, H. (1991). *Problems in providing future services to the mentally ill.* In V. Fransen (Ed.), *Mental health services in the United States and England: Struggling for change.* Princeton, NJ: Robert Wood Johnson Foundation.

17. *Substance Abuse and Mental Health Services Administration.* (2004). Homeless programs, branch programs for homeless people with serious mental illness: Homelessness. Center for Mental Health Services, Division of Services and Systems Improvement. Retrieved from mentalhealth.samhsa.gov/cmhs/homelessness/about.asp

18. *Substance Abuse and Mental Health Services Administration.* (2004) Highlights of organized mental health services in 2002 and major national and state trends. *Center for Mental Health Services, National Service Statistics. Retrieved from mentalhealth.samhsa.gov/publications/allpubs/SMA06-4195/Chapter19.asp*

19. Sullivan, M. (1997, February). State parity and licensure bills activate psychology advocates. *American Psychological Association.* Retrieved from http://www.apa.org/practice/pf/feb97/states.html

20. U.S. Department of Health and Human Services. (1999). *Mental health: A report of the surgeon general–Executive summary.* Rockville, MD: HHS.

21. U.S. Department of Health and Human Services. (2001). *Mental health: Culture, race, and ethnicity supplement.* Retrieved from mentalhealth.samhsagov/rec/execsummary-1.asp

22. Wang, P., Simon, G., Avorn, J., Azocar, F., Ludman, E., McCulloch, J., Petukhova, M., & Kessler, R. (2007). Telephone screening, outreach, and care management for depressed workers and impact on clinical and work productivity outcomes: A randomized controlled trial. *JAMA, 298*(12), 1401–1411.

Chapter 10

Long-Term Care

CHAPTER OBJECTIVES

After completing this chapter, readers should have an understanding of the following:

- The differentiation of long-term care from other types of health care services
- The history of long-term care in the United States
- The various payment mechanisms that influence access to and delivery of long-term care services
- The variety of new approaches to long-term care delivery currently available

INTRODUCTION

Long-term care refers to a range of health and social services that are needed to accommodate people with functional disabilities. They may be people of any age with conditions such as birth defects, spinal cord injuries, mental impairment, or other chronic debilitating conditions, but most often they are the very elderly whose ability to function independently is deteriorating. To assist these people, numerous services are provided that are based both in communities and in institutions. Long-term care services are expensive, and future costs are difficult to estimate. The government has no coherent long-term care policy, believing that the foundation of long-term care is the family, and that services should not replace family efforts but complement them. The basic policy questions for government are who should be eligible for services and who should pay for them. Questions surrounding long-term care—how it is delivered, evaluated, and financed—are among the most

critical health issues facing the nation. As the population lives longer, concerns grow regarding the number of elderly living with chronic disease and disability.

The tasks of keeping individuals mobile and as self-sufficient as possible for as long as possible are the focal point of long-term care.

People of any age who are unable to cope with the tasks of daily living for extended periods of time because of physical or mental impairment need social and health care services. The risks of functional disability increase with age, however, and the number of people age 65 and older in the United States has increased from 8 percent of the population in 1950, to 12.4 percent in 2005 (Saphir 1999; U.S. Census Bureau 2005). After 2010, survivors of the baby boom generation will start to reach age 65, causing a dramatic increase in that percentage of the population: An estimated 19.6 percent (over 71 million people) will be over 65 by 2030. Those 85 years and older are increasing faster than any other age group; this group is projected to double, from 1.4 percent of the population in 1995, to approximately 3 percent of the population in 2030 (ibid.). The 85 and older group consume the majority of long-term care services.

Families, friends, and neighbors help most people who are unable to cope with daily living tasks. For a growing number of others, "assisted living services" such as home care, adult day care, and other community-based services provide needed care without institutionalization. However, an increasing number of people, too frail to be left to outpatient care or left without family or friends, need some level of institutional care. This is typically available through long-term care facilities that include nursing homes, psychiatric and mental health facilities, and rehabilitation hospitals. The large majority of long-term care facilities are nursing homes that care primarily for the elderly. Continuing care retirement communities and personal care homes are newer approaches to caring for the elderly. New methods of financing care of the elderly include long-term care insurance and life insurance policies that offer accelerated or "living care" provisions that allow a portion of the life insurance benefit to be paid to a policyholder if long-term care is needed (Day 2007). However, individuals who are poor and uninsured remain with inadequate funds to provide for any form of long-term care, leaving primary responsibility to government funding.

NURSING HOMES

Nursing homes historically represented one of the more difficult problems in long-term care. With fair regularity, scandals erupted in homes that cheated patients, physically abused and neglected patients, provided inadequate medical and nursing care, and were fire hazards. To make matters worse, there were an insufficient number of beds in good nursing homes to deal with the growing number of people needing such care.

Nursing homes originated as county poorhouses (or almshouses) of the eighteenth and nineteenth centuries. Local governments established these institutions to care for people who were poor, to provide them with shelter, food, and clothing, and with work to help pay the costs of their care. As might be expected, many, if not most, of these people were older and had no families to care for them. Being older, many had disabilities. Over time, these almshouses became the community dumps for all of society's cast-offs, not only individuals who were poor and physically ill, but also who had mental illness and alcoholism. There was often no place for these people to go except the local poorhouses. Generally, conditions in these

homes were not good, for they had to get along on meager public appropriations and charity. The appropriations were meager because the public had little sense of identity with these institutions or with the people in them. The inmates were poor and noncontributing to the general welfare, and many were transient, without a previous history of community contributions. Why reward them with ideal facilities? Why tax the hardworking, thrifty citizenry to support those who were not that way? The politicians gave the almshouses the level of support the electorate wanted: bare minimum.

However, a society gets what it pays for. Scandals periodically erupted, as they do today, and public consciences were pricked. Over time, individuals with mental illness and retardation were removed and sent to more appropriate institutions, most of which were state-run rather than locally administered. In Maryland, the conditions in some county almshouses were so bad that the state set up a state-run chronic-disease hospital to care for people who are infirm in return for closing the county almshouses. In other states, improvements were made from time to time, and, as patients were reassigned, these county homes were left mainly with individuals who were aged, poor, and physically disabled who did not need hospital care but who were unable to subsist without some form of health service support (Raffel and Raffel 1994).

In subsequent decades, the state governments began to regulate these homes along with church, fraternal, and proprietary nursing homes, inspecting them and setting standards for performance. However, the hands of state regulation were generally lightly applied. Few states were prepared to close many of the county, voluntary, and proprietary homes because doing so would force the state to assume full responsibility.

As noted previously, nursing homes developed under other sponsorships. Church groups and fraternal organizations started homes for care of their members. These were mainly homes for people who were aged, but, over time, they had to develop supporting health services to meet the needs of their residents. These homes received strong support from their sponsoring bodies—not only direct financial aid but also much in-kind support in terms of gifts of equipment, volunteer maintenance, and harvesting services at farms. Sponsored homes also received a variety of volunteer direct patient care services, such as help in feeding patients, occupational and play therapy, and social visiting. It is widely acknowledged that the quality of service in church- and fraternal-sponsored homes was high, and the shortcomings often found in local government nursing homes and in some of the proprietary nursing homes were not found in voluntary homes.

The **proprietary** private (for-profit) nursing homes emerged during the 1930s, as a result of the Social Security Act of 1935, which provided welfare benefits for patients in nongovernmental institutions. The original exclusion of benefits for patients in public institutions (since repealed) apparently stemmed from congressional concern about conditions in county poorhouses and a desire to close them.

Many health professionals and civic leaders were concerned about the resulting rapid growth in the private nursing home sector, believing that high-quality care could not be developed and maintained if the homes depended on income derived primarily from welfare recipients, because these homes not only had to provide the needed care but also had to leave enough profit to make the owner's investment of money worthwhile. Resulting scandals in the proprietary sector supported the fears of these people. Not only were the payments insufficient both to maintain quality care and to ensure a reasonable return on the owner's investment, but also the very availability of large sums of money to pay for care in facilities that were in short supply proved to be an open invitation to the unscrupulous to enter the business. As it turned out, those who were poor, chronically ill, and needing nursing home care were also often at the bottom of the list for admission to proprietary homes. Even after the advent of Medicare and Medicaid, many of these homes gave preference to private applicants for admission, regardless of the need for care. The low payments by government programs did not permit a reasonable return on the owner's investment while still permitting quality of care. Many proprietary nursing homes also restricted the number of admitted patients who required a great amount of care, so as to avoid the greater costs of such care. As a consequence, long waiting lists developed in many states for admission of Medicare and Medicaid patients, particularly of those who needed the most care.

Aware of these circumstances, health professionals and civic leaders encouraged the development of nonprofit nursing homes. Congress responded by amending the Hill-Burton Act in 1948, to make construction grants available for public and nonprofit nursing homes, and for some states to also design new grant programs. The resistance of the proprietary sector to such grant programs was vigorous and highly political. One of the successful efforts of the proprietary sector was to get Congress to approve Federal Housing Authority (FHA)-guaranteed construction loans for proprietary nursing homes.

The distribution of nursing homes and beds among the public, proprietary, church and fraternal, and other nonprofit sponsorships shifts constantly, but the proprietary sector clearly dominates. In 2004, 61.5 percent of facilities were for-profit, 30.8 percent were nonprofit, and 7.7 percent were government-owned (National Center for Health Statistics 2006a).

The number of facilities that other organizations own as part of chains was also on the increase—10,800 in 1999, compared to 7,200 independent facilities (Jones 2002). However, that trend has leveled off and is even beginning to reverse, with 8,700 nursing homes in chains in 2004, compared to 7,400 independent homes (National Center for Health Statistics 2006b). This evidence of the trend toward integration that was prevalent during the 1990s leveled off in the early twenty-first century. The need for nursing home beds persisted for some years, but new homes were built, access to home health care increased, and occupancy rates began to fall (see Table 10–1). As baby boomers begin to age, the amount of chronic disease will increase. As family units become

TABLE 10-1 Number of Nursing Homes, Beds, Current Residents, and Occupancy Rates, for Selected Years

	1973–74	1977	1985	1995	1997	1999	2004
Total nursing homes	15,700	18,900	19,100	16,700	17,000	18,000	16,100
Bed	1,177,300	1,402,400	1,624,200	1,770,900	1,820,800	1,879,600	1,730,000
Current residents	1,075,800	1,303,100	1,491,400	1,548,600	1,608,700	1,628,300	1,492,200
Occupancy rate (%)	95.3	98.4	80.5	96.4	88.4	86.6	86.3

SOURCE: National Center for Health Statistics. 2006. National Nursing Home Survey.

smaller and all able people are working, the demand for facilities for care of the aged may again increase. The demand accelerated enormously with the implementation of Medicare and Medicaid, which paid for some of this care. The demand also increased as government and health insurance companies sought to reduce the lengths of stay in acute hospitals by moving patients to a less acute level of care. The aging of the baby boomers may spur another rise in demand for long-term care.

With the advent of Medicare and Medicaid, the federal government established definitions for the types of institutions that would fall within the framework of those eligible for reimbursement, as well as standards to govern and ensure quality of care in those homes eligible to participate. If a home for people who are aged wanted to be paid under Medicare or Medicaid for care to eligible patients, the home had to meet certain standards. The federal government originally recognized two types of homes as eligible: the skilled nursing facility and the intermediate care facility. The U.S. Department of Health and Human Services (HSS) provided the definitions:

A skilled nursing facility (SNF) is a nursing home that has been certified as meeting federal standards within the meaning of the Social Security Act. It provides the level of care that comes closest to hospital care with 24-hour nursing services. Regular medical supervision and rehabilitation therapy are also provided. Generally, a skilled nursing facility cares for convalescent patients and those with long-term illnesses.

An intermediate care facility (ICF) is also certified and meets federal standards and provides less extensive health-related care and services. It has regular nursing service, but not around the clock. Most intermediate care facilities carry on rehabilitation programs, but the emphasis is on personal care and social services. Mainly, these homes serve people who are not fully capable of living by themselves, yet are not necessarily ill enough to need 24-hour nursing care. (Jones 2002)

The nursing home reform legislation that was passed as part of the 1987 Omnibus Budget Reconciliation Act (OBRA '87) created the category of nursing home facility (NF) to describe a state-licensed facility providing skilled nursing and/or intermediate care services to residents on a twenty-four-hour basis. The terms *skilled nursing care, intermediate care,* and *residential care* are now used to describe the levels of care most nursing facilities provide (Jones 2002).

Demographics of Nursing Homes and Nursing Home Residents

There were 15,899 certified nursing homes and 1,716,102 certified nursing home beds in the United States in 2006 (National Center for Health Statistics 2007) (see Table 10–2). Another 300 uncertified facilities accounted for 21,000 beds (National Center for Health Statistics 2006b). Although nursing homes provided just one type of care for all residents at one time, most now designate units for patients with Alzheimer's and AIDS, and hospice units to care for residents with special needs.

A typical person in a nursing home is older, female, unmarried, and suffering from some type of dementia (see Figure 10–1). The length of stay for nursing home residents varies by the reason for admission. Those who are admitted for rehabilitation services may stay only two or three months and then return to living

TABLE 10–2 Certification Status of Nursing Homes and Number of Beds, Residents, and Occupancy Rates for Certified and Uncertified Facilities

	Nursing Homes	Beds	Current Residents	Occupancy Rate
Certified	15,800	1,708,900	1,475,600	86.4%
Medicare and Medicaid	14,100	1,599,600	1,379,700	86.3%
Medicare only	700	33,100	28,100	85.0%
Medicaid only	1,100	76,200	67,900	89.1%
Uncertified	300	21,000	16,600	*

*Data unknown

SOURCE: National Center for Health Statistics. 2006. National Nursing Home Survey.

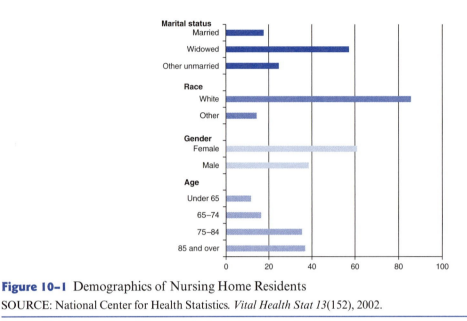

Figure 10–1 Demographics of Nursing Home Residents
SOURCE: National Center for Health Statistics. *Vital Health Stat 13*(152), 2002.

in the community. Those admitted because of a permanent condition may reside in the nursing home for the remainder of their lives, perhaps two or more years, depending on the age and diagnosis at admission. An average length of stay becomes misleading under such circumstances. Most patients in nursing homes need unskilled care—that is, help with activities of daily living and medical oversight rather than medical treatment. Nearly 90 percent of patients in nursing homes are 65 years of age or older. The remaining are younger people who cannot care for themselves because of chronic diseases or accidents (Jones 2002).

Occupancy rates in certified nursing homes showed a slight decline in the 1990s, from 89 percent in 1991, to 86.3 percent in 2004 (National Center for Health Statistics 2006b). Although there is much discussion about the need for long-term care with a growing elderly population, the care has moved to other sites, such as personal care homes, home care, and adult day care, all of which are discussed later in this chapter.

Hospital-Based Care

A number of hospitals have skilled nursing units (step-down units) within their facilities, developed in part to provide a more efficient use of their acute care beds. Certified hospital-based nursing homes increased from 8.7 percent of nursing facilities

in 1991, to 17.7 percent in 2005 (CMS 2006). Hospital-based nursing homes may have higher-quality care because they have more patients eligible for Medicare and higher staffing levels, and are more likely to be not-for-profit (Harrington et al. 1999).

Rural community hospitals are eligible to have "**swing beds**," beds that can handle acute cases one day and skilled nursing care cases the next. This allows a hospital some flexibility. It is a particularly inviting approach to a hospital that has low occupancy rates, and is doubly inviting if an area has a shortage of nursing home beds. Rather than close beds or keep them unoccupied, rural hospitals can use them to provide a stepped-down level of care, thus providing revenue otherwise lost and allowing patients to stay in their local communities. If the hospital is pressed for acute beds at any time, it then has the option of converting the long-term care beds back to acute beds. Nearly 45 percent of hospitals offered skilled nursing facilities in 2005, indicating an effort to garner funding from sources other than acute care (American Hospital Association 2007).

Nursing Home Costs

The costs of providing nursing home care have exploded; costs rose from $4 billion in 1970, to $121.9 billion in 2005 (see Table 10–3). In 2005, Medicaid financed 43.9 percent of nursing home costs; Medicare paid 15.7 percent, and other government sources paid about 2.7 percent, whereas private insurance paid for only about 7.5 percent. Residents paid out of pocket for about 26.5 percent, and private sources other than insurance covered the remaining 3.7 percent (National Center for Health Statistics 2007). These figures represent a small decrease in the Medicaid share and small increase in the Medicare portions since the 1990s (see Table 10–3).

Private long-term care insurance is now available, and the number of policies sold has increased from 515 in 1987, to 8.3 million as of 2001. However, this was still a small percentage of the estimated 35 million Americans over the age of 65 in the year 2000. At the inception of long-term care policies, a typical policy paid for nursing home care and limited home health care. Today's policies tend to include a much broader range of coverage, including both skilled and intermediate nursing home care, personal care, home- and community-based care, and case management (Merlis 2003).

Premiums for long-term care insurance vary enormously, from $325 per year to more than $7,000 per year for an individual, depending on age, medical condition, the amount of the daily benefit, the number of days not covered when the patient is first admitted, and whether or not the policy includes inflation protection (ibid.). Because most patients of long-term care require intermediate or custodial care, it is important to include those provisions as well as home health care in policies; it is also important to include people with mental disorders (for example, Alzheimer's disease).

Unfortunately, many people cannot afford, and few have the foresight, to obtain private insurance. About 24 percent of employers offer long-term care insurance plans to employees so that they can get group rates, but employees are usually required to pay the premium. The federal government began offering long-term care insurance in 2002 (Georgetown University 2003). Tax incentives (using pretax dollars for premiums or deducting premiums on tax returns) for purchasing long-term care insurance have not resulted in increased participation, except among people in higher income brackets. Unfortunately, many Americans do not realize that Medicare does not pay for most long-term care.

Medicare will pay for nursing home care only if patients require skilled nursing services or rehabilitation services on a daily basis. The care must follow a minimum three-day stay in a hospital, be ordered by a physician, and be periodically recertified as necessary for a maximum of 100 days. Because many nursing home residents require custodial rather than skilled nursing care, Medicare is not the primary payer of their care.

TABLE 10–3 Nursing Home Expenditures (in Billions) and Percentage by Source of Funds for Selected Years

	1960	1970	1980	1990	2000	2002	2003	2004	2005
					Amount in Billions				
Nursing home expenditures	$0.80	$4.00	$19.00	$52.60	$95.30	$105.70	$110.40	$115.00	$121.9
All sources of funds	100.00%	100.00%	100.00%	100.00%	100.00%	100.00%	100.00%	100.00%	100%
Out-of-pocket payments	77.30%	52.00%	37.20%	36.10%	30.00%	27.90%	27.60%	26.60%	26.50%
Private health insurance	0.00%	20.00%	1.20%	5.60%	8.20%	8.20%	7.80%	7.50%	7.50%
Other private funds	6.30%	4.80%	4.20%	7.20%	4.70%	3.80%	3.80%	3.70%	3.70%
Government	16.40%	43.00%	57.50%	51.10%	57.00%	60.10%	60.90%	62.20%	62.30%
Medicaid	---	23.30%	53.80%	45.80%	44.10%	44.60%	44.90%	44.80%	43.90%
Medicare	---	3.50%	1.60%	3.20%	10.80%	13.30%	13.50%	14.90%	15.70%

SOURCE: National Center for Health Statistics. 2007. *Health, United States, 2007 with chartbook on trends in the health of Americans.*

Prior to 1997, Medicare paid for skilled nursing home care (when deemed medically necessary) on a cost-plus basis, reimbursing the facility's costs plus a small margin for profit. The Balanced Budget Act of 1997, however, changed the method of payment to a prospective payment system modeled after inpatient hospital payments. Nursing homes are now paid a flat rate per day for patients eligible for Medicare. Many nursing homes have found maintaining a high level of care difficult under the decreased payment mechanism. However, that does not mean that the payment as calculated is unfair and totally responsible for the difficulties. Some organizations, particularly some of the large chains of nursing homes that went on a buying binge during the cost-plus payment era, simply overextended themselves and their credit lines. When skilled nursing home care was no longer lucrative, some began to divest. Others have been able to implement cost-containment features while struggling to maintain quality care, just as in other areas of health care delivery.

Medicaid finances long-term care for the elderly poor and those who have exhausted their savings as private-paying residents. Unlike Medicare, most Medicaid programs pay for both skilled and custodial care for people with long-term disabilities, but only if they are poor enough to qualify for coverage. Although funded by a combination of state and federal funds, Medicaid is run by the states, and eligibility for coverage and the services provided vary greatly among the states. Generally, Medicaid coverage is available only to people with very low incomes. This restriction has resulted in the practice of "**spending down**" among some elderly, which involves paying for care out of pocket until a person becomes poor enough to qualify for Medicaid.

Some elderly people try to transfer their assets, such as real estate and securities, to trusts and relatives to protect the assets from Medicaid spend-down provisions. However, most states now have provisions that allow them to look back some three to five years to retrieve the value of those transferred assets. People who pay out of pocket for nursing home care deplete their resources and qualify for Medicaid within a short time, because the national average cost for nursing home care is estimated at approximately $69,000 per year (American Health Insurance Plans 2006). Legislation has been enacted to protect spouses of residents of nursing homes from financial devastation, allowing them to keep the family home and/or certain assets and income to continue to provide for themselves independently.

Quality of Care, Quality of Life

Prior to 1965, little was done to regulate nursing homes, though state governments were responsible for the licensing of nursing homes. Since the implementation of Medicaid and Medicare, Congress set minimum standards for nursing home care under federal funding and charged the Health Care Financing Administration (now CMS) with the responsibility of monitoring, interpreting, and enforcing those standards. CMS contracts with each state to inspect nursing homes for quality, resident care processes, staff-resident interaction, and environmental and safety standards, to become certified for Medicare and Medicaid beneficiaries (Medicare 2007).

At the time of Medicare and Medicaid implementation, nursing home standards were liberally applied; that is, homes were approved even though they did not fully meet the standards. The decision by the government to apply standards liberally was political: The homes were already in business, and not to certify them and thus deny benefits to the population who thought they were getting benefits would be a political liability for the president and for the legislators who passed the legislation. However, another consideration undoubtedly operated: Getting marginal homes approved would, over time, provide an opportunity to force them to raise the quality of their services, and such improvement would be easier to bring about the more dependent the homes were on Medicare and Medicaid payments.

Reform and improvement efforts have had little success in a "suppliers' market" as the number of people needing care rises. Some states have placed moratoriums on building new facilities to contain costs, while more people need care than there are affordable beds to provide care. Meanwhile, nursing home operators attempt to contain costs by reducing numbers of qualified staff, providing minimal activities, and regimenting care. Needless to say, many nursing homes are not cheery places in which to live or work (Bryan 1986).

Because of the concern over quality of care in nursing homes, Congress requested a study by the Institute of Medicine in 1986. The study found the quality of care "appalling," despite standards for certification and growing competition among nursing home providers. Many residents received inadequate care, which often contributed to their deteriorating health (ibid.). The Institute of Medicine's study, among others, resulted in recommendations for new federal regulations. In 1987, Congress passed nursing home reform legislation as part of the Omnibus Budget Reconciliation Act (OBRA '87), which called for the following:

EXHIBIT 10-1

COMMENTARY
Who Will Care for the Frail Elderly?

"Although caring for elderly parents was a widespread practice in the nuclear families of previous generations, the duration of such care was considerably shorter commensurate with the much shorter lifespan. In the very near future, the "baby boomer" generation will begin to arrive at the geriatric threshold. Shortly thereafter, as they age and become frail, this generation will present a major societal challenge. According to the U.S. government, 15 million Americans used nursing facilities, alternative residential care, or home care services in 2000, and this is expected to increase to 27 million by 2050. Consequently, as the "baby boomers" progress to old age, the demand for direct care workers (i.e., registered nurses, licensed practical and vocational nurses, nurse aides, and home health and personal care workers) will increase dramatically, as the available workforce shrinks. In addition to a projected shortfall in direct care workers, medical schools will be hard-pressed to supply the projected 36,000 certified geriatricians necessary to care for the 70 million Americans who will be 65 or older in 2030.

How will the U.S. care for this huge wave of potentially disabled elderly? Who will pay for their care? How can we afford the additional societal and financial burden? These questions must be addressed now. Without careful planning and investment, the U.S. soon will face a rapidly growing group of frail elderly citizens whose misery will be evident throughout our society. Now is the time to begin discussion and debate—in the halls of Congress and in the halls of medical and nursing schools across the country—in order to address this impending crisis."

From Joseph S. Alpert, MD, and Pamela J. Powers, MPH. 2007. *Who Will Care for the Frail Elderly? The American Journal of Medicine, 120,* 470

Discussion Question

There has been no change in health care policy to prepare for the high probability of increased need for long-term care for the elderly as the baby boomers age. The first baby boomers (born in 1946) will become 75 in 2021, and they may need help with activities of daily living as they are forced to live with chronic illnesses.

1. How will society provide for this large group of the elderly?

- Comprehensive assessment to determine the functional, cognitive, and affective levels of residents to be used in care planning
- Specific requirements for nursing, medical, and psychosocial services to help residents attain and maintain the highest possible level of functioning, both mentally and physically
- Regulations protecting patients' rights

Specific regulations enforcing OBRA '87 have brought about data-collection processes that help consumers, as well as inspectors, evaluate and monitor nursing home care (AARP 2007). Most people dread the prospect of entering a nursing home largely because of the lack of privacy, the loss of autonomy, and the regimentation (see Figure 10–2). Regulations cannot address residents' needs to have a caring environment, to have a sense of community, and to be free of loneliness, boredom, and helplessness.

The Eden Alternative

The Eden Alternative is a different way of thinking about long-term care. The concept, founded by Dr. William Thomas, transforms nursing homes into human habitats that not only shelter but also nurture those who live and work within them. Dr. Thomas identifies three plagues of the elderly: loneliness, helplessness, and boredom. The treatment for these plagues is a natural environment filled with companion animals, plants, and children, as well as the spontaneity that fills most noninstitutionalized environments. When the elderly are given the opportunity to care for other living things, they respond in ways that pills and therapies cannot effect.

Adopting the Eden Alternative also means changing the approach to managing staff. Eden's premise is that "as management does unto staff, so shall staff do unto residents" (Thomas 1998). Staff must be empowered to take part in the process of change, see residents and other staff members as part of

SEE ME

What do you see, nurses, what do you see?
  Are you thinking, when you look at me—
A crabby old woman, not very wise,
  Uncertain of habit, with far-away eyes,
Who dribbles her food and makes no reply,
  When you say in a loud voice—"I do wish you'd try."

Who seems not to notice the things that you do,
  And forever is losing a stocking or shoe,
Who unresisting or not, lets you do as you will,
  With bathing and feeding, the long day to fill.

Is that what you're thinking, is that what you see?
  Then open your eyes, nurse, you're looking at ME...
I'll tell you who I am, as I sit here so still;
  As I rise at your bidding, as I eat at your will.

I'm a small child of ten with a father and mother,
  Brothers and sisters, who love one another,
A young girl of sixteen with wings on her feet.
  Dreaming that soon now a lover she'll meet;
A bride soon at twenty—my heart gives a leap,
  Remembering the vows that I promised to keep;
At twenty-five now I have young of my own,
  Who need me to build a secure, happy home;

A woman of thirty, my young now grow fast,
  Bound to each other with ties that should last;
At forty, my young sons have grown and are gone,
  But my man's beside me to see I don't mourn;
At fifty once more babies play 'round my knee,
  Again we know children, my loved one and me.

Dark days are upon me, my husband is dead,
  I look at the future, I shudder with dread,
For my young are all rearing young of their own,
  And I think of the years and the love that I've known;
I'm an old woman now and nature is cruel—
  'Tis her jest to make old age look like a fool.

The body is crumbled, grace and vigor depart,
  There is now a stone where once I had a heart,
But inside this old carcass a young girl still dwells,
  And now and again my battered heart swells.

I remember the joys, I remember the pain,
  And I'm loving and living life over again,
I think of the years, all too few—gone too fast,
  And accept the stark fact that nothing can last—
So I open your eyes, people, open and see,
  Not a crabby old woman, look closer—see ME!

Figure 10–2 See Me

SOURCE: This poem was found among the possessions of an elderly lady who died in the geriatric ward of a hospital. No information is available concerning her—who she was or when she died.

---

a "neighborhood" of caring, and be able to work in a more spontaneous and natural manner. Regimentation and scheduled events give way to individual choice, opportunity, and personal growth. The Eden Alternative benefits management with lower turnover and absentee rates (Bayne 1998).

An outgrowth of the Eden Alternative is the Greenhouse Project, which carries the Eden principles to new construction. The model advocates building smaller "cottages" for six to eight residents, giving them more choice while providing safe residence.

ASSISTED-LIVING FACILITIES

Faced with the increasing numbers of people needing long-term care, care providers are rethinking the concept of nursing homes. New forms and combinations of care have been implemented with new residential programs and types of personnel. The Eden Alternative is one new form of care. Assisted-living facilities are another option to provide care for those who cannot live independently but do not require skilled nursing care. Once referred to as personal care homes, they allow a combination of independent residency in an apartment-like setting but provide supervision and help with some of the functional limitations of residents, providing such services as group meals, laundry, cleaning services, and medication monitoring. Some assisted-living facilities are part of a broader "retirement community" that allows all levels of living, from independent apartments to skilled nursing care. Residents move to different levels of care as needed, with little disruption to their lives and families. Other assisted-living centers are freestanding facilities. Insurance usually does not cover the costs of assisted-living facilities. Residents pay personally, as they would for rent or a mortgage, or else they qualify for government subsidy in publicly supported facilities.

COMMUNITY-BASED CARE

Many of the elderly would prefer not to go into nursing homes if necessary services were available in the community. Studies in the 1980s showed that between 20 percent and 40 percent of the nursing home population could be cared for at less-intensive levels if adequate community-based care were available (Long-Term Care 1981). However, health care payment structures encouraged people to choose nursing home care, even when community services were available. Medicaid paid for nursing home care but not for community-based services, unless the state received a waiver from the federal government. Beginning in 1981, waivers were granted to some states to offer certain kinds of social services (for example, help with bathing, cooking, or cleaning) to people living at home, in the hope that nursing home care could be delayed or avoided and the high government expenditures for nursing home care could be reduced.

The federal government financed the most extensive study of community-based care from 1982 to 1984. It involved 6,300 elderly people, whose average age was 80, in ten states (U.S.

Department of Health and Human Services 1987a). The states were granted Medicaid waivers and funds to provide a broad base of community services to help elderly people who are impaired to remain in their own homes rather than enter nursing homes. Comprehensive case management called "channeling" was used, whereby a person, called a case manager, identified the participating person's specific problems and services needed and developed a plan of care. The case managers helped their clients access needed services, and they coordinated community services and informal help given by family and friends. They monitored the services to be sure that they were delivered and that they met the needs of the client. The results of the study showed that the community-based programs did not reduce nursing home costs and, in fact, increased the cost to the government. The community services had little effect on the number of admissions into nursing home. Most of the elderly studied would have remained in their own homes whether or not the community services were provided.

Mechanic (1987) points out that the reason for admission to a nursing home may be based on factors other than need, because many living in the community may have as great a need level. Rather, admission may be the result of the loss of a spouse or other significant support person(s), or a major illness or accident that makes such people lacking support unable to care for themselves.

The services provided in the "channeling" project did not replace the care that family and friends gave, but it complemented that care and enabled informal caregivers to maintain their efforts rather than become overwhelmed. The channeling long-term care study "indicates that the expansion of case management and community services beyond what already exists does not lead to overall cost savings. But it does yield benefits in the form of in-home care, reduced unmet needs, and improved satisfaction with life for clients and informal caregivers who bear most of the burden. Whether these benefits are commensurate with its costs is a decision for society to make" (U.S. Department of Health and Human Services 1987b). The results of the National Long-Term Care Demonstration (as this study is called) agree with other community care demonstrations.

Kemper (1987) suggests that policy makers should move beyond asking whether expanding community care saves money and should address the issues of how much community care society is willing to finance, who should receive it, and how to deliver it efficiently. A synthesis of twenty-seven studies of home and community care for the chronically ill elderly, including the ten-state, multimillion-dollar National Long-Term Care Demonstration, concluded that the health benefits were small. Longevity and mental functioning were unaffected. Physical functioning either remained the same or decreased, apparently because clients became dependent on the home care aid. Only life satisfaction or "contentment" was favorably affected, but even this improvement was small and dissipated after several months, despite continuing care. Most of those using home care services were not at risk of entering a nursing home, and although nursing home use was reduced in some studies, the cost of home care offset any savings from the reduced use of nursing homes.

One of the demonstration projects for comprehensive community care that survived is the Program of All-Inclusive Care for the Elderly (PACE). The participants of PACE continue to live at home (for the most part) while receiving services developed by an interprofessional care team addressing the needs of the particular participant. While developing the plan for social and medical services, the program must include all Medicare and Medicaid eligible services in addition to other required services. PACE providers receive a capitated fee and can require no cost sharing on the part of the participant. Much like a managed care organization, the PACE provider is at financial risk for participants' care without limits on amount, duration, or scope of services (CMS 2005a).

The results of the 1980 studies make it hard to justify home care on the basis of health benefits or cost savings. However, expanding home care is still popular, not only because it is "the right thing to do" (Weissert 1991), but also because the move to prospective payment for hospital care and the incentive to decrease the length of stay in the hospital setting has made home care available to more than the potential nursing home population. Many patients of all ages, discharged from the acute care setting of the hospital, continue to require an intermittent level of skilled nursing care. Home care can provide that care without additional institutionalization for patients.

HOME HEALTH CARE

Home health care agencies typically provide care for individuals in the community who are disabled. They supply people confined to their homes with a combination of medical services (part-time skilled nursing care, physical therapy, speech therapy, occupational therapy, medical social services, and some medical supplies and equipment) and personal care services (helping clients bathe and dress, changing bed linens, and cooking). In most cases, the services supplement the care the clients receive from family and friends. Although most of the agencies' clients are elderly, there are also younger clients who are recovering from an illness or accident, from a stay in the hospital, or from chronic medical conditions and need prolonged care but do not require hospitalization. The Centers for Disease Control and Prevention (CDC) reports that the number of people served by home health care agencies rose from 1.2 million in 1992, to 2.4 million in 1996, but decreased to 1.3 million in 2000 (National Center for Health Statistics 2005).

Home care agencies operate under various names, have varying organizational ties, and offer differing services. They can be independent, hospital-operated, or health department–managed agencies. The number of home health agencies has increased from 2,924 in 1980, to a high of 10,807 in 1997, and down to 6,928 in 2003. The decrease coincides with the changes in Medicare reimbursement for home health services. Of home health agencies, 63 percent were for-profit, 10 percent were nonprofit, and 17 percent were government-owned in 2003 (National Association for Home Care and Hospice 2007).

The earliest home health care agencies were visiting nurse agencies, which were created in the late 1800s to bring needed care to communities that had no hospital. A nurse, usually one with public health training, would visit homes to provide care to patients and support to the family. Today, visiting nurse agencies represent only 8 percent of all freestanding home health agencies in the United States, and they continue to provide care to some 4 million patients annually (Visiting Nurse Association of America 2007).

Home health care expanded, particularly in the 1980s, and includes such services as skilled nursing care; personal care; medication preparation and management; equipment delivery, setup, and management; respiratory, physical, speech, and infusion therapy; and even hospice care—all provided to patients in their own homes. The Joint Commission accredits over 3,400 home health care organizations. Accreditation meets the organization's needs in demonstrating quality care, obtaining state licensure, and meeting certification requirements for the Medicare and Medicaid programs and other insurers (Joint Commission 2007).

Expenditures in home health care reached $13 billion in 1990, and increased to $47.4 billion in 2005. Public programs financed almost 75 percent of the 2005 costs. Medicare paid almost $18 billion, and Medicaid paid over $8 billion for home health care in 2005. Patients' out-of-pocket expenditures accounted for about $5 billion, whereas private insurance paid only $5.7

TABLE 10-4 Home Health Care Expenditures by Source of Funds for Selected Years

	2005	2003	2000	1998	1997	1995	1992
	Expenditures in Millions of Dollars						
Home health care	47,451	38,025	30,514	33,221	34,544	30,529	18,170
Private funds	11,997	10,876	13,607	16,519	13,810	11,630	7,548
Consumer payments	10,900	9,971	12,377	15,045	12,535	10,378	6,524
Out-of-pocket payments	5,120	4,778	5,451	6,678	5,459	4,509	2,842
Private health insurance	5,780	5,193	6,926	8,367	7,076	5,869	3,682
Other private funds	1,097	905	1,229	1,474	1,275	1,253	1,024
Public funds	35,454	27,148	16,907	16,702	20,734	18,898	10,622
Federal funds	26,463	20,428	12,328	12,556	16,728	15,325	8,055
Medicare	17,879	13,688	8,556	9,422	13,850	12,964	6,446
Medicaid	8,348	6,574	3,663	3,047	2,802	2,307	1,569
Other	236	167	109	87	77	53	39
State and local funds	8,991	6,720	4,579	4,146	4,005	3,573	2,567
Medicaid	7,166	5,171	3,093	2,538	2,328	2,006	1,369
Other	1,825	1,549	1,486	1,608	1,677	1,567	1,198

SOURCE: CMS. 2005. National Health Expenditures by Type of Service and Source of Funds, CY 2005–1960.

billion (see Table 10–4). The remainder came from other private sources (CMS 2005b).

The growth in home health expenditures is a result of liberalized Medicare payments, an increase in the number of home health providers, and an increased demand for services. However, the 1997 Balanced Budget Act placed greater restraints on home health care reimbursement from Medicare. Services previously paid on a fee-for-service basis are now paid under a prospective payment system, just as hospital payments and skilled nursing facility payments. Tighter funding led to consolidation of organizations whereas technology led to the development of telemedicine to bring an even higher level of care to those unable to leave their homes.

ADULT DAY CARE

Another long-term care program that enables some elderly to remain in the community is adult day care. Adult day care programs can maintain or improve client overall functioning, increase social interactions, offer respite care for family caregivers, or even allow caregivers to remain employed. They differ from senior centers in that they serve adults who are physically impaired or mentally confused and require supervision, increased social opportunities, and assistance with personal care or other daily living activities. There are over 3,500 adult day care centers nationally, serving primarily a population of people suffering from dementia (National Adult Day Services Association 2008).

Adult day care programs are operated by hospitals, nursing homes, and social agencies. Only 22 percent are for-profit, with the remaining 78 percent being nonprofit or public organizations. Medicare does not pay for adult day care; although Medicaid does cover it in some states, it can be a financial burden and available to only those in higher income brackets. More private long-term care insurance policies are now including "community care," including adult day care, as a covered service. As noted earlier, however, the number of the elderly covered under such policies is small. Nationally, adult day care centers charge anywhere from $25 to $100 a day, much less than the cost of nursing home care. Transportation can be a problem that makes adult day care a much less promising investment than home care for some (National Adult Day Services Association 2008).

In 1993, the Robert Wood Johnson Foundation awarded a number of grants in hopes of stimulating innovation in the adult day care field. The goal of the program was to demonstrate that adult day care centers could provide beneficial services to clients and their families at affordable prices (Gunby 1993). The grant programs recognized that high-quality activity programs help reduce depression in the participants and help them maintain function. Adult day care centers can become more responsive to caregiver needs by offering a wider range of services, such as longer hours, hours on weekends and in evenings, and overnights. The average age of the adult day care participant is 72 years of age. Two-thirds of the participants are women, and 59 percent of the participants require assistance with two or more activities of daily living. Lack of reimbursement by Medicare and Medicaid programs means adult day care is available to a limited number of those who need the services (National Adult Day Services Association 2008).

HOSPICE CARE

Although earlier models of care for the dying existed, St. Christopher's Hospice in England is often cited as the model for hospice development in the United States. The first pilot program ran in a chronic-disease hospital in Massachusetts. The program, which emphasized symptom and pain control, focused on the psychosocial needs of both patients and the family. In 1974, the first freestanding hospice, Connecticut Hospice Inc., was established in New Haven, Connecticut. Connecticut Hospice Inc. started as exclusively home care, but it built an inpatient facility three years later to deliver a full range of care (Mor and Masterson-Allen 1987).

A number of factors contributed to the development of hospice. The late 1960s and early 1970s saw a growth in the awareness of the experience of dying. Particularly important was the influence of Elisabeth Kubler-Ross's book, *On Death and Dying* (1969), on the stages of dying. It brought attention to the patient as a person and detailed the experience of dying for both the patient and the caretaker (Paradis and Cummings 1986). Advanced technology and training in medicine as a science had produced an impersonal medical delivery system that lost sight of the patient's personhood. Although the hospital originated as a place to die, cure now became the focus. New technologies sought to defy death as a normal process. The controversial Karen Quinlan court case brought discussion of patients' rights to terminate treatment to the forefront. Legislation in various states supported patient autonomy and decisions to withhold or withdraw treatment (Mor and Masterson-Allen 1987). Hospice provided the **palliative care** and the psychosocial support needed by terminally ill patients who opted out of technological intervention near the end of life.

Hospice ideals often came into conflict with the views of established medical systems. Particularly controversial was the limited role of the physician in hospice care. Physician input was necessary for proper symptom and pain control, but this input was only part of a team effort to deliver care in the hospice environment. Nurses, chaplains, social workers, volunteers, and family all were seen as equally important. This idea was in direct conflict with the amount of power and control that physicians experienced in traditional health care settings. Particularly challenged was the role of physician paternalism. No longer were physicians expected to make decisions in the best interest of the patients. Physicians were expected to communicate honestly with patients about their prognoses and treatment options and allow the patients to participate fully in all treatment decisions (Abel 1986).

Hospice also challenged traditional hospital practices that often isolated patients at a time when they most needed support. Patients in hospice were allowed to have family and/or friends with them at all times, wear their own clothing, choose their meals, and encounter as few restrictions as possible. Staff spent unrestricted time with patients, delivering more spiritual and emotional care than medical care (ibid.).

Hospice was first established as a nonprofit, voluntary endeavor. Volunteers provided care, and funds were secured through service organizations, philanthropies, and individual contributors (Paradis and Cummings 1986). Earliest models were independent, providing care in the home or a freestanding facility totally separate from the hospital or established home health agency. Subsequent models have been based in a home health agency or hospital. Existing home health agencies began providing hospice care, contracting with hospitals and/or nursing homes to provide inpatient care when home-based care was no longer feasible. Hospital-based hospice might consist of separate units, scattered beds throughout the facility, or teams trained to deliver hospice care in the home (ibid.). Variations exist even within these three major models.

As the delivery of hospice care became more widespread, securing funds became more important. Largely through the efforts of the National Hospice and Palliative Care Organization, efforts were made to provide funding through federal grants and third-party payers. Increased dependence of hospice on government and on private reimbursement mechanisms brought with it increased requirements to conform to certain standards and behaviors. Although some hospice organizers wanted no part of the influences of regulators, even at the expense of funding opportunities, others sought integration into the established medical care system as a matter of survival. In its efforts to seek third-party reimbursement, particularly Medicare reimbursement, the National Hospice Organization worked closely with the Joint Commission to develop the accreditation process for hospice standards. These standards subsequently became very influential over hospice care. The Joint Commission now requires hospitals to accredit their hospice programs or risk losing hospital accreditation (Paradis and Cummings 1986).

Medicare regulations, finalized by the Health Care Financing Administration (now CMS) in 1983, provided for payment for hospice services to certified hospice providers. In this set of certification requirements, the transformation of hospice takes place. Certified hospice programs are subject to the following requirements:

- A care plan must be established for each person admitted to the hospice program, and care must be provided in accordance with that plan.

- All the core services must be directly provided with hospice employees (specific regulations limit the subcontracting of services).

- All aspects of the care plan must be managed regardless of the setting in which the patient resides (the hospice manages the plan even if the patient is intermittently admitted to a hospital or nursing home) (Tierney and Wilson 1993).

- At least 80 percent of care must be provided in the patient's home and only 20 percent in inpatient settings.

- Reimbursement was capped at $9,000 for six months of services, emphasizing the difficulty in predicting the length of a patient's life (Bulkin et al. 1992).

Medicare reimbursement brought funding in a more steady and predictable stream than what could be provided through contributions or grants. However, it also brought about regulation that limited the availability of hospice care to some patients. The mere prospect of waiving one's rights to hospital care can be too frightening to opt for hospice care. The requirement that 80 percent of the patient's care be provided in the patient's home makes patients who have no family support structure ineligible for care (Hoyer 1990; Jones 1988). Although Medicare funding brought hospice care into mainline medicine, it also effected change from the original conception of hospice care. However, the influence worked both ways. The hospice movement encouraged physicians to discuss death with their patients and brought family and other support systems closer to dying patients.

Current Medicare payment requirements are as follows:

- The patient's doctor and the hospice medical director must certify that the patient has a life-limiting illness and death may be expected in six months or less if the disease runs its normal course.

- The patient signs a statement choosing hospice care instead of routine Medicare-covered benefits for the illness.

- The patient must receive care from a Medicare-approved hospice program.

Care is no longer restricted to a patient's home. As well, a wide range of services are available to the patient, including physician and nursing care, therapy, medications for symptom relief, homemaker services, counseling, and grief support for the patient and family. The only noncovered service is medication not related to symptom relief (Caring Connections 2007).

REHABILITATION FACILITIES

Rehabilitation hospitals or centers provide acute and/or residential care to people suffering from traumatic brain injury, stroke, disabling diseases, cognitive disorders, and a full array of other problems resulting in functional disability. Services provided can include physical therapy, occupational therapy, speech therapy, and counseling or psychological therapy, as well as nursing care and personal care. Length of treatment might be anywhere from a few months to permanent residence in the facility. Rehabilitation centers admit people who are otherwise medically stable, and their goal is to get patients to the highest level of functioning possible for discharge back to the community and maintenance on an outpatient basis, or to slow the debilitation process as much as possible as patients remain in the residential portion of the facility.

Some rehabilitation centers specialize in treatment for one category of diagnosis, such as spinal cord injury or drug and alcohol rehabilitation. Others provide a wide range of care. Because of the wide range of diagnoses and services provided, providing an average cost of care is difficult. The patient's diagnosis, variety of therapies needed, treatment response times, and comorbidities (other illnesses) will determine costs and length of stay.

Although the discussion here applies to facilities specializing in rehabilitation therapy, it is important to remember that rehabilitation services might also take place within nursing homes, acute care hospitals, outpatient facilities, and the patient's home. The term *rehabilitation facility* might also be applied to mental health and substance abuse organizations discussed elsewhere.

CONTINUING CARE COMMUNITIES

Continuing care communities became popular about twenty years ago as an arrangement providing for the needs of the elderly, including nursing care. These communities require a large entrance fee of between $50,000 and $100,000 or more (often obtained through the sale of a home), and a monthly payment to contribute to operating costs (often financed by pension or assets). For this fee, housing and nursing care is ensured, along with housekeeping and some meals. People with high-risk health problems are either excluded or required to pay more. Medicare pays only for acute medical care that may be necessary. People are encouraged to enter after retirement while still in good health. Accommodations are usually apartments and, when residents can no longer cope in apartments, an assisted living facility. Until recently, nonprofit groups ran most communities, but now for-profit communities are being developed, some of which do not require a large entrance fee but charge a monthly fee according to the amount of care needed. Continuing care communities are available only to those with adequate financial resources who want the security they provide. However, there are some government-subsidized housing complexes with facilities and services for the elderly poor who cannot manage housekeeping and personal tasks. Often these senior housing communities have long waiting lists.

SUMMARY

Long-term care refers to a wide range of health and social services that are needed to compensate for the functional disabilities of people of any age. Although many people with chronic conditions that prevent them from functioning independently are under 65 years old, most are the very old who are no longer able to independently cope with the activities of daily living. For those people, nursing home care is an option, and its cost

is financed almost entirely by Medicaid and by out-of-pocket payments of residents. Private insurance pays for only about 8 percent of nursing home costs.

Community-based and private organizations provide home care to enable people who are functionally disabled to remain in the community. Home care may delay, but probably does not eliminate, nursing home admissions; it does, however, appear to improve the quality of life of caregivers and recipients. Other long-term care services include rehabilitation hospitals, adult day care, and hospice care.

Historically, quality of care delivered in long-term care, primarily nursing homes, has been of great concern. Legislation has focused on quality of services delivered in most long-term care settings, but as in other venues, regulation does not ensure personal and patient-centered care.

The state and federal governments (via Medicaid and, to a lesser extent, Medicare) finance the majority of long-term care. Medicare pays for nursing home and rehabilitation care as long as a patient needs skilled nursing care. Medicaid pays for custodial care after a patient has no personal resources to cover the costs. Medicare will pay for hospice care and medically necessary home health care. However, such services as adult day care, assisted-living facilities, and residence in a continuing care facility must be paid with personal funds.

The costs have risen sharply, and the demand for services continues to increase, making a prime policy issue of the question of who should pay for long-term care. Many policy makers believe that neither government nor the private sector alone can provide long-term care and are seeking new ways of financing it, especially in light of the pending growth in the elderly population. One approach being tested is to encourage all people to purchase long-term care insurance just as they would health or life insurance. Financing is only one major problem; other problems include determining the appropriateness and quality of services. As with other health care organizations, the Joint Commission is the primary accrediting organization for long-term care providers. State agencies may also be involved in licensing and accreditation.

ACTIVITY-BASED LEARNING

- Medicare provides a website to help people choose a nursing home. At www.medicare.gov, search for "nursing home compare." The information provides quality information, accreditations status, and any type of regulatory deficiencies.

On the website, find information on some nursing homes in your area. Are you surprised by any of the information?

- Log onto the website for the Eden Alternative (www.edenalt. com). Are any of the nursing homes in your state registered Eden facilities? Is there an Eden facility nearby? If there is, arrange to visit the facility to experience the difference.

- The American Health Care Association provides information and advocates for people needing long-term care. Access the association's website (www.ahca.org) to see its suggestions for choosing a quality nursing home. What are some of the points it suggests looking for in nursing home care?

A QUESTION OF ETHICS

- Is it ethical for the elderly to pass their wealth on to their children so that they may qualify for Medicaid coverage of nursing home care if it is needed?

- The term *sandwich generation* has been used to describe adults torn between the responsibilities of caring for minor children while at the same time caring for their elderly parents. What responsibility do children have for meeting the long-term care needs of their parents?

- Quality of life versus quantity of life issues are often discussed in relationship to the appropriateness of medical interventions in acute care settings. Quality of life is also the central theme in discussions of patient self-determination and the choice of hospice care. As the costs of long-term care rise and the numbers needing care increase, how do we decide if cost of care rather than quality of life is the driving mechanism in an individual's care during their final years?

REFERENCES

1. Advancement of Retired Persons (AARP). (2007). *The 1987 Nursing Home Reform Act fact sheet*. Retrieved from www. aarp.org/research/legis-polit/legislation/aresearch-import-687-FS84.html

2. Abel, E. (1986). The hospice movement: Institutionalizing innovation. *International Journal of Health Services*, 16(1), 71.

3. American Hospital Association. (2007). *TrendWatch chartbook 2007: Trends affecting hospitals and health systems*. Retrieved from www.aha.org/aha/research-and-trends/chartbook/2007chartbook.html

4. Bulkin, W., Wald, F., & O'Brien-Butler, J. (1992, May/June). Regulations vs. ideals: A case history of a hospice closure. *American Journal of Hospice & Palliative Care*, p. 18.

5. Bayne, M. (1998, December). Spotlight on the Eden Alternative. *Contemporary Long-Term Care*, p. 92.

6. Bryan, J. (1986, June). View from the hill. *American Family Physician 33*(6). Retrieved from web.lexis-nexis.com

7. Caring Connections. (2007). Paying for Hospice. Retrieved from www.caringinfo.org/CaringForSomeone/Hospice/PayingForHospice.htm

8. CMS. (2006). *Data compendium 2006 edition*. Retrieved from www.cms.hhs.gov/datacompendium/18_2006_data_compendium.asp

9. CMS. (2005a). *Program of All Inclusive Care for the Elderly (PACE) overview*. Retrieved from www.cms.hhs.gov/pace/

10. CMS. (2005b). National health expenditures by type of service and source of funds, CY 2005–1960. Retrieved from www.cms.hhs.gov/NationalHealthExpendData/02_NationalHealthAccountsHistorical.asp

11. Day, T. (2007). *Paying the cost of care*. Retrieved from www.longtermcarelink.net/eldercare/paying_the_cost_of_care.htm

12. Merlis, M. (2003). *Private long-term care insurance*. Georgetown University Long-Term Care Financing Project, Health Policy Institute, Washington, DC.

13. Gunby, P. (1993). Adult day care centers vital, many more needed. *JAMA, 269*(18), 2341.

14. Harrington, C., Carrillo, H., Thollaug, S., & Summers, P. (1999, January). *Nursing facilities, staffing, residents, and facility deficiencies, 1991 through 1997*. Retrieved on November 29, 1999 from www.hcfa.gov/medicaid/ltchomep.htm

15. Hoyer, R. (1990). Public policy and the American hospice movement: The tie that binds. *Caring, 9*(3), 30.

16. Joint Commission. (2007). *Home care: Fast track*. Retrieved from www.jointcommission.org/AccreditationPrograms/HomeCare/

17. Jones, A. (2002). *The National Nursing Home Survey: 1999 summary*. National Center for Health Statistics. *Vital Health Stat, 13*(152).

18. Jones, P. (1988). How has the Medicare benefit changed hospice? *Caring*, p. 8.

19. Kemper, P. (1987). Community care demonstrations: What have we learned? *Health Care Finance Review, 8*(4), 87.

20. Long-term care: In search of solutions. (1981). Washington, DC: National Conference on Social Welfare.

21. Mechanic, D. (1987). Challenges in long-term care policy. *Health Affairs, 6*(2), 22.

22. Medicare. (2007). *Nursing homes: About nursing home inspections.* Retrieved from www.medicare.gov/Nursing/AboutInspections.asp

23. Mor, V., & Masterson-Allen, S. (1987). *Hospice care systems: Structure, process, costs and outcome.* New York: Springer.

24. National Adult Day Services Association. (2008). Adult day services: Overview and facts. Retrieved from www.nadsa.org/adsfacts/default.asp

25. National Association for Home Care and Hospice. (2007). *Basic statistics about home care, 2004.* Retrieved from www.nahc.org/04HC_Stats.pdf

26. National Center for Health Statistics. (2007). *Health, United States, 2007 with chartbook on trends in the health of Americans.* Hyattsville, Maryland.

27. National Center for Health Statistics. (2006a). *National Nursing Home Survey.* Retrieved from www.cdc.gov/nchs/nnhs.htm

28. National Center for Health Statistics. (2006b). *Health, United States, 2006 with chartbook on trends in the health of Americans.* Hyattsville, MD. Retrieved from www.cdc.gov/nchs/data/hus/hus06.pdf

29. National Center for Health Statistics. (2005). *Health, United States, 2005 with chartbook on trends in the health of Americans.* Hyattsville, Maryland. Retrieved from www.cdc.gov/nchs/data/hus/hus05.pdf

30. Paradis, L., & Cummings, S. (1986). The evolution of hospice in America toward organizational homogeneity. *Journal of Health and Social Behavior, 27,* 370.

31. Raffel, M., & Raffel, N. (1994). *The U.S. health system: Origins and functions* (4th ed.). Albany, NY: Delmar Publishers.

32. Saphir, A. (1999, September 27). Forever young: Long-term care industry must reinvent itself to keep boomers, minorities happy. *Modern Healthcare,* p. S28.

33. Thomas, W. (1998). *Long-term care design: Building homeness into existing long-term care facilities.* Eden Alternative Literature.

34. Tierney, J., & Wilson, S. (1993, March/April). The effect of the Medicare regulations on hospice practice: Enhancing staff performance. *American Journal of Hospice & Palliative Care,* p. 26.

35. U.S. Census Bureau. (2005). *Population profile of the United States, population distribution in 2005.* Retrieved from www.census.gov/population/pop-profile/dynamic/PopDistribution.pdf

36. U.S. Department of Health and Human Services. (1987a). *National long-term care demonstration.* Washington, DC: HHS.

37. U.S. Department of Health and Human Services. (1987b). *The evaluation of national long-term care demonstrations: Final report executive summary.* Washington, DC: HHS.

38. Visiting Nurse Association of America (2007). *About VNAA.* From www.vnaa.org/vnaa/g/?h=HTML/AboutVNAA

39. Weissert, W. (1991). A new policy agenda for home care. *Health Affairs, 10*(2), 67.

Chapter 11

Public Health—The Health of the Community

CHAPTER OBJECTIVES

After completing this chapter, readers should have an understanding of the following:

- To understand the history of the U.S. public health system
- To understand the transition of public health to community health
- To introduce the concept of health care safety nets
- To understand the role of public health in emergency readiness

INTRODUCTION

Public health activities emphasize prevention of disease, disability, and premature death by the organized efforts of government. So much has been accomplished through public health interventions during its early years that the general public and government funding processes often take public health functions for granted. In 1988, the Institute of Medicine (IOM) recognized the responsibilities of public health agencies "to serve as stewards of the basic health needs of entire populations, but at the same time avert impending disasters and provide personal health care to those rejected by the rest of the health system" (p. 3). Pressure is on public health agencies to do more with less—in both financial and human resources. The very concept of public health as a function of government means that public health professionals who use their expertise to analyze, track, and control disease, must also convince political powers to act. The systems by which this is accomplished are varied from state to state and region to region, making the function of public health personnel more difficult.

By 2002, the IOM began to see the "health of the public" as a function of more than government agencies. The Committee on Assuring the Health of the Public in the 21st Century referred to a public health system that included government agencies, community groups and agencies, health care providers, educators, and other community sectors (Institute of Medicine 2003). This has added to public health capacity but has also brought the issue of coordination of services to the forefront.

THE HISTORY OF PUBLIC HEALTH

The first public health activities in the United States began in the early nineteenth century in the large cities and focused on sanitation. At that time, the major health threats were epidemics of such infectious diseases as smallpox, typhoid fever, and diphtheria. Local boards of health were formed to combat these epidemics, and their main function initially was to improve sanitation. They developed ordinances regarding waste disposal, street drainage, removal of filth, drainage of swamps, and other measures that would improve the sanitary environment. Quarantine of homes and ships, and much later, immunizations, were also important functions of local boards of health aimed at preventing the spread of infectious diseases.

In 1869, the first state board of health was formed in Massachusetts. By 1900, all states had boards of health. Their main functions remained the same as those of local units, but they focused on the statewide control of infectious or communicable diseases and the enforcement of sanitary regulations. They accomplished this mainly by encouraging the further development of local boards of health and then working through them, as well as by directly handling the issues that extended beyond the jurisdiction of a single local board or that required the organizational efforts and legal authority of the state government.

Departments of public health with full-time professional staffs headed by a medically trained health officer evolved to support the work of the health boards. In the early 1900s, the work of health departments began to broaden. The New York City Department of Health set up neighborhood health centers in slum areas to offer maternal and child health care services for the poor to deal with their high maternal and infant mortality rates; to detect (and in some cases treat) tuberculosis, the leading cause of death in 1900; and to control venereal (sexually transmitted) diseases. The expansion of the public health departments into personal health care, particularly maternal and child health, initially drew opposition from the medical profession, which considered it an intrusion into its domain.

Local and state public health departments were strengthened in 1935, by the infusion of federal monies, which earmarked grants for maternal and child health and for general public health activities. By the 1960s, the earlier threat of communicable diseases had largely been replaced by new concerns for chronic and degenerative diseases associated with modern life, such as heart and lung diseases, cancer, stroke, and mental illness. Public health officials made smoking as well as alcohol and drug abuse important public health issues, with programs geared to prevention and with financing by local, state, and federal funds. Since then, communicable diseases have again become prominent with the rise and rapid spread of **human immunodeficiency virus (HIV)** and **acquired immunodeficiency syndrome (AIDS)**, the reemergence of tuberculosis, the outbreak of **severe acute respiratory syndrome (SARS)**, and the threat of bird flu (avian influenza).

Although physicians have always done some preventive work, including checkups and the education of their patients on matters relating to their health, the bulk of their activities are focused on crisis intervention—on dealing with the vast array of concerns and complaints registered by patients when they consult their physicians. This is not to suggest that physicians are not concerned with prevention (the focus on managed care and health care cost containment has increased attention on healthy lifestyles in more recent years), but it does point out two fundamental facts.

First, the major preventive thrusts are beyond the organizational capacity of individual physicians. What is required is a communal effort organized under the regulatory powers of the state. Individual physicians can do little, for example, to ensure purity of water and air, the elimination of noxious substances from the environment, protection of people from a large number of communicable diseases, protection from unsafe social and occupational environments, and safety of marketable products such as drugs, foods, and automobiles. Physician authority is limited, but physicians can, as experts in matters relating to health, advise those who have authority (state government along with its agencies) to order and to take all necessary steps to protect society. Individual physicians and medical societies have given this kind of advice throughout history.

Second, despite the importance of prevention, the fact remains that society will always demand that the crises of life that call for physician intervention—injured children, complicated pregnancies, heart attacks—be addressed and that prevention, if necessary, be deferred. Medical crises come first, and society demands physician intervention with whatever resources are appropriate.

Having actively supported the creation of government health agencies, physicians in various states have nonetheless, from time to time, been in conflict with these health departments—sometimes in disagreement about how health department programs should develop professionally, sometimes in reaction to what private physicians felt was government intrusion into their domain. The American Medical Association (AMA), for example, though long supportive of many federal health initiatives, took issue with the Sheppard-Towner Act (1921)[1] and unsuccessfully opposed the grant program for development of child health programs in the states. At the time, the AMA saw

---

[1]The Sheppard-Towner Act of 1921 provided federal funding (with matching state funds) to reduce maternal and infant mortality. It was fiercely opposed by the American Medical Association (AMA), and some members of Congress, as too socialistic. Some of the influential pediatricians in the AMA who were in favor of the bill broke off from the organization and created the American Academy of Pediatrics. The law was allowed to lapse in 1929 (www.4woman.gov/TimeCapsule/century/appendix_a.htm).

this as the opening wedge for the provision of all medical care by government. On the other hand, the AMA recognized and supported the need for government action to provide medical care for the poor, but has vigorously opposed proposals for compulsory national health insurance.

Similar patterns appear at the state level. In some states, a happy and progressive relationship developed between the medical societies and the health departments. In Maryland, leaders in the medical society and in private practice worked closely with the state health department for many years to develop some of the most progressive public health programs in the nation. The qualities of leadership and political skill on the part of medical and government leaders often made the difference, along with some of the key issues of the time to which we all occasionally respond but over which we have little control. In a 1974 survey of local health departments, Miller et al. (1977a) found that in only one of ten of the large city health departments and in only one in five of the small local health departments was the medical society viewed by the department as a constraint on the development of services.

STATE HEALTH AGENCIES

State health agencies play a key role in the health of the U.S. citizens, and they perform a wide variety of public health services.

Administrative Organization

The traditional public health functions include the following:

- Communicable disease control
- Maternal and child health services
- Environmental sanitation
- Health education
- Laboratory services
- Vital statistics

Until recently, these were placed administratively in state health or public health departments. In some areas, there has been a tendency to remove some of the environmental health activities and place them in new environmental protection agencies. However, a state government's health responsibilities go far beyond these basic six functions. Not only have the basic six functions spawned a large number of related program activities far beyond the original range of services, but the states have also been responsible for care of those with mental illness

and retardation, and for professional and institutional licensure. The right to practice medicine, nursing, pharmacy, dentistry, and many other professional activities is a right granted by the issuance of a license from a state government, not from the federal government or a professional association, or by virtue of a university degree.

How a state government organizes its public health functions varies. History, personalities, federal grant programs, and chance, all play a role. Some states place all activities in a single agency. Some states place them in separate agencies. In any one state, the organizational pattern may change from time to time as new problems arise and as new opportunities are seized.

Leadership in state public health agencies also varies. Although early state agencies depended largely on medical professionals to head their organizations, times are changing. In some states, more emphasis is now placed on management skills as indicated by the background of the state health officers' credentials (see Table 11–1).

There are three basic models. In the first, a board of health with policy or administrative functions over the agency heads the health agency. The board is typically appointed by the governor

TABLE 11–1 Educational Degrees for State Public Health Officials, 2006

Degree	Total	Percentage
Medical doctor (MD)	16	28.07%
Master of public health (MPH)	3	5.26%
MD/MPH	15	26.32%
Registered nurse (RN)	2	3.51%
Master of social work (MSW)	2	3.51%
Doctor of dental science (DDS)	1	1.8%
Master of business administration	4	7.02%
Master of arts education (MA Ed)	1	1.8%
Doctor of public health	1	1.8%
Jurist doctor	2	3.51%
PhD	1	1.8%
None listed	9	15.79%

SOURCE: www.statepublichealth.org/index.php?template=sho.php.

and approved by the state senate. Board members are usually nonsalaried and, when the boards have policy or administrative roles to play, physicians tend to be in the majority. In addition to overall direction of the agency, boards of health (including boards that have only advisory functions) very frequently have authority to enforce public health laws by holding hearings on violations, hearing appeals on health officer actions, and by issuing board orders for compliance with the laws. Board orders must be enforced by law enforcement agencies, although the recipient of a board of health order can, of course, appeal it in the state courts. Many boards either appoint key agency personnel or have a strong influence in their appointment. Historically, there have been good and bad boards of health, progressive as well as nonprogressive boards. Some boards have been highly politicized by the types of people appointed to them; other boards have been highly professional with no partisan politics involved.

The second model of health agency governance has a governor-appointed secretary or commissioner of health. Like boards, this type of leadership can be good or bad, depending on the quality of the appointed official and the quality of the governor. If a governor avoids tough issues, if a governor tends to appoint based on political favors rather than competency, then the board system might be preferred. On the other hand, if the board isn't progressive, then a strong governor with a competent secretary of health would be preferred. The political style of a state often dictates how well each of the systems works. There is a tendency in recent years to move away from policy boards to the cabinet system of government in which the health agency head is the secretary of health.

A number of states have sought to create a third model—umbrella organizations bringing several human services agencies of state government together under one secretary. These superagencies (frequently called a Department of Human Services) do not include a set pattern of agencies, though health, mental health and retardation, education, and welfare are most common. Other agencies may also be included, such as rural health and corrections. The rationale for these superagencies stems from the fact that many of the clientele of one agency are clientele of one or more of the other agencies, and by placing these agencies under one authority, improved coordination would take place resulting in more effective and more efficient services. There are considerable anecdotal data to suggest that this theory is true. However, the superagency model may also result in each division guarding its own area.

A health professional, for example, may be very supportive of new initiatives in education or corrections as long as they are not at the expense of the health budget.

A 2001 survey of state public health agencies revealed differences in the structure and boards between 1990 and 2001. Table 11–2 lists those changes.

State Health Activities

Hanlon (1974, 299) cites a 1961 unpublished survey of activities engaged in by fifty state health departments. There were 103 different activities, some (environmental health, health education, maternal and child health, nursing) engaged in by all fifty departments. At least forty departments reported other activities including communicable disease control; dental health; engineering; hospital survey, planning, and construction; licensure; laboratories; tuberculosis control; and vital statistics. The categorization of activities was based on the organization charts for fifty state health departments. Other activities may have taken place in these organizations but not given a place on the organizational chart or embedded within areas of the organizational chart.

Miller et al. (1977b) conducted a similar analysis in 1977, but used state laws instead of the organization charts. They identified forty-four public health areas specified in state laws. The authors discuss the problems that flow from the language of the statutes. For example, although only 60 percent of the states authorized immunizations by statutory language, 100 percent authorized communicable disease control activities. The authors assumed that immunizations in 40 percent of the remaining states are authorized under the broader mandate of communicable disease control. Analysis by state laws also makes it unclear whether the programs are operated directly by a central department of state government (typically, state psychiatric and mental retardation hospitals, or by licensure of professional personnel, hospitals, nursing homes, and other health facilities), decentralized to regional offices of the state agency, or carried out by local government health agencies. Often, the state agency sets performance standards under which local programs operate in return for which some state monies are allocated to supplement local government resources. State standards often govern the operation of nongovernmental agencies; these standards must be met to be eligible for a license or for payment under some state-administered programs.

Some programs for which there is shared responsibility entail state service along with complementary local services. Standards

TABLE 11–2 Structure of U.S. State Health Agencies, Boards, and Councils of Health, 1990 and 2001

	1990, No. (%)	2001, No. (%)
Structure of state public health agency		
Freestanding, independent agency	31 (60.8%)	25 (55.6%)
Component of superagency	20 (39.2%)	20 (44.4%)
State board or council of health		
Yes	35 (70.0%)	26 (60.5%)
No	15 (30.0%)	17 (39.5%)
Responsibilities of board or council of health[a]		
Promulgate public health rules	13 (37.1%)	17 (65.4%)
Advise governor and legislature on state health policy issues	12 (34.3%)	13 (50.0%)
Formulate state health policy	22 (62.9%)	10 (38.5%)
Develop public health agenda	...[b]	6 (23.1%)
Provide public health information	24 (68.6%)	4 (15.4%)
Evaluate data	1 (2.9%)	4 (15.4%)
Establish public health budget	2 (5.7%)	4 (15.4%)
Conduct research	1 (2.9%)	2 (7.7%)
Individual or entity responsible for appointment of board/council members		
Governor	35 (100.0%)	23 (88.5%)
Other	1 (2.9%)	2 (7.7%)
Director of superagency	0 (0.0%)	1 (3.8%)
Legislature	0 (0.0%)	0 (0.0%)
Composition of board or council of health		
Public health professionals	26 (74.3%)	21 (80.8%)
Private citizens	14 (40.0%)	18 (69.2%)
Consumer representatives	7 (20.0%)	14 (53.8%)
Business professionals	20 (57.1%)	11 (42.3%)
Other	...	9 (34.6%)
Education professionals	1 (2.9%)	5 (19.2%)
Agency directors	3 (8.6%)	5 (19.2%)

NOTE: Data for 1990 derived from the 1991 Centers for Disease Control and Prevention (CDC) report, *Profile of State and Territorial Public Health System.*
[a] 1990 comparison data may underestimate the number of boards and councils performing these responsibilities, because data gathered from the narrative highlights reported by the CDC may not have included all of the activities occurring within the state.
[b] Not available.

SOURCE: Beitsch, L., Brooks, R., Grigg, M., and Menachemi, N. 2006. *American Journal of Public Health* 96(1):167–72.

are typically minimal standards—if one proposes to provide a service, it must at least meet those standards. In a sense, standards are a floor below, in which a program is not considered acceptable. They are rarely optimal standards at the outset because few, if any, could reach such levels without significant funding. Standards in public health, as in other areas, have been evolutionary in nature, initially the bare essentials that most could meet or that so clearly affected the public's health that no government could resist establishing them. After they are established, public health standards become a mechanism for improving marginal programs. Often, the standards by themselves are not enough; an added inducement is the offer of a grant of money for development or operation of a program that meets the standards. Grant money for local programs comes from the state government and also from the federal government. Sometimes federal monies have paid all of the costs of the program. Sometimes federal monies have paid only part of the costs. The federal strategy has been to offer to pay a sufficient proportion of the costs to stimulate the desired state or local action.

The mix of programs, the sophistication of programs, and the population served by programs vary considerably from state to state and from unit to unit within a state. Most states serve all the people through environmental health programs, ensuring the quality and safety of the environment through such activities as inspections of facilities.

It is easy to demonstrate the value of immunizations as well as water quality control measures. It is more difficult to demonstrate and persuade people of the value of many other public health measures. To do so often requires able professional and political leadership and an informed public. Controversy arises over such issues as mandatory versus voluntary HIV testing, distribution of condoms for AIDS prevention, and eligibility levels for Medicaid programs.

Although all states engage in environmental health activities, the degree and extent of activity varies. Similarly, all states have some personal preventive service programs, particularly in areas relating to maternal and child health, school health, and immunizations. Moreover, most have program activities relating to children with special health care needs, with a variety of diagnostic and treatment services available. In some states, however, access can be a problem, particularly when the state may require referral from a private physician or makes access to the service difficult through lack of public information about the service, infrequency of services, and remoteness of service. Some of these barriers are intentional, some accidental.

In a great many states, public health agency services have moved far beyond the traditional areas of environmental, personal preventive, mental health, and mental disabilities services. These states, directly or through local public health agencies, offer many of the services that hospitals and private physicians provide in other states. Where this occurs, most of the personal preventive and the medical care services are provided to the poorer people of the state. However, some programs are available to all citizens, regardless of income status. This, again, varies considerably from state to state.

Public health services have also evolved over the years, particularly since 2000. Many new areas of concern have emerged, some because of the prevalence of chronic diseases, emergence of new diseases, and emergence of new threats to the public. Table 11–3 indicates some of those new areas of public health concern.

LOCAL HEALTH ACTIVITIES

There are about 3,000 local health departments and 3,000 local boards of health in the sixty state, territorial, and tribal health departments in the United States (Institute of Medicine 2003). There are five different types of local agencies: single county, city, combined city/county, town/township, and district/regional. The majority of agencies are county agencies, as seen in Figure 11–1 (National Association of City and County Health Officials 2006).

Local health departments have activity in many areas including data collection and analysis (vital records and statistics, reportable diseases), **epidemiology** and surveillance (chronic disease and communicable disease), health code development and enforcement, health planning, inspection activities (food control, health and recreational facility safety/quality), health education, water supply safety, sewage disposal systems, solid waste management, vector and animal control, water pollution, AIDS testing and counseling, child health, chronic disease, family planning, immunizations, prenatal care, sexually transmitted diseases, tuberculosis, and **women, infants, and children (WIC)** food supplement programs.

The larger the population that the local health department serves, the greater range of services provided. A high percentage of the larger departments also provide services in the areas of air quality surveillance and control, hazardous waste management, occupational health and safety, dental health, services for children with a handicap, laboratory services, and primary

TABLE 11-3 States with Responsibilities in Emerging Areas of Public Health Practice: United States, 2001

Emerging Responsibility	States with Responsibility	
	No.	%
Bioterrorism	42	89.4
Vaccine for children program	41	87.2
Injury control epidemiology	41	87.2
Injury control and prevention	41	87.2
Breast and cervical cancer screening	41	87.2
Chronic disease epidemiology	40	85.1
Tobacco control and prevention	39	83.0
Cancer epidemiology	39	83.0
Environmental epidemiology	37	78.7
Disaster preparedness	36	76.6
Parental epidemiology	36	76.6
Violence prevention	32	68.1
Emergency medical services/regulation and service provision	30	63.8
Quality improvement or performance management	29	61.7
Toxicology	27	57.4
Radon control	26	55.3
Breast and cervical cancer treatment	21	44.7
Institutional review board	21	44.7
State Title XXI Children's Health Insurance Initiative	13	27.7

SOURCE: Beitsch, L., Brooks, R., Grigg, M., and Menachemi, N. 2006, January. Structure and functions of state public health agencies. *American Journal of Public Health*, 96(1).

care. Where the local health department does not provide appropriate public health services, the state health department typically provides them, particularly laboratory, environmental, and mental health services.

Those in charge of local health departments are typically called local health officers or county health officers. Slightly more than half of them are medically qualified, but only one-third of these have had advanced graduate training in public health or related areas. The larger departments tend to have physicians with advanced training in public health in charge.

It is important for us to appreciate more fully what health departments do, for it should go without saying that, were it not for organized public health efforts, our nation would not be as stable, as successful, or as livable as it is. The work of local health officers and their collaborators makes our society one in which it is safe to live and that is conducive to the healthy development of individuals.

The pattern of local health department organization varies from state to state. How much autonomy the local department has from the state authority varies from state to state and even

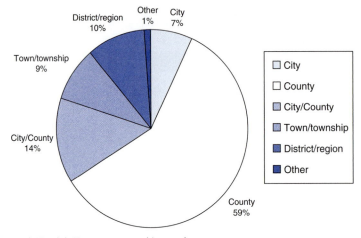

Figure 11–1 Types of Local Health Departments/Agencies

SOURCE: Suen, J. and Magruder, C. *National profile: Overview of capabilities and core functions of local public health jurisdisctions in 47 states, the District of Columbia, and 3 U.S. territories.* Journal of Public Health Management Practice, 2004, 10 (1), 2–12.

within the state, depending on the extent of state support, the dynamism of local health officers, the relative political strength of the different local governments, as well as the administrative style of the state health agency leaders.

State health departments set minimum standards for local department operations. Typically, local units submit their budgets and plans to the state authority for review and approval. With state approval, local departments are then approved to receive state funds. In many states, local units can, if they wish, exceed the standards set by the state and use their own resources to accomplish that end. The level of state support varies but is usually based on a minimum program expected of the local unit and funds distributed according to some kind of formula.

THE FEDERAL GOVERNMENT AND PUBLIC HEALTH

Public health involves interplay among federal, state, and local governments. The federal government provides some direct health services, but its chief role has been that of stimulating the development of new and improved services by providing monies to encourage the actions it wants to see developed. Indeed, except in some circumscribed areas, the federal government has no constitutional authority to provide direct health services for people, this being the domain of the states and the private sector.

The Congressional Role in Health

For government to do anything requires money that must be raised by some form of taxation. The use of that money, as well as the raising of it, must have a legal base; somewhere in the U.S. Constitution there must be a clause that justifies a law and, in turn, an appropriation, for government to do what it does. This applies to all areas of government activity. The U.S. Supreme Court is arbiter when otherwise irresolvable disputes arise about whether the activity of the government is in accord with the authorities granted to the government by the Constitution.

The *Powers of Congress* part of the Constitution (Article 1, Section 8) provides authority to raise and support armies, to provide and maintain a navy, and to make all laws "necessary and proper" for carrying out those powers. This justifies the allocation of monies for military, naval, and air force hospitals and health services. It requires only a slight extension of logic to justify the Department of Veterans Affairs (VA) work in health, whether it is the building of a hospital or clinic for treatment of veterans with service-connected disabilities or the support of medical education to ensure an adequate supply of physicians so that there will be enough to meet the staffing needs of the VA system. Similarly, the federal government can justify the medical school for the armed forces that was built on the grounds of the National Naval Medical Center in Bethesda, Maryland. The Uniformed Services University of the Health Sciences and the F. Edward Hébert School of Medicine were established by Congress in 1972, to train health care professionals for the Department of Defense and the U.S. Public Health Service (Joyce 2007).

The Constitution also grants to Congress the power to regulate foreign and interstate commerce. This justifies much of the federal activity regarding regulation of foods, drugs, product and occupational safety, and some environmental health activities, because they move in, or affect, interstate or foreign commerce. The power to control federal lands, along with the presidential power to make treaties (with the advice and consent of the Senate), are the sources of federal activity in providing health services for Native Americans and Alaskan natives. Other direct service activities also rely on these clauses for legitimacy. By far, the greatest federal influence comes from the distribution of monies to the states, local governments, and nongovernmental agencies. Sometimes these grants of money can be justified as "necessary and proper" for carrying out the specific constitutional powers already cited. An even more significant basis for grant monies derives from the power of Congress "to lay and collect taxes, duties, imports, and excises, to pay the debts and provide for the common defense and general welfare of the United States" (Article I, Section 8).

The "general welfare" clause justifies support for medical research, Medicare, Medicaid, health employee training, and so on. The power to make monies available for certain general welfare activities also permits the writing of regulations that set out the conditions that must be met to receive the money. The regulations are applications of the law that the administering agencies in the executive branch write and published in the **Federal Register**, a daily (Monday through Friday) official publication of the U.S. government. Because regulations have force of law, they must follow the intent of Congress. Frequently, litigation revolves around whether a regulation has followed the intent of Congress. The courts determine this, drawing not only on the law itself, but also on congressional committee reports that indicate the thinking of the Senate, the House, and sometimes the conference committee on the bill.

Health Responsibilities of the Executive Branch

A number of major federal agencies are concerned with health services. Principal among these are the Department of Defense, with a large network of facilities to care for members of the armed forces and their dependents; the Department of Veterans Affairs, with a network of hospitals, nursing homes, and services to care for veterans of the armed forces; the Department of Labor,

with its Occupational Safety and Health Administration; the Environmental Protection Agency; and the Department of Health and Human Services.

Department of Health and Human Services

The Department of Health and Human Services (HHS) is the principal health agency of the federal government and has a budget second only to the Department of Defense (see Figure 11–2). The department's programs are administered by eleven operating divisions, including eight agencies within the U.S. Public Health Service and three human services agencies (Administration on Aging, Administration for Children and Families, and the Centers for Medicare and Medicaid Services).

The eight U.S. Public Health Service agencies are:

1. *The National Institutes of Health (NIH)* is a medical research organization that provides over $27 billion in grants for research projects studying a wide range of disease process and interventions. It includes twenty-seven different institutes and centers such as the National Cancer Institute, National Institute on Aging, National Institute of Child Health and Human Development, National Institute of Environmental Health Sciences, National Institute of Mental Health, and the National Center on Minority Health and Health Disparities, to name just a few.

The mission of the NIH is the "pursuit of fundamental knowledge about the nature and behavior of living systems and the application of that knowledge to extend healthy life and reduce the burdens of illness and disability" (NIH 2007a). It accomplishes this by conducting basic science and clinical research in its own laboratories and clinics (including the Warren Grant Magnuson Clinical Center and a new facility opened in 2004, the 870,000-square-foot Mark O. Hatfield Clinical Research Center). The major thrust of the NIH (about 80 percent of the funding), however, is the support of research in universities, medical schools, hospitals, and other research institutions, mostly on the basis of applications submitted by scientists who seek to carry out some type of biomedical research. The applications for research grants are reviewed not only by NIH scientists for their scientific merit and appropriateness to the NIH mission, but also by advisory panels of experts who are not employees of the federal government. The monies support the time of investigators who are typically located where new physicians are being trained, where medical and other biomedical specialists are being trained, and where physicians are responsible for

Public Health Agencies	FY 2005 BUDGET	EMPLOYEES
National Institutes of Health	$ 28.6 billion	17,543
Indian Health Services	3.8 billion	16,251
Food and Drug Administration	1.8 billion	10,446
Centers for Disease Control and Prevention	8.0 billion	8,837
Agency for Toxic Substances and Disease Registry	76.0 million	365
Health Resources and Services Administration	7.4 billion	2,034
Substance Abuse and Mental Health Services Administration	3.4 billion	558
Agency for Healthcare Research and Quality	319.0 million	296
Other Health and Human Services Agencies		
Center for Medicare and Medicaid Services	489.0 billion	4,943
Administration for Children and Families	47.0 billion	1,382
Administration on Aging	1.4 billion	126

Figure 11–2 U.S. Public Health Agencies under the Department of Health and Human Services: 2005 Budget and Number of Employees
SOURCE: U.S. Department of Health and Human Services, www.hhs.gov/about/whatwedo.html (retrieved March 8, 2006).

patient care. The interaction of investigators with these medical providers undoubtedly contributes daily to the quality of training and to the quality of medical care.

Research is, of course, a never-ending process. The NIH, therefore, has a role in ensuring that promising young researchers are trained, and that there are adequate research facilities in the country. NIH monies go into these activities. Another principal activity of the NIH is to ensure access to knowledge, and to promote the dissemination of new knowledge. This effort is centered in the National Library of Medicine, a library noted not only for its extensive references, over 150 major medical journals, current audiovisual materials, and over 200 abstracts and indexes in the Reading Room, but also for **Medline**, **MedlinePlus**, and **PubMed** (National Library of Medicine 2007).

The Fogarty International Center provides a focus for the NIH in international cooperation in all aspects of biomedical research. It serves as a base for the exchange of knowledge on biomedical research, medical education, research training, and health services through conferences and seminars, provision of postdoctoral fellowships for research in the United States and overseas, support of scientific exchanges between the United States and other countries, and sponsorship of special studies and reports that are of international significance (NIH 2007b).

2. *The Food and Drug Administration (FDA)* is a regulatory agency of the Department of Health and Human Services

and is, without a doubt, the nation's largest and oldest consumer protection agency. It began as the Division of Chemistry and then the Bureau of Chemistry with primarily a scientific function. In 1906, with the passage of the Federal Food and Drugs Act, the bureau began its regulatory functions. The bureau's name was changed to the Food, Drug, and Insecticide Administration in 1927, and its nonregulatory functions were moved to other departments. The name was changed to the Food and Drug Administration (FDA) in 1930 and, after several assignments under other government agencies, was placed in the Department of Health and Human Services in 1980 (U.S. Food and Drug Administration 2007).

The FDA's mission statement, found on its website (www.fda.gov/opacom/morechoices/mission.html), states the following:

The FDA is responsible for protecting the public health by assuring the safety, efficacy, and security of human and veterinary drugs, biological products, medical devices, our nation's food supply, cosmetics, and products that emit radiation. The FDA is also responsible for advancing the public health by helping to speed innovations that make medicines and foods more effective, safer, and more affordable; and helping the public get the accurate, science-based information they need to use medicines and foods to improve their health.

To carry out its mission, the FDA inspects food processing plants and tests foods and food additives in its laboratories to make certain they are safe for public consumption. Its inspectors check for false and misleading labeling of foods and for deceptive packaging.

Perhaps the FDA's best-known role is that relating to drugs. Before any new drug can be marketed, manufacturers must provide the FDA with evidence of its safety and effectiveness. In its laboratories, the agency also regularly tests every batch of most antibiotics and all insulin before they go on sale. The FDA also regulates drug labeling, reporting of adverse reactions, drugs in **clinical trials** (informed consent, dosage, and reporting), prescription versus over-the-counter drugs, and drug advertising. In an enhanced effort to ensure the safety of pharmaceuticals, the FDA has a new "Drug Safety Initiative" to directly provide information on a wide range of drugs to consumers and health care providers. The "Index to Drug-Specific Information" (available at www.fda.gov/cder/drug/drugsafety/DrugIndex.htm) provides specific information about each drug such as uses, precautions, side effects, directions for use, and so on.

In addition to its role relating to pharmaceuticals, the FDA has a variety of other functions and authorities relating to medical devices, biologicals (blood products, vaccines, tissues, and human cells), cosmetics, animal food and drugs, and radiologic devices.

From time to time, the FDA's standards have been subject to criticism from drug manufacturers because of what they feel are sometimes inordinate delays in securing FDA approval. They point to the frequent availability of many drugs on the European markets (where regulations are also rigorous) long before the FDA grants approval. Not all agree with the industry's complaint in this regard. The FDA's role has been most prominent in recent years, as it has worked with the pharmaceutical industry on problems that have developed with drugs previously certified as safe. Recent cases can be cited regarding arthritis medications, Vioxx and Celebrex, and weight loss medications containing Fen-Phen.

3. *Centers for Disease Control and Prevention (CDC)* programs seek to prevent and control infectious and chronic diseases; to prevent disease and death associated with environmental and workplace hazards; and to reduce health risks through education and information. The CDC is based in Atlanta, Georgia, although its personnel and some of its units are found in different parts of the country and in different parts of the world. The CDC is organized into coordinating centers

for environmental health and injury prevention, health information services, health promotion, infectious diseases, global health, terrorism preparedness and emergency response, and the National Institute for Occupational Safety and Health (CDC 2007a).

The CDC is perhaps best known for tracking the causes of infections and communicable diseases. It was founded in 1946, to find the cause of malaria, and has since provided national leadership in preventing and controlling HIV infection, sexually transmitted diseases, and tuberculosis. The work of identifying and controlling infectious disease is heavily based on epidemiology and laboratory studies at the federal, state, and local levels. Much of the work of prevention is done through vaccination programs for children and adults. However, the CDC also has a wide range of programs for health promotion such as preventing birth defects, promoting healthy lifestyles, and fostering understanding of human genomic discoveries in relationship to health and disease prevention (CDC 2007b).

Within the CDC is the National Center for Health Statistics (NCHS), which works closely with state and local health departments to collect data on the health of the American people. The health statistics allow NCHS to document the population's health status, identify possible health disparities, monitor trends in health care delivery, support health research, and provide input to and evaluate health policy (CDC 2007c).

Since the aftermath of the World Trade Center attacks on September 11, 2001 (often referred to as "9/11"), the government and private agencies have placed emphasis on emergency response to mass casualties, **bioterrorism**, and chemical emergencies. Since Hurricane Katrina in late August 2005, additional emphasis has been placed on natural disaster warning and recovery. The Coordinating Office for Terrorism Preparedness and Emergency Response provides direction to the CDC for these important initiatives.

4. *Indian Health Service (IHS)* runs a comprehensive medical care system serving the needs of more than 1.5 million Native American Indians and Alaskan natives belonging to more than 557 federally recognized tribes in 35 states (Indian Health Services 2005). The mission of the IHS is the following:

   [I]n partnership with people, to raise their physical, mental, social, and spiritual health to the highest level. The IHS goal is to ensure that comprehensive, culturally acceptable personal and public health services are available and accessible to all American Indian/Alaska Native people. (Indian Health Services 2006)

Health care services for Native Americans are a federal responsibility established in 1787, based on Article I, Section 8 of the U.S. Constitution and early treaties between the federal government and the numerous Native American tribes. The Indian Self-Determination and Education Assistance Act of 1993 and the Indian Health Care Improvement Act (1994) give tribes the option of administering and managing health care programs in their own communities or continuing to remain part of the federally administrated program. The federal system consists of 33 hospitals, 59 **health centers**, and 50 **health stations**, in addition to health care provided by some private health care practitioners. American Indian tribes and Alaskan native corporations administer 15 hospitals, 221 health centers, 9 residential treatment centers, 97 health stations, and 176 Alaskan village clinics (Indian Health Services 2007).

The IHS also provides scholarships to people training in health care professions to help meet the staffing needs of IHS programs. Preference is given to qualified Native Americans in application and selection; however, others may apply. In return for scholarships, loans, or summer employment, students must agree to work in IHS programs for specified periods of time after completing their training.

5. *Health Resources and Services Administration (HRSA)* is assigned the task of helping to improve the nation's health delivery system by providing grant support for a variety of educational and health service activities. Its mission is to "provide national leadership, program resources and services needed to improve access to culturally competent, quality health care" (HRSA 2007).

HRSA functions through its various bureaus, which mirror their areas of focus. The Bureau of Health Professions focuses on coordinating, developing, and utilizing the nation's health professionals. The National Practitioner Data Bank, a national registry of actions taken against medical practitioners by disciplinary agencies, operates under the auspices of the bureau. The Healthcare Systems Bureau has several areas of responsibility, including organ and cell transplantation, facilitation of preparedness programs for response to mass casualty incidents, support for health care facility construction and renovation, reduction of numbers of people without insurance, and management of national programs for childhood vaccine and smallpox vaccine injury compensation. The *HIV/AIDS Bureau* provides support for people living with HIV/AIDS who have no or inadequate

insurance. It also houses the Office for the Advancement of **Telehealth** and the Center for Quality.

Perhaps one of the best-known bureaus is the Maternal and Child Health Bureau, which works "to improve the physical and mental health, safety and well-being of the maternal and child health population . . . with special health care needs" (HRSA 2007). The Bureau of Primary Health Care targets issues of assessing the health care needs of underserved populations, providing services to the underserved, and moving toward eliminating health care disparities. The bureau also targets special problems by providing such services as Black Lung Clinics Program and the National Hansen's Disease Program.

Along with its bureaus, HRSA has many support areas such as the Office of Minority Health and the Office of International Health Affairs. The Office of Rural Health Policy is somewhat self-explanatory in that it works to strengthen the delivery of health services to people in rural areas (see Figure 11–3).

6. The *Agency for Healthcare Research and Quality (AHRQ)* was formerly known as the Agency for Health Care Policy and Research. The agency is "charged with improving the quality, safety, efficiency, and effectiveness of health care for all Americans" (AHRQ 2005). It carries out its mission primarily through research that provides information on quality, safety, and organizational excellence to health care providers, consumers, public and private insurers, and policy makers. Among its most recent research focus areas is "translating research into practice (TRIP)" as an initiative to translate research results into what are referred to as evidence-based tools that practitioners can use to provide more effective care to patients. *Effective*, in this sense, means care resulting in improved patient status in a cost-effective manner.

Another focus area is patient safety. Research is necessary to understand why errors occur and what strategies can be developed to avoid errors. The strategies in the area of patient safety, as in TRIP, are also evidence-based practice.

7. The *Substance Abuse and Mental Health Services Administration (SAMHSA)* focuses on programs and funding to improve "the lives of people with or at risk for mental [disorders] and substance abuse disorders" (SAMSHA 2007). It works through federal, state, and local government agencies and with faith-based organizations to facilitate prevention in the at-risk population and recovery of people with mental illness and substance abuse problems. The hope is to allow people in treatment

	Bureaus	Offices
Health Resources and Services Administration	Primary Health Care	Administrator
	Maternal and Child Health	International Health Affairs
	Health Professions	Legislation
	Healthcare Systems	Communications
	HIV/AIDS	Equal Opportunity and Civil Rights
	Clinician Recruitment and Service	Planning and Evaluation
		Minority Health and Health Disparities
		Center for Quality
		Operations
		Federal Assistance Management
		Rural Health Policy
		Health Information Technology
		Regional Operations

Figure 11-3 Health Resources and Services Administration Bureaus and Offices
SOURCE: Delmar, Cengage Learning.

to remain in the community and live full lives. As with other government agencies, the focus is on research to practice and evidence-based treatment. SAMHSA supports programs, policy, and knowledge development through funding of a wide range of programs. For example, in 2006, $13.5 million was awarded in grants to community-based organizations for family-centered substance abuse treatment for adolescents.

8. The *Agency for Toxic Substances and Disease Registry (ATSDR)* serves to protect the public from the effects of hazardous substances in the environment. Its functions include assessment of waste sites, health surveillance and registries, emergency response to hazardous substance releases, research, information development and dissemination, and education and training regarding hazardous substances (ATSDR 2007).

ATSDR was created by the Comprehensive Environmental Response, Compensation, and Liability Act of 1980 (CER-CLA), more commonly known as the Superfund law. The law was essentially a response to the Love Canal problem in New York State in the 1970s. About 1,300 uncontrolled waste sites have been identified and placed on the National Priorities List for remediation (see http://www.atsdr.cdc.gov/hazardouswastesites.html). These uncontrolled waste sites are a major environmental threat to human health. Despite the enormity of the problem, funding for cleanup faces cutbacks, even as more sites are added to the National Priorities List.

The U.S. Public Health Service Commissioned Corps

The mission of the U.S. Public Health Service Commissioned Corps is "protecting, promoting, and advancing the health and safety of the nation" (U.S. Public Health Service Commissioned Corps 2007a). The Corps is one of the uniformed services of the United States, and traces its history in 1798, to the founding of marine hospitals to care for merchant seamen. In 1874, the marine hospitals were formalized into the Marine Hospital Service headquartered in Washington, DC. The Marine Hospital Service became the Commissioned Corps in 1889. Opened only to physicians originally, the Corps expanded to include dentists, pharmacists, nurses, sanitary engineers, and other health personnel. Over time, its functions expanded beyond treatment of merchant seamen to include infectious disease control, quarantine functions, and processing of immigrants. Because of its broadened responsibilities, the Corps was officially renamed the Public Health and Marine Hospital Service in 1902 and then the Public Health Service in 1912. Today, the Public Health Service functions under the Department of Health and Human Services and consists of the Office of Public Health and Science, ten Regional Health Administrators, and eight operating divisions. Members of the Commissioned Corp work in a variety of agencies throughout the Department of Health and Human Services (U.S. Public Health Service Commissioned Corps 2007b).

The Office of the Surgeon General, under the direction of the surgeon general, oversees the Commissioned Corps. The president appoints the surgeon general who reports to the

EXHIBIT 11-1

Love Canal

Love Canal was a planned community on the eastern edge of Niagara Falls, New York. William T. Love once envisioned a navigable waterway between the upper and lower Niagara Rivers that would provide power to the area in which industry and homes would be developed. The project never came to fruition, and the land was used as a recreational area until it was sold in 1920, when the canal became a municipal and chemical disposal site.

It was primarily used by Hooker Chemical Company until it reached maximum capacity, was filled with layers of dirt, and was sold to the city for one dollar. The site became an area for post-World War II housing. The Love Canal neighborhood eventually included about 800 private, single-family homes, 240 low-income apartments, and the 99th Street Elementary School located near the center of the landfill.

By the 1970s, numerous reports of toxic odors, inexplicable health problems, and seeping chemicals brought attention to the site. On the first day of August 1978, the lead paragraph of a front-page story in the New York Times read:

> NIAGARA FALLS, N.Y.—Twenty five years after the Hooker Chemical Company stopped using the Love Canal here as an industrial dump, 82 different compounds, 11 of them suspected carcinogens, have been percolating upward through the soil, their drum containers rotting and leaching their contents into the backyards and basements of 100 homes and a public school built on the banks of the canal.[1]

A record amount of rainfall had occurred and the leaching began shortly afterward. Corroded waste disposal drums were breaking through the ground, puddles of noxious substances were found in backyards and on the school grounds, and children playing outdoors had burns on their hands and faces. There were high rates of miscarriages and birth defects in the area. On August 7, 1978, the governor of New York announced that it would buy the homes affected by the chemicals. By month's end, 98 families had already been evacuated, and eventually 221 families moved. President Jimmy Carter declared the site a national disaster site in May 1980.

Two rings of homes that originally surrounded the Love Canal were torn down, and the land on which they stood, along with Love Canal, were buried under a 40-acre cap with a liner and extensive barrier drain collection system, which is operated and maintained by New York State. An extensive, fenced buffer area separates the site from the remainder of the area. The site is surrounded by monitoring wells and routine monitoring that, to date, shows that this containment system is working effectively.[2]

In September 1988, 200 homes in the northern section of Love Canal were declared "habitable" by the U.S. Environmental Protection Agency. A public corporation took ownership of the abandoned properties, fixed up the homes, and resold them. The area is now known as Black Creek Village.[3]

Discussion Question

The Love Canal was a lesson to be learned but it was not the last major environmental threat.

1. Go to http://www.atsdr.cdc.gov/hazardouswastesites.html, and identify areas with which you may be familiar.

[1] From www.epa.gov/history/topics/lovecanal/01.htm
[2] From www.epa.gov/history/topics/lovecanal/07.htm
[3] From www.cnn.com/US/9808/07/love.canal/

---

assistant secretary for health for a four-year term (see Table 11–4). Although the surgeon general has a number of duties, the central activities lie in the duty "to protect and advance the health of the nation through educating the public; advocating for effective disease prevention and health promotion programs and activities; and provide a highly recognized symbol of national commitment to protecting and improving the public's health" (Office of the Surgeon General 2007).

The Office of the Surgeon General has changed in its influence over the years, as has its relationship to other units in government. Until 1968, the surgeon general reported directly to the secretary of health, education, and welfare (the predecessor of the secretary of health and human services). In 1968, President Johnson abolished the Office of the Surgeon General, and the surgeon general became an advisor to the assistant secretary of health. In fact, during this time period, a report to Congress questioned the need

TABLE 11-4 Recent History of U. S. Surgeons General

Surgeon General	Appointed by	Dates of Service	Area of Emphasi
Jesse Steinfeld	Pres. Nixon	1969–1973	Cancer treatment
Julius Richmond	Pres. Carter	1977–1981	Access and equity through neighborhood health centers
C. Everett Koop	Pres. Reagan	1982–1989	Smoking cessation, AIDS prevention
Antonia Novello[i]	Pres. G. H. W. Bush	1990–1993	Health of women, children, and minorities; underage drinking
Joycelyn Elders[ii]	Pres. Clinton	1993–1994	Universal health coverage, sex education
David Satcher	Pres. Clinton	1998–2002	Promoting healthy lifestyles
Richard Carmona	Pres. G. W. Bush	2002–2006	Risks of secondhand smoke; obesity
Kenneth Moritsugu	(Acting surgeon general)	2006–2007	Organ and tissue donation, health promotion, bioterrorism
Steven K. Galson	(Acting surgeon general)	2007–	Disease prevention, eliminating health disparities, public health preparedness, and improving health literacy

[i] First female and first Hispanic surgeon general.

[ii] First African American surgeon general; she was forced to resign because of controversial statements regarding sex education.

for the position of surgeon general and the Public Health Service Commissioned Corps. Then Surgeon General Steinfeld opposed such a move and garnered enough support in Congress that the recommendations of the report were not implemented. In 1972, the surgeon general again became advisor to the secretary of health; in 1977, the positions of assistant secretary of health and surgeon general were combined; and in 1981, they were separated again. In 1987, the Office of the Surgeon General was reestablished; the surgeon general reported to the assistant secretary of health and became responsible for the Commissioned Corps.

C. Everett Koop, in office from 1982 to 1989, was largely responsible for revitalizing the Commissioned Corps. He was also a very high profile surgeon general with his attacks on tobacco use and, later, with his work to prevent the spread of AIDS. He wrote "Understanding AIDS," the public health brochure that was mailed to all 107 million households in the United States in 1988, the largest public health mailing ever done (U.S. Department of Health and Human Services 2007).

The 2006 public health priorities of the Office of the Surgeon General (created under Richard H. Carmona) are disease prevention (overweight and obesity, HIV/AIDS, birth defects, injuries), eliminating health disparities, public health preparedness, improving **health literacy**, organ donation, children and healthy choices, and bone health and osteoporosis. Since October 2007, Rear Admiral Steven Galson has served as acting surgeon general. He has named four areas of focus in addressing public health concerns: disease prevention, eliminating health disparities, public health preparedness, and improving health literacy (U.S. Department of Health and Human Services 2008).

Medical Care, Public Health, and the Health of the Community

Although it may have many formal definitions, medical care is focused on a provider–patient relationship. One patient with a disease or illness receives care from a physician or team of health care providers to cure or at least stop the progression of the illness or disease. Public health, as we have reviewed it here, focuses on government's efforts to prevent disease and promote health for the general public as a whole. Some say public health is community health. However, community health includes publicly funded health centers as well as privately held health centers providing care to underserved and uninsured populations. Community health includes faith-based organizations. The care provided in such centers includes prevention, treatment, education, training for health care providers, and promotion of the delivery of high-quality services.

The 1996 welfare reform legislation reduced federal funding of social services but included a provision for "charitable choice," which allows faith-based organizations to receive state funding for social programs. Funds were available for such initiatives from Temporary Assistance for Needy Families (TANF), a program that replaced Aid to Families with Dependent Children (AFDC) (Schuerger 2004). In 2001, President Bush created the White House Office of Faith-Based and Community Initiatives to work with the Department of Health and Human Services (HHS) in inviting faith-based and community-based organizations to participate in funding opportunities for providing human services to populations in need. HHS was to work to remove barriers that the new participants might encounter in competing for funds.

The general public had mixed reactions to the inclusion of faith-based organizations in government grants. The new legislation and regulations stimulated the debate about separation of church and state. However, many community-based and faith-based organizations have been able to provide additional services to needy populations not provided by government through the new funding stream.

Although community-based and faith-based centers provide health care services in an ambulatory care setting, safety net hospitals provide inpatient care to the most vulnerable. **Safety net hospitals** are not always public hospitals, but are defined by the fact that they provide care to those without insurance and from low-income populations—groups that otherwise would have no source of care. The Institute of Medicine defines safety net hospitals as having the following characteristics:

- By legal mandate or explicitly adopted mission, they maintain an "open door," offering patients access to service regardless of their ability to pay; and

- A substantial share of their patient mix is uninsured, Medicaid, and other vulnerable patients (Institute of Medicine 2000).

Some safety net hospitals are public hospitals (such as San Francisco General Hospital Medical Center and Cook County Hospital in Chicago), but many are nonprofit facilities (such as Community Medical Centers of Fresno and the University of Chicago Hospitals and Health Systems). Oftentimes, the location of the hospital in a poor neighborhood rather than its ownership status makes it a safety net hospital. Hospitals located in poor neighborhoods develop a mission to serve their neighbors regardless of ability to pay. They earn the name "safety net," indicating a status as providers to the underserved, and as a service to the larger community that would be hard-pressed to provide care for this population were it not for the safety net provider.

EMERGING ISSUES OF PUBLIC AND COMMUNITY HEALTH

Historically, public health has involved tracking and controlling communicable diseases, air and water quality issues, and sanitation. Although these are still very important functions of public health, new problems and issues are under the purview of public health and community health. Heart disease, cancer, and stroke remain the leading causes of death (CDC 2004). However, people are living longer, but they are not necessarily living healthy. Chronic diseases are on the rise, with diabetes, obesity, and depression affecting both adults and children at increasing rates. Many researchers, health officials, and other community members are concerned about increases in diabetes and obesity in children. Schools are evaluating the nutritional value of their lunches, and some are even prohibiting soft drink and snack machines in their facilities. Other focus areas are the sedentary habits of children, such as time spent playing computer games and watching television versus the time spent in physical activities such as outdoor games, sports, and walking.

Communicable diseases have not disappeared. New diseases, including HIV, severe acute respiratory syndrome (SARS), new flu strains, and the reemergence of tuberculosis, are all areas of concern. It takes the work of local and state health departments in conjunction with the CDC to track outbreaks and determine the causes and ways to stop new outbreaks.

Emergency preparedness has also become a very strong focus of public health. Every state and local jurisdiction should have an emergency preparedness plan in place to deal with all types of incidents, including floods, earthquakes, and acts of terrorism. The CDC publishes the *Public Health Emergency Response Guide for State, Local, and Tribal Public Health Directors* as a guide for formulation of a plan and for training (U.S. Department of Health and Human Services 2006). The attack on the Twin Towers of the World Trade Center in 2001 and subsequent threat of **anthrax** and the devastation of the Gulf Coast from Hurricane Katrina in 2005, have all made the importance of emergency preparedness plans apparent. The CDC publishes guidelines not only for public health organizations, but also for individuals, health care facilities, and businesses.

SUMMARY

Public health remains a core function of the United States health care system. The amount of attention paid to public health has vacillated throughout history, yet its functions have continued and expanded. Water and air safety continue to be vital responsibilities of public health. Many infectious diseases have been contained (small pox, measles, polio), and yet others have emerged, providing new challenges to the public health system. Health departments promote vaccination of appropriate sectors of the population to control infectious disease, yet not everyone in the target populations receives vaccinations. Not all state and local health departments receive the necessary funding to function at their highest levels. Much of the funding is dependent upon the emphasis that public health receives from the federal government.

Several different agencies of all three levels of government and in communities work in diverse areas of public health needs. The federal level provides most of the grants and regulatory functions for public health. State and local health departments provide most of the hands-on functions. The needs of the growing numbers of those without insurance place a heavy burden on public health services and the safety net hospitals around the United States. Public health concerns have moved from acute and infectious illness to a focus on the increase in chronic illnesses, especially diabetes and obesity among adults and children. Perhaps one of the greatest challenges in our time is to coordinate these efforts of various levels of government and efforts of community groups to provide the most efficient and effective set of comprehensive services to some of the neediest of our population.

ACTIVITY-BASED LEARNING

- How much do you know about your local health department? Referring back to Figure 11–1, what is the jurisdiction of your local health department? Where is it based and what are its functions?

- How much do you know about your state health department? What is its organizational structure, who heads it, and what are its responsibilities?

- Does your local or state health department have an emergency preparedness plan?

A QUESTION OF ETHICS

The responsibilities at the various levels of public health are numerous.

- Given this fact, has appropriate attention been paid to the funding and organization of the various health departments and agencies?

- In 2007 and 2008, various consumer products were recalled for safety issues. Is the FDA failing in its responsibilities or has the federal government failed consumers through lack of funding to the FDA?

- Does providing funding to faith-based community organizations violate the separation of church and state?

REFERENCES

1. AHRQ. (2005). *AHRQ at a glance*. Retrieved from www.ahrq.gov/about/ataglance.htm

2. ATSDR. (2007). *About ATSDR*. Retrieved from http://www.atsdr.cdc.gov/about/index.html

3. Centers for Disease Control and Prevention (CDC). (2007a). *About CDC*. Retrieved from www.cdc.gov/about/default.htm

4. CDC. (2007b). *CDC organization*. Retrieved from www.cdc.gov/about/cio.htm

5. CDC. (2007c). *About the National Center for Health Statistics*. Retrieved from www.cdc.gov/nchs/about.htm

6. CDC. (2004). *Leading causes of death*. National Center for Health Statistics. Retrieved from www.cdc.gov/nchs/fastats/lcod.htm

7. Hanlon, J. J. (1974). *Public health administration and practice* (6th ed.). St. Louis, Mosby.

8. Health Resources and Services Administration (HRSA). (2007). Strategic plan FY 2005-2010. U.S. Department of Health and Human Services. Retrieved from www.hrsa.gov/about/strategicplan.htm#vision

9. Indian Health Service. (2007). Indian Health Service introduction. Retrieved from www.ihs.gov/PublicInfo/PublicAffairs/Welcome_Info/ThisFacts.asp

10. Indian Health Service. (2006). Fact sheet. Retrieved January 2006 from www.ihs.gov/PublicInfo/PublicAffairs/Welcome_Info/ThisFacts.asp, p. 1.

11. Indian Health Service. (2005, February). Retrieved from www.ihs.gov/PublicInfo/PublicAffairs/Welcome_Info/IHSintro.asp

12. Institute of Medicine. (2003). *The future of the public's health in the 21st century.* National Academy Press: Washington, DC.

13. Institute of Medicine. (2000, March). *America's health care safety net: Intact but endangered* (M. Lewin and S. Altman, Eds.). Washington, DC: National Academy Press.

14. Institute of Medicine. (1988). *The future of public health.* National Academy Press: Washington, DC.

15. Joyce, R. E. (2007). Medical school: no tuition, plus pay and benefits while attending. Retrieved from www.spear.navy.mil/profile/profile/mar01/pages/pages16-19.html

16. Miller, C. A., Brooks, E. F., DeFriese, G. H., Gilbert, B., Jain, S. C., & Kavaler, S. (1977a). A survey of local public health departments and their directors. *American Journal of Public Health*, Vol. 67, p. 935.

17. Miller, C. A., Brooks, E. F., DeFriese, G. H., Gilbert, B., Jain, S. C., & Kavaler, S. (1977b). Statutory authorizations for the work of local health departments. *American Journal of Public Health,* Vol. 67, p. 940.

18. National Association of City and County Health Officials. (2006). 2005 *national profile of local health departments.* Retrieved from www.naccho.org/topics/infrastructure/documents/NACCHO_report_final_000.pdf

19. NIH. (2007a). *About NIH.* Retrieved July 18, 2007 from www.nih.gov/about/index.html#mission.htm

20. National Institutes of Health (NIH). (2007b). *About Fogarty.* The Fogarty International Center. Retrieved from www.fic.nih.gov/about/index.htm

21. National Library of Medicine. (2007). Especially for: Retrieved from www.nlm.nih.gov

22. Office of the Surgeon General. (2008). Public Health Priorities. U.S. Department of Health and Human Services. Retrieved from www.surgeongeneral.gov/priorities/index.html

23. Office of the Surgeon General. (2007). *Duties of the Surgeon General.* U.S. Department of Health and Human Services. Retrieved from http://www.surgeongeneral.gov/about/duties/index.html

24. Office of the Surgeon General. (2007). *C. Everett Koop.* U.S. Department of Health and Human Services. Retrieved from www.surgeongeneral.gov/library/history/biokoop.htm

25. SAMSHA. (2007). About us: Agency overview. Retrieved from www.samhsa.gov/about/background.aspx

26. Schuerger, K. 2004. *Information packet: Faith-based and community initiatives.* National Resource Center for Foster Care & Permanency Planning. Retrieved from www.hunter.cuny.edu/socwork/nrcfpp

27. U.S. Department of Health and Human Services. (2008). Office of the Surgeon General Public Health Priorities. Retrieved from www.surgeongeneral.gov/priorities/index.html

28. U.S. Department of Health and Human Services. (2006). Public health emergency response guide for state, local, and tribal public health directors. Retrieved from www.bt.cdc.gov/planning/pdf/cdcresponseguide.pdf

29. U.S. Food and Drug Administration. (2007). FDA history. Retrieved from www.fda.gov/oc/history/default.htm

30. U.S. Public Health Service Commissioned Corps. (2007a). About the Commissioned Corps: *Mission.* Retrieved from www.usphs.gov/AboutUs/mission.aspx

31. U.S. Public Health Service Commissioned Corps. (2007b). About the Commissioned Corps: *History.* Retrieved from www.usphs.gov/aboutus/history.aspx

PART THREE

The Changing Health Care Environment

Chapter 12

Information Management Systems

CHAPTER OBJECTIVES

After completing this chapter, readers should have an understanding of the following:

- Why health care organizations feel the need to develop information systems in the clinical setting, particularly an electronic medical record

- The variety of approaches to information systems in health care

- The difficulties encountered in adopting and maintaining health information management systems

- The continuing need to develop health information management systems

INTRODUCTION

Hospitals and medical practices have long used information systems for business functions such as accounts receivable, accounts payable, payroll, and electronic billing. Clinical computerized applications are not as widespread. Certainly, some organizations use computer systems in specific areas, such as laboratories or patient scheduling, but their use in direct patient care is in early development, and their value has not been established. Variation in clinical practices and rapidly changing technology make standardization (which is required for any good database) difficult. In addition, as one nurse-manager phrased it, "Physicians always refer to an aversion to cookbook medicine—aversion to canned responses." Physicians often view medicine as an art and do not see inputting data into a computer as relevant to treating and caring for patients. One physician involved in the clinical use of computers suggested that not many physicians are sophisticated computer users, and they may not recognize the value of what computers can do to aid in clinical practice (Barsukiewicz 1998).

Attitudes toward health information management systems (HIMS) have changed, specifically toward **electronic medical records (EMR)**, not only a process of replacing paper record with information on a computer, but a process that organizes the information in such a way as to make the information analyzable to add to the quality of care provided to the patient. The EMR is also known as a CMR (computerized medical record) and EHR (electronic health record). In 1991, the Institute of Medicine issued a report suggesting the following three ways in which computers might help decrease health care costs:

1. Improved information can reduce redundant testing and other services resulting from unavailable or lost results.

2. Administrative costs can be reduced by electronic submission of (reimbursement) claims and automatic reports.

3. The productivity of practitioners can be increased by reducing time spent waiting for missing or unavailable charts, reviewing poorly organized or illegible data, and sifting through redundant data. (Institute of Medicine 1991)

Managed care's approach to delivering health care emphasizes case management and so-called cradle-to-grave patient care, providing the incentive for a single, comprehensive, computerized medical record as a natural vehicle for shared information. The paper medical record alone does not facilitate the key tasks of managed care: identifying best practices, coordinating care, ensuring compliance with established clinical pathways (protocols), and getting specialists' feedback to primary care practitioners. Advances in computer hardware and software now make possible an automated medical record that is widely accessible, comprehensive, and up-to-date and is, at the same time, capable of providing analyzable data (Institute of Medicine 1991).

EMRs can enhance communication within and outside the organization. Within organizations, various departments can link order confirmation and test results directly to patient records. Staff can clarify orders, ask and answer questions regarding patient care, and access resources. Externally, physicians can link with one another and with other facilities to share information about mutual patients. Providers can link with payers and vice versa. Coordinated care avoids duplicated efforts on the part of patients and providers, and it decreases response time to patient care needs. In clinical applications, HIMS must be able to meet diverse technical information-processing requirements, as well as diverse user needs.

THE NEED FOR AN ELECTRONIC MEDICAL RECORD

As more Americans live with multiple chronic diseases, coordination of care is of primary concern. Safety is at risk when patients are on a regimen of multiple medications. Medication errors are the largest contributors to patient injury and death by medical error. The EMR can contribute to a decrease in patient injury through warnings to clinicians of patient allergies and adverse medication interactions. Electronic medical records (EMRs) can also incorporate best practices and evidence-based guidelines to aid patients and practitioners in clinical decision making (Institute of Medicine 2001).

As Exhibit 12–1 illustrates, there are multiple reasons for the drive toward the EMR. Traditional paper records may include a large amount of information about patients and their treatment

---

EXHIBIT 12–1

In the Dark—The Case for Electronic Health Records

Cara B. Litvin, M.D.

I sighed as I flipped again through the paperwork sent with my first admission of the night. All I found was a partially legible discharge summary. The patient, a young man who was ventilator dependent and in a vegetative state since receiving a gunshot injury six months previously, had been transferred from a nursing home after a workup revealed a new deep venous thrombosis in his leg.

From the limited notes provided by the nursing home, I ascertained that the gunshot had initially caused a subarachnoid hemorrhage. It was my job, as a night-float admitting resident, to determine whether it was safe to start anticoagulation for his thrombosis. I rummaged through his papers again. All I could find regarding his brain hemorrhage was the handwritten statement "Recent head CT stable."

I was angry that physicians had sent this patient without adequate documentation. In the corporate world, a business transaction would not be finalized if crucial information were missing, but transfers like this are commonplace in medicine. I called the nursing home and reached a doctor who had never heard of my patient. He agreed to look up the record and call me back. A few minutes later, someone else from the nursing home paged me and said he couldn't find any mention of a previous head CT. I pressed him for more information. After a second perusal of the record, he discovered that a "brain" CT had been performed a few days earlier. My spirits rose as I waited for the report. "Oh," he said, "we don't have a report. We're not an acute care facility, so it takes several days for us to receive reports." Defeated, I hung up.

Half an hour later, I was wheeling my ventilated patient to the CT scanner for new views of his brain. These days, we can find the answer to almost any question immediately by doing a Google search, but unfathomably, it is still not possible for

(continues)

EXHIBIT 12–1 (Continued)

a physician in Manhattan to obtain a timely report of a study performed in another New York borough.

I waited for a corrections officer to open the gates to the prison floor of the hospital so I could see my next admission—a prisoner from Rikers Island who had been sent to a different hospital for stabilization and was being transferred here for treatment. The nurse warned me, "There's not much there," as I looked through the chart. The discharge summary from the transferring hospital was one of the briefest I had ever seen: "Admitted for altered mental status, s/p respiratory distress, and intubated. Treated with broad-spectrum antibiotics. Extubated 2 days ago and now stable for transfer."

A set of basic laboratory tests from a couple of days earlier was included with the paperwork, but there were no culture reports, no mention of which antibiotics had been used, and no chest radiography reports. A ten day course of critical care had been summed up in three sentence fragments and one set of lab tests. I spent another twenty minutes drawing labs and cultures and then ran back to the emergency room to see another new admission, still without a clear plan for the patient I had just left.

Later that night, I looked over the chart for my sixth admission. A 72-year-old patient with schizophrenia who spoke only Cantonese had been referred from a Chinatown clinic for admission. Because only the words "PPD positive" had been written on the referral sheet, he had been isolated in the emergency room. I wasn't sure whether the tuberculosis positivity was a new finding, and the patient appeared comfortable on the stretcher. He was not coughing, and his lungs were clear. Without any family members present to provide clarification, I tied a mask on him and walked him outside his isolation room to a translator phone. Even through the translator, I could barely get a history. I looked for evidence of a recent skin test on his forearms but found nothing. He was afebrile, and his chest radiograph was normal. I couldn't understand why his primary care doctor had thought he needed to be admitted. Once again, I felt as though I were practicing medicine in the dark.

Very few of my patients that night had come directly from the emergency department. Most were transfers and referrals, which meant that another physician had already evaluated them that day. But deplorable documentation had left me at a loss. I knew the teams I would be signing out to in the morning would probably be able to track down more information, but it was unfair to all of us—especially to the patients—that care was suboptimal simply because records were not available.

The hospital where I work is dedicated to underserved patients and has limited resources, so it is not surprising that our information systems are lacking. But the private hospital where residents in my program do rotations has a similar story—discharge summaries are nonexistent and clinic notes are unobtainable. Even at a prestigious specialty referral center where old charts are scanned and can be viewed on any computer, it is often difficult to piece together a patient's history, largely because it is hard to decipher the handwritten progress notes.

It is only during our rotations at the Veterans Affairs (VA) hospital that we glimpse how information can be conveyed effectively. Since the early 1990s, the VA has been a pioneer in adopting information technology, using an integrated electronic health record (EHR) system to promote high-quality care. The VA now outperforms Medicare and most private health plans on many quality measures.[1] Prescriptions, lab tests, studies, consults, reports, and progress notes from all visits by patients to any VA hospital are stored in EHRs. Although interns sometimes complain about having to scroll through a vast electronic chart to write an admission note, care is enhanced by this system.

Information is vital to the provision of high-quality care, yet too often, improving information systems is not seen as a priority. Throughout training, the practice of evidence-based medicine is emphasized. We are expected to be familiar with all the current literature on medications, procedures, and imaging methods, but our currency is irrelevant when a flawed communication system limits our ability to translate knowledge into clinical practice.

In recent years, the technological lag of the medical world has finally been noticed, and the concept of a national EHR system has gained popularity. The use of EHRs is still relatively limited: One study showed that only about one in four doctors use such systems, and
(continues)

EXHIBIT 12-1 (Continued)

fewer than one in ten use them as efficiently as possible.[2] Barriers include the cost of implementation (an EHR system can cost more than $20,000 per physician[3]), the lack of communication standards, inadequate data exchange, insufficient user training, and privacy concerns.[4] Nevertheless, the Bush administration has set a goal of having EHRs for most Americans by 2014,[5] and a bipartisan effort has been made to promote the adoption of health information technology. The achievement of such a goal will require not only extensive funding and research on implementation but also recognition among physicians that medicine is an information science.

At six in the morning, I headed to the emergency room to see my last admission, a 52-year-old Bangladeshi patient who had immigrated about five years earlier and had been followed in our hospital and clinics. Our hospital record system, though not as fully integrated as the VA system, provides access to typed discharge summaries, clinic notes, and the results of tests performed at our institution. I was able to scan through the records on the computer, so I knew most of the man's history before I met him. He said he had exertional chest pain. I knew that he had been admitted several times within the past year reporting a similar problem but that two stress tests had been negative. In fact, the record contained a clinic note from the previous week indicating that he had reported similar symptoms to his primary care physician. Although he had risk factors for coronary disease and needed to be taken seriously, I was reassured by his previous workup.

The patient mentioned that the day before, he had seen a doctor who was not part of our system. "He told me to go to the nearest hospital, but even though I had to take a long subway ride to get here, I knew that coming here would be better for me because you would have all my records," he said. I smiled. The patient had lived in the United States for

only five years, but he had already zeroed in on one of the greatest flaws of the U.S. health care system.

Dr. Litvin is a resident in the Department of Medicine at New York University Medical Center, New York.

[1] Jha, A.K., J.B. Perlin, K.W. Kizer, and R.A. Dudley. 2003. Effect of the transformation of the Veterans Affairs health care system on the quality of care. *New England Journal of Medicine* 348:2218–27.

[2] Jha A.K., T.G. Ferris, K. Donelan, et al. 2006. How common are electronic health records in the United States? A summary of the evidence. *Health Affairs* (Millwood) 25:496–507.

[3] Kaushal R., D. Blumenthal, E.G. Poon, et al. 2005. The costs of a national health information network. *Annals of Internal Medicine* 143:165–73.

[4] Baron R.J., E.L. Fabens, M. Schiffman, and E. Wolf. 2005. Electronic health records: just around the corner? Or over the cliff? *Annals of Internal Medicine* 143:222–6.

[5] A new generation of American innovation. Washington, DC: The White House, 2004. (accessed May 24, 2007, at http://www. whitehouse.gov/infocus/technology/economic_policy200404/chap1. html.)

Discussion Questions

This story of one doctor's day tells about the need for electronic medical records.

Think of Electronic Health Records in terms of costs, utilization and quality.

1. What are the advantages of the system, as well as the barriers to creating useful systems?

2. What are some other industries that use electronic systems that the health care industry could use as a model?

3. What would have to change and what could stay the same?

---

by a physician and/or clinic. The problem is that the paper medical records do not travel with patients and are not available to all practitioners who provide care to those same patients. Patients generally see multiple health care providers. Those with a regular primary care physician often also visit specialists and have tests at various locations. Those without a regular source of care may

visit multiple clinic sites or emergency departments. Lack of access to medical records contributes to possible duplication of tests or disconnected care. Duplication of tests unnecessarily adds to the cost of care. Paper medical records may also have illegible entries and large amounts of paperwork that are difficult to sort through. A more basic fact is that paper medical records may get misplaced or misfiled, making their retrieval a long and sometimes impossible task. Computerized medical records are easily retrievable.

EMRs, on the other hand, can be accessible to multiple providers who have permission to view and post to the records. Recent test results may be available, as well as medical history, treatment plan, and recent interventions including medications. This is assuming, of course, that the EMR is a searchable database rather than just scanned handwritten documents in a computer. The greatest advantage to an EMR is access to medication information and an interactive medication warning system. If a patient has medication allergies or is on multiple medications that may interact with a medication the physician wishes to prescribe, the computer will provide a warning to the physician to avoid any adverse effects to the patient.

Medication Errors

Because medication errors are the most prevalent of all medical errors causing harm to patients, a medication warning system is a great advantage. The Institute of Medicine (IOM; 2001) recommends six major aims for health care delivery, the first of which is safe health care. The **Leapfrog Group** has as the first of its aims to "[r]educe preventable medical mistakes and improve the quality and affordability of health care." Leapfrog's focus is to help employers purchase better health care plans for their employees by encouraging health care organizations to report on quality initiatives. One of the first quality initiatives supported by Leapfrog is the adoption of computerized physician order entry (CPOE) by hospitals. According to Leapfrog, "With CPOE systems, hospital staff enter medication orders via computer linked to prescribing error prevention software. CPOE has been shown to reduce serious prescribing errors in hospitals by more than 50 percent" (Leapfrog Group 2007).

Best Practices

Preventing errors, however, is not the only advantage of EMRs. There is much variation in treatment protocols for the very same illness or disease. Variation has often been attributed to physician training and local standards of care. Physicians will tend to treat patients in the way they were trained in a particular medical residency. As those physicians move on to perhaps another community to practice medicine, they will adopt the standards by which other physicians in the community practice. However, there is no evidence or data as to which manner of treatment is more effective, efficient, and cost-effective. True EMRs have the potential to track data that follows the outcomes of treatment so that researchers may study which treatment is the most effective

for the lowest cost. That is not to say that cost is the driver. It is simply saying that, if two methods of treatment are equally effective, then the one that costs less is the most cost-effective.

Tracking treatment outcomes without a computer database is very difficult. True research on treatment outcomes has the potential to lead to a higher quality of care.

This process of data collection and analysis is often referred to as evidence-based medicine. Once treatment protocols based on outcomes measures can be determined, decision support systems may be incorporated in the electronic medical record to aid physicians to provide evidence-based medicine in their treatment of patients.

BARRIERS TO IMPLEMENTATION OF INFORMATION TECHNOLOGY

Although the advantages of EMRs are well recognized, implementation is difficult. Many organizations have multiple computer systems to handle the separate functions of billing, laboratory analysis, and business functions. Getting these multiple systems to "talk" to one another is a huge endeavor. Getting these systems connected to a new EMR is even a larger endeavor. The costs of implementation are immediate; benefits are long-term and difficult to quantify. The additional burden of getting systems within organizations to "talk" with systems in other organizations is costly, and no one has determined who is responsible for those costs.

Costs of EMR Implementation

The financial costs of EMR implementation are difficult to determine. Blumenthal and Glaser (2007) indicate that the range for purchasing and installing an EMR is between $15,000 to $50,000 per physician. Adoption is higher among those in larger group practices (see Figure 12–1), whereas those in small or solo practice have difficulty committing the necessary capital (Blumenthal and Glaser 2007, 2,531). Hospitals face proportionately greater costs. Although it may be easy to see the advantages of the EMR, the cost is a barrier. Gains from EMRs may take years to realize whereas the outlay is immediate.

Along with the direct financial cost, there are indirect costs. Productivity of physicians and staff decreases during implementation, and training with it often taking months to return to the productivity level prior to implementation. Maintenance of hardware and upgrades of software are continuing expenses

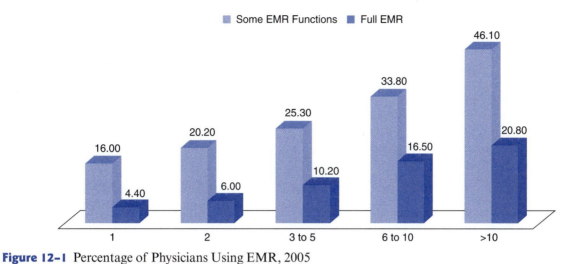

Figure 12-1 Percentage of Physicians Using EMR, 2005

SOURCE: Blumenthal, D., and J. Glaser. 2007. Information technology comes to medicine. National Ambulatory Medical Care Survey. *The New England Journal of Medicine*, 356 (24):2,531. Copyright 2007 Massachusetts Medical Society. All rights reserved.

throughout the lifetime of the EMR system. Given the questions of costs, the Rand Corporation estimated that, if 90 percent of physicians and hospitals adopted the EHR, capital expenditure of $121 billion of a period of fifteen years would yield $531 billion in savings over the same period (ibid.).

Resistance to Change

Many organizational behaviorists have studied resistance to change. The implementation of EMR is no different than any other organizational change in that it will bring problems among physicians and staff including fear, uncertainty, and distrust of the change. The issues that many physicians report are loss of eye contact with patients, lack of typing skills that will slow down the process, falling behind schedule, and a disruption of the patient–physician relationship (Schnipper et al. 2006; Barsukiewicz 1998). Some physicians also fear that the EMR's treatment protocols will result in "cookbook" medicine and limit both patient and physician individual decision making.

Despite these fears, Mulvehill et al. (2005) found that template-guided documentation took no longer than undirected documentation, yet significantly improved billing processes and was positively received by physicians and residents. Establishing template-guided documentation is often the first step to implementing EMR.

Confidentiality

Patients are concerned in general about the confidentiality of their medical records. Having a medical record on a computer seems to increase those concerns, with fears of others being able to "hack into" the records. Even if these fears are unfounded, they must be addressed.

The Health Insurance Portability and Accountability Act (HIPAA) of 1996 addressed computerization of medical records in Title II and encouraged "the development of a health information system through the establishment of standards and requirements for the electronic transmission of certain health information" (Public Law 104-191, 1996). In passing HIPAA, Congress focused primarily on setting standards for electronic technology that went beyond individual organizations developing an EMR for patient care. The focus was on electronic *transmission* for information sharing across providers of care.

Medical records have traditionally been protected through various state and federal laws. However, electronic transmission became more of an issue and includes use of medical records by insurance companies, researchers, and providers of care. HIPAA not only addressed standards such as code sets, it also called for security in exchanging information, and privacy of medical information. When addressing security, any health care provider, health plan (insurance or other), and **data clearinghouse**, must implement "a series of administrative, technical, and physical security procedures for **covered entities** to use to assure the confidentiality of electronic protected health information" (CMS 2008). Among other things, the security role sets standards to ensure that only those who should have access to personal health records actually have access. The privacy rule helps set standards for who should have access. In addition to electronic health records, the privacy rule also applies to written and oral information. The security rule only applies to electronic transmission of information. The Office for Civil Rights oversees and enforces the privacy rule. CMS oversees and enforces the security rule (Department of Health and Human Services 2007).

The privacy rule protects all "individually identifiable health information." *Health care providers must provide patients with statements revealing the situations under which information will be revealed. These situations are limited to treatment activities, payment requests, and information sharing with another provider participating in the patient's care. Authorization from the patient (a signature on the disclosure statement or equivalent) must be obtained. Other disclosures of information must be specifically addressed with the patient unless required by law or a public health agency. Health care information that is not individually identifiable does not require patient authorization. Identifiers may include such things as name, address, date of birth, social security number, employer, and any other information that may make the information easy to connect to a particular patient.*

To assure the safety and privacy of health information, organizations must appoint a privacy officer and document-specific policies and procedures for all employees to follow. Periodic employee training must take place. Heavy monetary fines and imprisonment may be imposed for lack of compliance (Office of Civil Rights 2003).

The Technology

In the mid-to-late 1990s, the technology housing the EMR was fairly limited to a desktop or laptop computer. Either hardware configuration made data entry while interacting with the patient nearly impossible. Physicians were concerned about their own "typing" ability, the time data entry took, and the loss of eye contact with patients during the data entry process. Entering information in the computer in a typical patient exam room meant turning attention away from the patient and toward the computer. A traditional paper record allows physicians to look at patients while making notes and only occasionally glancing away.

Advances in technology have now made available notebook computers that use "touch-and-click" data entry, handheld computers that can upload the day's patients, allow new entries, and then download to the main system. Some work has also been done with voice recognition software so that no keyboarding is necessary. All of these advances, however, come with a larger price tag that we have already indicated is a barrier to implementation.

The wide range of hardware and software also has a great bearing on connectivity. As mentioned earlier, many organizations already have various business and laboratory applications in their organizations. Connecting these systems to share information is a major undertaking. The EMR should be able to transmit treatment information directly to billing systems. Laboratory systems should be able to transmit information to the EMR. If they do not, then time and resources are wasted in manually connecting the information.

REGIONAL HEALTH INFORMATION ORGANIZATION

The purpose of a regional health information organization (**RHIO**) is to share information between health care providers across the community. Although in the previous section, we discussed the difficulties of connectivity between information systems, RHIOs were developed to bridge those difficulties and move to information sharing across organizations. Funding for these projects have come from a variety of partnerships, usually involving some federal, state, and private collaboration. Sharing information across organizations is important because, according to reports:

- In 2002–03, 41 million Americans changed their residence (20 percent of these to another county; another 20 percent to another state).

- 21 percent of children age 4 or less moved during the same period

- 11 percent of a Medicaid managed care population sought care in an emergency department (ED) more than once a year

- The average use for this group was five visits per year...and not to the same ED (Frisse 2005)

The MidSouth eHealth Alliance is a RHIO developed in the Memphis area. Participating hospitals and clinics share their information with one another through a database not accessible to anyone not part of the alliance. Patients' information is kept confidential, following all federal and state regulations regarding confidentiality. In fact, patients may opt out of participation in the database by signing a form at the point of care.

Emergency departments took the first step in sharing information, for the first time having readily available information about a patient who may have been treated at another emergency department for the same condition. This added to continuity of care and avoidance of duplication of treatment. Again, only those organizations that contribute to the alliance may access information from the database.

Although not all RHIOs developed in the last few years have been successful, many have been successful, and new ones are forming. RHIOs face the same challenges regarding cost, emerging technology, and voluntary participation that individual organizations face.

PATIENT HEALTH RECORDS

The personal health record (PHR) can help patients to manage their own health. PHRs allow patients access to their EMR to view, and sometimes modify, their information; to e-mail their physician; and to get referrals, prescription refills, and schedule appointments. PHRs are in earlier stages of development than EMRs. Insurance companies are the most frequent organizations to offer PHRs to their clients so that they can view claims, receive reminders of preventive care, and find physician participants in their plan (Blumenthal and Glaser 2007).

INFORMATION ON THE WEB

The Internet provides a wealth of information. It is not uncommon for patients (or family members or friends) to research information when faced with symptoms of illness or special health choices. Many sites are available to help in medical decision making, but caution must be taken to make sure that the information is reliable. Some typical sites are the following:

- Medicinenet.com is written by a network of doctors to provide medical education to the public.

- WebMD.com is also a medical information site that strives to provide information on a wide range of medical situations.

- Healthfinder.com, hosted by the U.S. Department of Health and Human Services, provides reliable up-to-date health information on their website.

- The American Hospital Directory (http://www.ahd.com/) provides information about hospitals, including services provided, financial reports, Joint Commission accreditation status, utilization data, and so on.

- Medicare provides a website to help people choose a nursing home (Nursing Home Compare). The site provides such information as ownership, Medicare or Medicaid participation, bed size, and so on.

Anyone using the information from the Internet must remember that it is educational information and is meant to supplement discussion with a physician. No website is meant to diagnose or treat medical conditions but simply to educate.

SUMMARY

Information management is an important part of today's health systems. Although the medical community has long used computerized systems for such things as billing, patient demographics, and business functions, managing patient clinical information is still done primarily in a paper medical record.

Evidence is available showing that a computerized or electronic medical record (EMR) can enhance the quality of health care delivery. IOM studies have indicated that computerized physician order entry systems can greatly reduce the incidence of medication errors. Other studies have shown that EMRs can reduce costs by preventing duplication of services and can improve quality of care by providing more coordinated services through available patient records.

Even with the evidence of higher quality of care, health care organizations have been slow to adopt EMRs. The barriers are many: cost, physician resistance, resistance to change in general, connectivity with other business and laboratory functions, among others. The technology can be cumbersome and pose a barrier to the patient–physician relationship. Although benefits seem real, implementation costs are immediate, and savings come over time.

Patients may someday have access to their own records but, in the meantime, have access to educational materials through various websites that help them to have more informed conversations with their providers.

ACTIVITY-BASED LEARNING

- As mentioned in the chapter, a small number of physicians have adopted EMRs in their practices. Is there a physician practice in your area that has adopted EMRs? Arrange to visit the practice to see the capabilities of the EMRs.

- Check the Leapfrog Group website (www.leapfrog.org). Click on the "consumer" tab, choose an area in which you might be interested, and review hospital performance in that area.

- Go to WebMD and research an illness. Was the information helpful to you?

A QUESTION OF ETHICS

- If an EMR can really help improve the quality and safety of health care delivery, does the U.S. government have a duty to help hospitals and physicians implement the system?

- RHIOs allow patients to opt out of having their information shared in the database. Is there a risk to allowing the opt-out feature?

REFERENCES

1. Barsukiewicz, C. (1998). Computerized medical records: Physician response to new technology. Unpublished doctoral dissertation, Pennsylvania State University.

2. Blumenthal, D., & Glaser, J. (2007). Information technology comes to medicine. *The New England Journal of Medicine, 356*(24), 2527–2534.

3. CMS. (2008). Security standard: Overview. Retrieved from www.cms.hhs.gov/SecurityStandard

4. Department of Health and Human Services. (2007). Security 101 for covered entities. HIPAA Security Series. Retrieved from www.cms.hhs.gov/EducationMaterials/Downloads/Security101forCoveredEntities.pdf

5. Frisse, M. (2005). Tennessee Regional Demonstration Project. Volunteer eHealth Initiative, Vanderbilt University.

6. Institute of Medicine. (1991). *The computer-based patient record: An essential technology for health care.* Committee on Improving the Patient Record. Washington, DC: National Academy Press.

7. Institute of Medicine. (2001). *Crossing the quality chasm: A new health system for the 21st century.* Committee on Quality of Health Care in America. Washington, DC: National Academy Press.

8. Leapfrog Group. (2007). The Leapfrog Group fact sheet. Retrieved from www.leapfroggroup.org/about_us/leapfrog-factsheet

9. Mulvehill, S., Schneider, G., Cullen, C., Roaten, S., Foster, B., & Porter, A. (2005). Template-guided versus undirected written medical documentation: A prospective, randomized trial in a family medicine residency clinic. *Journal of the American Board of Family Practice, 18*(6), 464–469.

10. Office of Civil Rights. (2003). Summary of the HIPAA Privacy Rule, OCR Privacy Brief. U.S. Department of Health & Human Services. Retrieved from www.dhhs.gov/ocr/privacy/index.html

11. Public Law 104–191. (1996). Health Insurance Portability and Accountability Act of 1996, Title II, subtitle F, Sec. 261. Retrieved from aspe.hhs.gov/admnsimp/pL104191.htm#261

12. Schnipper, L., Tsurikova, R., Melnikas, A., Volk, L., & Middleton, B. (2006). Barriers to electronic health record use during patient visits. *AMIA Annual Symposium Proceedings*, 499–503.

Chapter 13

Current Issues in Health Care Delivery

CHAPTER OBJECTIVES

After completing this chapter, readers should have an understanding of the following:

- The importance of quality of care
- The need for outcomes measurement
- Innovative approaches that organizations take to address issues of quality of care
- The challenges of health care reform

INTRODUCTION

The discussion of quality of health care services is evident in every aspect of health care delivery. Although we would all hope that quality has always been at the forefront of concern, we are more aware of quality when working in an environment of very strong cost containment. Is it possible to provide high-quality care while striving to reduce the costs of health care delivery? The managed care market rose to the forefront because of its promise to deliver care cost-effectively without reducing quality. Certainly, the fee-for-service environment and cost-plus reimbursement mechanism for reimbursing hospitals fostered a system that paid little attention to efficiencies. However, spending more money does not automatically translate into higher quality of care. Therefore, greater efficiency could be applied to reduce costs while still maintaining the quality of care provided. However, quality is an intangible. Because it is difficult to define, it is difficult to measure, yet measuring quality has been the thrust of health care policy in recent years.

Along with quality of care, reform for health insurance coverage for all Americans is a high-priority issue. Many proposals have been put forth, but we have seen no sweeping changes as of yet. Will the Obama administration make a difference?

THE EMPHASIS ON QUALITY

The Institute of Medicine (IOM; 2001) published a report on health care quality. A statement from the executive summary is quite clear: "Between the health care we have and the care we could have lies not just a gap, but a chasm."

The IOM recommendation on the quality of health care emphasizes six areas for improvement: safety, timeliness, efficiency, effectiveness, patient centeredness, and equitable care. The issue of safety has already been addressed in Chapter 12, with the emphasis on computerized systems to prevent medical errors. However, safety can also be improved by process analysis. Looking at care processes improves safety and also addresses efficiency. A process is a sequence of tasks and activities. Review of those tasks and activities may reveal areas for improvement, such as increasing capacity, reducing costs, and/or reducing variability. Medical errors can be reduced by process improvement; seldom do people make the errors, but a system can allow errors to happen.

Process Improvement

There are many approaches to process improvement. Root cause analysis may identify problematic issues. It identifies a problem and then looks at any possible contributing factors. Actual contributing factors are then subject to change to improve the process.

Six sigma is an improvement tool with a systematic problem-solving method based on rigorous statistical analysis. Sigma is a measure of **variation** (also known as standard deviation). Six sigma represents virtual perfection. Six sigma goals include the following:

- Making it easier for the person to do the right thing than the wrong thing

- Making mistakes obvious to the person immediately so that some correction can be made on the spot

- Allowing the person to take corrective action or stop the flow before any irreversible step occurs

The criteria for six sigma are three to four errors per million opportunities. It is not difficult to see that the criteria would improve safety and efficiency in health care delivery.

This "lean process" also focuses on improving quality while dramatically changing the operational processes to become faster and more flexible with less waste.

Effective Care

Variation in the process and outcomes of medical practice has long been the norm because of the complexity of medicine and the complexity of the conditions with which each patient may present. New advances in clinical epidemiology and in computer technology, however, have spawned the opportunity to learn from variation and determine those processes that produce the best outcomes defined as patient status (Blumenthal 1996). It is now possible to accumulate and analyze multiple types of data from billing records, patient encounters, and even computerized medical records.

In the short term, **outcomes measurement** provides health plans and employers with information regarding hospital perfor-

mance and, in some cases, individual physician performance. Outcomes measurement in the long term may provide more standardized care. Consumers will have access to information on the appropriate regimen of care for a specific group of common afflictions. Variations will still exist, mainly because of the variations in patients' conditions (age, comorbidities, lifestyle, and so on). However, patients will be more informed about options for care and about the expected outcomes of each option.

On a national level, the National Committee for Quality Assurance (NCQA) was created in 1990, to accredit and review health maintenance organizations. Through its process of evaluating HMOs, it provides objective information on sixty measures in the areas of quality, access to care and patient satisfaction, membership and utilization of services, financial performance, and general management. As of August 31, 2007, NCQA had accredited 221 commercial health plans, 59 Medicaid plans, and 74 Medicare plans. The data come largely from the Health Plan Employer Data and Information Set (HEDIS), created by employers and health plans to standardize information for comparative purposes. Although this information consists of performance data regarding HMOs, it says much about the providers who are part of the HMO network. HMOs are compared for their childhood vaccination rates, diabetic eye exam rates, use of beta-blocker treatment after heart attack, postpartum visits after a live birth, asthma control, cholesterol screening, and so on. Beginning in 2008, NCQA also began accrediting preferred provider organizations (PPOs) (NCQA 2007).

The Leapfrog Group (also mentioned in Chapter 12) is an employer initiative toward health care quality improvement that emphasizes safety, quality, and affordability. Through its group purchasing commitment, Leapfrog members agree to educate employees about comparative ratings of providers and urge providers to report performance measures. Leapfrog's initial focus is on having providers implement computerized physician order entry, employ **intensivists** (physicians who work in the hospital intensive care unit), and use evidence-based hospital referrals. In 2001, Leapfrog surveyed hospitals in six urban and suburban areas; in 2007, they are in thirty-three regions (Leapfrog Group 2007).

Outcomes are important measures for employers to consider when choosing health plan options for their employees, and important measures for consumers to consider when choosing a health care provider. However, outcomes are not the only measure of quality.

Patient-Centered Care

Standardized treatment makes it more difficult for health care providers to differentiate themselves in a competitive environment. Certainly, in very specialized care, some providers come to mind almost immediately. Sloan-Kettering Cancer Center, Johns Hopkins Hospital, and the Mayo Clinic are but a few of the names that most of us readily recognize. However, not all of us have access to these specialized centers either because of geographic location or because our personal situation does not lend itself to seeking treatment at such institutions. Most of us choose from a more local selection of providers. If all hospitals provide nearly the same spectrum of care (for example, general surgery, diagnostic imaging, laboratory tests, therapies) with similar health outcomes, what criteria help determine the hospital we choose? If all physicians follow similar protocols for care, how do we choose a particular physician? Health care providers are beginning to pay more attention to how they provide treatment—not just the treatment itself—and have become more aware of the service component of health care delivery as a means of attracting patients in a competitive environment.

The Service Component of Physician Practices

Prior to the 1980s, when there was little recognition of competition among physicians, medical offices and clinics often operated on a schedule convenient to the physicians rather than the patients. Patients often found themselves taking time off from work or taking their children out of school to accommodate the practitioner's office hours. Competition has changed much of that. Physicians' offices are now open longer hours to provide evening and sometimes weekend appointments. Amenities such as convenient parking, proximity to referral physicians, on-site laboratories, and prescription dispensing have become the norm for medical practices—all as a service to patients. Comfortable waiting rooms, patient education materials, television, playrooms, and a wide variety of magazines await patients' arrivals.

Perhaps the largest service incentive, however, has been the focus on quality management. Employees now go through continuous quality improvement seminars to learn to service patients rather than treat patients. Management, too, learns to work with, rather than supervise, employees. Mentoring, nurturing, and encouraging creativity, autonomy, and personal growth are tools that managers learn as leadership skills to build a better environment for employees in health care organizations. As management learns to treat employees in a more caring and involved manner, staff learns to treat patients in a more caring manner.

Chapter 12 provided information on how health care organizations are implementing computer systems, and electronic medical records (EMRs), in particular, to streamline medical record keeping and to provide comprehensive information regarding patient care. EMRs, however, also offer a new opportunity for service to patients through links to patient education. Physicians, on the basis of a particular patient's diagnosis, can link to appropriate websites or internal files to print information that patients can take home. The educational material may include important follow-up instructions, background information on a particular illness, and important notes on preventing recurrence and/or further progression of the problem. Patients, who often find verbal instructions and information overwhelming at the time of an encounter with a physician, find the take-home materials invaluable (Barsukiewicz 1998; Watson 2000). The EMR may also allow patients to interact with their provider via e-mail or other electronic forms of communication.

The IOM's six areas of quality included timely care. Perhaps one of the biggest complaints of patients regarding visits with physicians is the long wait. Wait time includes time from the call for an appointment to the date of the appointment. Wait time also includes time spent waiting to actually meet with the doctor once the patient has arrived at the practice. True quality and patient satisfaction requires that all health care providers begin reviewing their schedules and booking only the number of patients that they can actually see in a day, rather than overbooking. This may be a very ripe area for process improvement.

The Service Component of Health Services Organizations

Chapter 10 discussed efforts in long-term care to bring a more natural and spontaneous environment into the nursing home setting through implementation of the Eden Alternative. Eden is not the only approach to bringing a better quality of life to long-term care residents. Another approach is the Pioneer Network, which "embraces resident-centered care including an environment of neighborhoods instead of nursing units and schedules determined by residents" (Trocchio 2000, 1). In the Pioneer Network approach, residents live a more natural lifestyle, determining for themselves when they want to get up, what and when they want to eat, and what they want to do for the day. There is anecdotal evidence that the Pioneer Network approach, as with the Eden Alternative, reduces dependency on drugs, reduces staff turnover, and contributes to a healthier and happier environment for both residents and staff.

Hospitals are also seeking a better environment for their patients, whether in the inpatient or outpatient setting. Baptist Memorial Hospital in Collierville, Tennessee, was built with a service focus in mind. Although the hospital provides inpatient and outpatient services, the physical structure of the facility is such that the two types of services are somewhat separated for patients receiving care. Patients and others visiting the facility are greeted by a large, airy central lobby with a beautiful fountain, foliage, skylights, and comfortable seating. Immediately adjacent to the central lobby is a dining room, a community medical library open to the public, and a cardiac rehabilitation center. Surrounding the central lobby area are the diagnostic services and the outpatient surgery area. What is not immediately evident is the fact that this central lobby area serves as the waiting area for each of the services surrounding it.

Inpatient services are provided on the second floor in self-contained twelve-bed nursing wings, each containing a dedicated nursing station, supply room, and equipment. In the maternity wing, large and comfortable birthing rooms are actually labor, delivery, recovery, and postpartum rooms all in one. Physicians' offices are on the second and third floors of the hospital, providing for integrated care. The hospital was built with patient comfort and convenience in mind. Inpatients essentially are cared for in dedicated areas separate from outpatient activities. Outpatients move through the facility without having the feeling of being in a hospital. The beauty of the setting is a "therapy" in itself.

One might question the cost of a beautiful setting with fountains and restful, peaceful décor. In building a new facility, however, material costs were very much a part of the strategic plan, and efforts were made to use materials and space in an aesthetically pleasing, efficient, and cost-effective manner (R. Lassiter, pers. comm., 2000). The result is a facility (use of the word **hospital** no longer seems appropriate) that is patient-centered and reflects the changes taking place in health care delivery today.

The incentive to change hospital care into a more patient-centered process in more pleasant surroundings is not limited to new construction. Facilities can be found in many areas that have made changes to incorporate a service focus into health care delivery. Many hospitals have developed means of providing more patient-friendly care, from greeters at the main entrance to

escorts who help patients find needed services. Preregistration to cut down on waiting times and paperwork is now the norm for most inpatient and outpatient services. Some hospitals in busy and congested areas have incorporated valet parking into their patient services.

A more formal program dedicated to transforming hospital care into natural, comforting, and homelike environments is known as the Planetree project. Planetree was founded in 1978, on the concept that a homelike environment, encouraging family involvement and integrating a more holistic approach to care, enhances the healing process (Planetree 2007). The following is a description from its website (www.planetree.org) and brochure:

> Planetree's approach is holistic and encourages healing in all dimensions—mental, emotional, spiritual, and social, as well as physical. It seeks to maximize health care outcomes by integrating complementary medical therapies such as mind-body medicine, therapeutic massage, acupuncture, yoga, and energy therapies . . . with conventional medical therapies . . . and recognizes the importance of architectural and environmental design in the healing process.

Planetree facilities are designed with spaces for patients and families to have both quiet places when they desire solitude and inviting meeting places when they want to socialize. The conventional hospital room is not always conducive to either. The Planetree project incorporates lounges, kitchens, libraries, chapels, and gardens into the facility. Music, storytelling, and art complement the warmth of the environment, and humor is incorporated to create patient-centered care (Planetree 2008). Although Planetree has not become the majority form of inpatient care, it is more than just a dream. Over seventy-five organizations in the United States and internationally are official Planetree affiliates at the writing of this text. Perhaps the most difficult aspect of implementing a concept such as Planetree is the cultural change that must take place. Staff training, education, and commitment to the concept are long-term processes, much like commitment to total quality improvement projects that focus on customer service and increasing quality in any organization.

Increased Quality through Equitable Care

As discussed in Chapter 4, not all Americans receive the same access to health care. There are many reasons for unequal access, but equity is deeper than simply being able to see a physician or receive care in a hospital or clinic. Equity also applies to the ability to receive the highest quality of care without regard to race, ethnicity, gender, or religion. We have read about disparities in longevity, treatment regimens, and early diagnosis. These disparities are a focus of current quality initiatives as well as public health initiatives.

Increased Quality through Interdisciplinary Team Patient Care

The Institute for Healthcare Improvement (IHI) and partner hospitals launched the 100,000 Lives Campaign in 2004. The campaign encouraged hospitals to join by instituting programs to avoid errors and save patient lives. The program ran from December 2004 to June 2006, and enlisted over 3,100 hospitals that saved an estimated 122,000 lives. Programs were designed so that they could be replicated at other facilities to improve patient safety throughout communities. A new initiative, the 5 Million Lives Campaign, has a goal to enroll more than 4,000 hospitals to prevent medical harm over the next two years (IHI 2007).

Oftentimes, poor patient care is a result of failed communication among providers. Handoffs between care providers are ripe for treatment errors. The IHI has many programs to improve patient care. One such program is Innovation Communities, and one such initiative is "Taking Action to Transform Care at the Bedside" (ibid.). This team approach to patient care increases quality through increasing communication between caregivers. Care team members make rounds together, meeting patients and discussing the treatment plan with the patient and with one another. Everyone is "on the same page" and fully understands the treatment plan. Teams include doctors, nurses, pharmacists, social workers, and others who may be involved in the patient care. Under the team approach, physicians are no long the lone directors of patient care creating orders for others to complete at other times of the day. The team works together for the benefit of patients.

The effort to transform care at the bedside has these primary aims: to provide safe and reliable care, vitality and teamwork, patient-centered care, and value-added care processes. One result from the initiative has been the use of rapid response teams to bring care to patients before a crisis occurs. Learn more about rapid response teams in Exhibit 13–1.

QUALITY AND THE COST OF CARE

Not all improvements in quality of care can be achieved without increasing the cost of care. Certainly when we discuss equity in access to care, those without health insurance need to be recognized. Providing universal health care coverage is not a quality measure that can be achieved without consideration of cost.

At the writing of this text, the 2008 presidential election is taking place. Prior to the issues of the failing economy, health care reform was a major campaign issue. Both candidates proposed their approaches to increased health care coverage. Portions of their proposals were taken from previous legislative proposals whereas some are new. The effort to reform health care goes back to 1945, when President Truman proposed a national health insurance fund (Harry Truman Library and Museum 2008). However, national health insurance is not part of either candidate's proposal although there is some evidence that a single-payer national health system could save some $350 million a year. The savings would come mainly from streamlining the payment system (Physicians for a National Health Program 2008).

President Barack Obama's current proposal will include:

- Requiring health insurance plans to cover preexisting conditions
- Creating tax credits to allow small businesses to provide health insurance for their employees
- Lowering costs for businesses by covering a portion of the catastrophic health costs they pay in return for lower premiums for employees
- Limiting overcharging for malpractice insurance
- Investing in strategies to reduce medical errors
- Imposing a payroll tax on large employers who do not provide health insurance for their employees
- Establishing a health insurance exchange that will make it possible for individuals to purchase health insurance at a reasonable cost
- Providing a tax credit for the cost of premiums to everyone who needs it

Of course there are more details to the plan, too much to include here (Obama 2008).

EXHIBIT 13–1

Patient Care Case Study

At 18 months old, Josie King climbed into a hot bath and suffered first- and second-degree burns. She was rushed to one of the most prestigious hospitals in the country, Johns Hopkins. After ten days in the pediatric intensive care unit, Josie was recovering well, having received constant medical attention.

Josie was then sent to the intermediate care floor, doing well enough that discharge was expected within a few days. Her older brother and two sisters were planning a homecoming celebration. During the days that followed, Josie's mom, Sorrel, noticed that Josie seemed thirsty all the time; yet Sorrel was told not to let Josie drink. Sorrel became concerned because Josie was just not acting and looking well. Two different nurses told Sorrel, after looking at Josie, that she was doing fine. Sorrel went home to get some needed rest.

Upon returning in the early morning, Sorrel knew that Josie was not fine and demanded that the doctor come. Josie's medical team arrived, administered Narcan (a drug used to reverse the effects of narcotic depression). Sorrel was told she could give Josie fluids, and a verbal order stated no narcotics were to be given to Josie. Josie began to perk up, was more alert, and was keeping the liquids down. In the early afternoon, a nurse came in and administered a syringe of methadone to Josie, over the objections of Sorrel who was told the order for no narcotics had been changed.

As Sorrel rubbed Josie's feet, Josie's heart stopped. Sorrel screamed for help, and a crowd of nurses and doctors came rushing into the room. The next time Sorrel saw Josie, she was hooked up to life support. The family made a very difficult decision, days later, to remove Josie from life support as they held her in their arms. Josie died of a medical error in one of the best hospitals in the world.

The King family's sorrow and anger propelled them forward to do something that would prevent this from ever happening to a child again. Sorrel began speaking at various hospitals to tell her tragic story. Tami Merryman, vice president of the Center for Quality Improvement and Innovation at the University of Pittsburgh Medical Center (UPMC), heard Josie's story and remembered Sorrel's words, "'If I would have been able to call a rapid response team, I believe Josie would be here today." Tami knew they had to do something for their patients.

UPMC created Condition H in case of an emergency or if the patient was unable to get the attention of a health care provider. Condition H allows patients and families a way to call for immediate help when they feel they are not getting adequate attention or when they become concerned about what is happening. A rapid response team arrives at the patient's bedside within minutes when Condition H is called.

Patients and families are given education information on Condition H when they are admitted, and additional information is available in each patient room. The point is that the patient or family member is often best able to recognize when a patient's condition has changed. They are given the ability to call for the rapid response team. The system has not been abused, it is not a waste of resources, and data suggests that 69 percent of the calls would have led to potentially harmful patient situations if Condition H had not been called. Other hospitals across the country are now implementing rapid response initiatives similar to Condition H.

Discussion Questions

1. Name some of the points in this story where the system broke down and caused the medical error.

2. What are some things that could have been done differently?

SOURCE: Presented with permission from Sorrel King and the Josie King Foundation (www.josieking.org).

Senator John McCain's proposal for health care reform would include:

- Promoting competition to improve the quality of health insurance at lower prices
- Providing a tax credit to individuals and families to offset the cost of health insurance
- Making insurance more portable
- Promoting health savings accounts
- Covering patients with preexisting conditions

Again, this is not McCain's entire plan, but it is impossible to include everything in this text (McCain 2008).

It remains to be seen if any of these proposals or pieces of these proposals will be implemented as part of health policy in the near future. Neither candidate can move their plans along without the cooperation of Congress. Although health care costs remain as a priority in most Americans' minds, putting a plan into place that will satisfy the wide range of interests involved is a gargantuan task.

SUMMARY

Not all organizations are successful in implementing quality incentives. A successful organization is one with strong and dedicated leadership. Health care organizations in particular have been slow to change, and the turmoil caused by cost containment, the move to managed care contracting, a high degree of government regulation, and increased competition have left organizations struggling to find new ways to differentiate themselves, yet hesitant to take on long-term, major projects in an era of uncertainty.

Quality of care is not something that can be put aside for later. The IOM has emphasized the need for quality care in areas of patient safety, efficiency, effectiveness, patient-centered care, timely care, and equitable care. Organizations have taken a variety of approaches to improve care, some voluntarily and some induced by competition. Public reporting of various outcomes measures provide employers, insurers, and patients with information to make more informed choices when choosing physicians, hospitals, and other health care providers.

Although information might be more readily available, not all Americans can use the information to choose providers. People who are uninsured oftentimes do not have a regular source of care and must resort to emergency departments or clinics for care. Reducing or eliminating the number of people without insurance has been an area of focus for health policy makers for a long time. It remains to be seen if a new administration in Washington will be able to address the problem with any measure of success.

ACTIVITY-BASED LEARNING

- Access the Planetree website (www.planetree.org), and find the list of affiliates. Are any of them in your area? Is it possible to visit a Planetree site? If not, access the website of one of the affiliate organizations. Do you see a difference in the Planetree organization compared to your other health care organization(s)?

- Hospitals and medical centers try very hard to differentiate themselves through promotional materials and advertising. Pick a local hospital or medical center and investigate new services or facilities that they have incorporated into their organizations to attract consumers and differentiate themselves in the realm of providing quality health care.

A QUESTION OF ETHICS

- Given the struggles in containing the costs of health care and given the increasing numbers of Americans who find themselves without health insurance, should organizations be investing in physical changes to their facilities to attract new patients through a more comfortable environment?

- Is the incorporation of holistic and alternative medicine with traditional medicine good medicine, in your opinion?

REFERENCES

1. Barsukiewicz, C. (1998). *Computerized medical records: Physician response to new technology* (Doctoral dissertation, Pennsylvania State University, 1998). Dissertation Abstracts International, 59, 08B:3996.

2. Blumenthal, D. (1996). Quality of care: What is it? *New England Journal of Medicine, 335*(12), 891–894.

3. Harry S. Truman Library & Museum. (2008). This day in Truman history. Retrieved from www.trumanlibrary. org/anniversaries/healthprogram.htm

4. Institute for Healthcare Improvement (IHI). (2008). Transforming care at the bedside: Overview. Retrieved from www.ihi.org/IHI/Programs/StrategicInitiatives/ TransformingCareAtTheBedside.htm

5. IHI. (2007a). Learning and innovation community: Taking action to transform care at the bedside. From http:// www.ihi.org/IHI/Programs/InnovationCommunities/ TransformingCareattheBedside.htm?TabId=1

6. IHI. (2007b). Protecting 5 million lives. From www. ihi.org/IHI/Programs/InnovationCommunities/ TakingActiontoTransformCareattheBedside.htm

7. Institute of Medicine (IOM). (2001). *Crossing the quality chasm: A new health system for the 21st century*. Washington, DC: National Academy Press.

8. Leapfrog Group. (2007). The Leapfrog Group fact sheet. Retrieved from www.leapfroggroup.org/about_us/leapfrog-factsheet

9. McCain, J. (2008). Straight talk on health system reform. Retrieved from www.johnmccain.com/content/default.aspx?guid=8475c713-a541-4b97-a2aa-800e35da37bb

10. National Committee for Quality Assurance (NCQA). (2007). *About NCQA.* Retrieved from http://www.ncqa.org/tabid/675/Default.aspx

11. Obama, B. (2008). Health care at a glance. From www.barackobama.com/issues/healthcare.bg

12. Physicians for a National Health Program. Our Mission: Single-Payer National Health Insurance. Retrieved from www.pnhp.org

13. Planetree. (2008). About Planetree. Retrieved from http://www.planetree.org/about.html

14. Planetree. (2007). Planetree: Welcome. Retrieved from www.planetree.org/about/welcome.htm

15. Trocchio, J. (2000). Pioneer Network seeks innovation, culture change in long-term care. *Catholic Health World, 16*(13), pp. 1, 5.

16. Watson, M. (2000, October 15). Doctors plan paperless practice. *The Commercial Appeal*, pp. C1, C4.

Acronyms in Common Use

AAFP	American Academy of Family Physicians
AAMC	Association of American Medical Colleges
AANA	American Association of Nurse Anesthetists
AAPA	American Academy of Physician Assistants
ABMS	American Board of Medical Specialties
ACAOM	American College of Acupuncture and Oriental Medicine
ACGME	Accreditation Council for Graduate Medical Education
ACNM	American College of Nurse-Midwives
ACS	American College of Surgeons
ADA	American Dental Association
ADLEX	American Dental Licensing Examination
AFDC	Aid to Families with Dependent Children
AHA	American Hospital Association
AMA	American Medical Association
ANA	American Nurses Association
ANCC	American Nurses Credentialing Center
AOA	American Osteopathic Association
APC	Ambulatory payment classification
ASC	Ambulatory surgical centers
AUPHA	Association of University Programs in Health Administration
CAAHEP	Commission on Accreditation of Allied Health Education Programs
CAHEA	Committee on Allied Health Education and Accreditation
CAHME	Commission on Accreditation of Healthcare Management Education
CCME	Coordinating Council on Medical Education
CDC	Centers for Disease Control and Prevention
CEO	Chief executive officer
CHAMPUS	Civilian Health and Medical Program of the Uniformed Services
CLIA '88	Clinical Laboratory Improvement Amendments of 1988
CMS	Centers for Medicare and Medicaid Services
CON	Certificate of need
CPOE	Computerized physician order entry
CRNA	Certified registered nurse anesthetist
CT	Computed tomography
DC	Doctor of chiropractic
DDS	Doctor of dental surgery
DHSS	Department of Health and Social Services
DHEW	Department of Health, Education, and Welfare
DMD	Doctor of dental medicine
DO	Doctor of osteopathy
DPM	Doctor of podiatric medicine
DRG	Diagnosis-related group
E&M	Evaluation and management
ECFMG	Educational Commission for Foreign Medical Graduates
ED	Emergency department
EENT	Eye, ear, nose, and throat
EMR	Electronic medical record (also CMR, EHR)
EMT	Emergency medical technician

EPSDT	Early Periodic Screening, Diagnosis, and Treatment
ER	Emergency Room
ERISA	Employee Retirement Income Security Act
ESRD	End-stage renal disease
FHA	Federal Housing Administration
FLEX	Federal Licensing Examination
FMG	Foreign medical graduate
FMGEMS	Foreign Medical Graduates Examination in Medical Sciences
FSMB	Federation of State Medical Boards
GAO	General Accounting Office
GDP	Gross domestic product
GHA	Group Health Association
GME	Graduate Medical Education
GNP	Gross national product
GP	General practitioner
HSA	Health savings account
HCFA	Health Care Financing Administration
HDHP	High-deductible health plan
HIMS	Health Information Management System
HIP	Health Insurance Plan of New York
HIPAA	Health Insurance Portability and Accountability Act of 1996
HMO	Health maintenance organization
ICF	Intermediate care facility
ICU	Intensive care unit
IHI	Institute for Healthcare Improvement
IMG	International medical graduate
IPA	Individual Practice Association
JAMA	Journal of the American Medical Association
JCAHO	Joint Commission on Accreditation of Healthcare Organizations
LCSB	Liaison Committee for Specialty Boards
LCME	Liaison Committee on Medical Education
LPN	Licensed practical nurse
MBA	Master of business administration
MHA	Master of health administration
MCAT	Medical College Admission Test
MD	Medical doctor
MOC	Maintenance of certification
MPP	Medicare Participating Physician
MRI	Magnetic resonance imaging
MSKP	Medical Sciences Knowledge Profile
MUC	Medically underserved community

NACNEP	National Advisory Council on Nurse Education and Practice
NAPLEX	North American Pharmacist Licensure Examination
NBME	National Board of Medical Examiners
NCSBN	National Council of State Boards of Nursing
NCCOAM	National Certification Commission for Acupuncture and Oriental Medicine
NCHS	National Center for Health Statistics
NCLEX-PN	National Council Licensure Examination for Practical Nurses
NCLEX-RN	National Council Licensure Examination for Registered Nurses
NF	Nursing home facility
NICU	Neonatal intensive care unit
NLN	National League for Nursing
NLNAC	National League for Nursing Accreditation Commission
NMA	National Medical Association
NPDB	National Practitioner Data Bank
NRMP	National Resident Match Program
OB-GYN	Obstetrics and gynecology
OBRA	Omnibus Budget Reconciliation Act
OD	Doctor of optometry
OMB	Office of Management and Budget
OPG	Outpatient payment groups
OPPS	Outpatient prospective payment system
PA	Physician assistant
PACE	Program of All-Inclusive Care for the Elderly
PAS	Professional activity study
PCP	Primary care physician
PHC4	Pennsylvania Health Care Cost Containment Council
PhD	Doctor of philosophy
PHR	Personal health record
PHO	Physician-hospital organization
POS	Point-of-service plan
PPO	Preferred provider organization
PPS	Prospective payment system
PRO	Peer review organization
PSRO	Professional Standards Review Organization
PTA	Physical therapist assistant
RBRVS	Resource-based relative value scale
RHIO	Regional Health Information Organization

RN	Registered nurse	UCR	Usual, customary, and reasonable allowances
SAMHSA	Substance Abuse and Mental Health Services Administration	USIMG	United States Citizen International Medical Graduate
SCHIP	State Children's Health Insurance Plan	USMLE	United States Medical Licensing Examination
SNF	Skilled nursing facility		
SSI	Supplementary Security Income	VA	Veterans Administration
TANF	Temporary Assistance for Needy Families program	VQE	Visa Qualifying Examination
		WHO	World Health Organization

Glossary

Abuse: unreasonable or unnecessary care.

Accept assignment: health care provider agrees to the fee schedule of the third-party payer.

Acquired immunodeficiency syndrome (AIDS): the progression of HIV to a level where other opportunistic diseases begin to destroy the body.

Actuary: person who evaluates the likelihood of events to minimize the financial impact of risk and uncertainty.

Acupuncture: therapy involving stimulation of anatomical points on the body, most commonly by penetration of the skin with needles.

Allopathic physician (MD): physician trained in a traditional medical school.

Ambulatory care: medical care that does not require an overnight stay.

American Osteopathic Association (AOA): accrediting body for programs leading to a DO and osteopathic facilities. It is also a member organization serving osteopathic physicians.

Anthrax: a serious disease caused by *Bacillus anthracis*, a bacterium that forms spores. In the United States in 2001, anthrax was deliberately spread through the postal system by sending letters with powder containing anthrax. This caused twenty-two cases of anthrax infection.

Apothecary: In colonial times, an apothecary practiced as a doctor. Apothecaries made house calls to treat patients, made and prescribed medicines, and trained apprentices. Some apothecaries were also trained as surgeons and male midwives. In more recent times, an apothecary is a reference to a pharmacist or pharmacy.

Aseptic techniques: sterile techniques.

Asymmetry of information: a condition in which the provider of services has more information than the buyer of the services, causing the buyer to enter into a transaction based on trust.

Auscultation: diagnostic procedure for listening to sounds within the body, such as a heart beat. Originally performed by pressing the ear to the body, it is now done with a stethoscope.

Baby boomers: those born between 1946 and 1964. "Boom" refers to the increase in births after World War II.

Behavioral disorders: the way people behave.

Bioterrorism: an attack using the deliberate release of viruses, bacteria, or other germs (agents) to cause illness or death in people, animals, or plants.

Capitation: a fixed monthly payment to a health care provider in return for a range of services rendered to a consumer. The payment is often a payment per patient per month for primary care physicians.

Cardiac catheterization: procedure performed to obtain diagnostic information about the heart or its blood vessels.

Certificate of need (CON): a regulatory process in some states that requires Agency approval before any new facilities or services costing over a specific dollar amount may be created. Certified registered nurse anesthetist (CRNA): Nurse trained beyond the RN level to independently provide anesthetics to patients.

Chiropractic: the treatment of illness by manipulation of the spinal column and body joints, physiotherapy, and dietary counseling without the use of drugs or surgical intervention.

Chronic conditions: conditions that can be treated to stop or slow the progression but cannot be cured.

Clinical trials: research studies using human volunteers to answer specific health questions. They are often used to determine whether experimental treatments or new ways of using known therapies are safe and effective under controlled environments.

Cognitive disorders: the way people think.

Community hospital: nonfederal, short-term hospital where general and specialty care are provided.

Community rate: An insurance rating given to a specific group of people based on risk and cost factors.

Concurrent review: review of the patients' records while in the hospital to determine the appropriateness of continued hospitalization.

Co-payments (co-pays): a fixed amount of money a patient must pay for each type of health care service (for example, $20 per physician visit). Coinsurance: a percentage of the cost that a patient must pay for each health service (for example, 20 percent of the cost). Community rating: determining the premiums for health insurance by statistically determining the risk of illness among a broad community of persons.

Cost shifting: charging higher prices to private insurers to make up for shortfalls in uncompensated care.

Covered entities: those people and organizations subject to the regulations found in HIPAA.

Data clearinghouse: entities that process nonstandard information into a standard format.

Deductibles: a certain amount of money a patient pays toward health care costs before the health insurance plan starts to pay.

Defensive medicine: the physician's tendency to order more tests to confirm a diagnosis and needed treatment to avoid lawsuits.

Dentist: a trained professional who diagnoses and treats diseases, injuries, and malformations of teeth, gums, and related oral structures.

Deprofessionalization: a term used to describe the loss of some of the autonomy of a professional when others can perform similar services and the gap in knowledge between provider and consumer (patient) is decreased.

Diagnosis-related groups (DRG): a method of paying for health services in hospitals based on the diagnosis and treatment plan of a patient at admission.

Doughnut hole: colloquialism for the gap in Medicare coverage for prescription drug costs.

Dual eligible: individuals who are entitled to Medicare Part A and/or Part B and are eligible for some form of Medicaid benefit. For individuals with low incomes, Medicaid will pay some Medicare premiums, deductibles, and/or coinsurance.

Educational Commission for Foreign Medical Graduates (ECFMG): developed an exam regarding medical knowledge and language reading for international medical graduates.

Electronic medical record: replacement of a patient's typical file from paper to computer. The EMR is not simply a process of placing information in a computer, but organizing it in such a way as to make the information analyzable to add to the quality of care provided to the patient. The EMR is also known as a CMR (computerized medical record) and EHR (electronic health record).

Emotional disorders: the way people act with others.

Endodontics: The branch of dentistry that deals with diseases of the tooth root, dental pulp, and surrounding tissue.

Epidemiology: The scientific study of factors affecting the health and illness of individuals and populations. As a cornerstone of public health research, it is a method of identifying risk factors for disease and determining treatment approaches for disease.

Experience rating: determining the premiums for health insurance by reviewing the history of illness of the group being insured.

Federation Licensing Examination: national licensing exam based on NBME questions.

Federal Register: the official daily publication for rules, proposed rules, and notices of federal agencies and organizations, as well as executive orders and other presidential documents; published by the Office of the Federal Register, National Archives and Records Administration (NARA).

Fiduciary: people who hold plan assets in trust for beneficiaries and administer benefits under those plans; therefore they have a special legal duty to act in the best interests of those beneficiaries.

Fiscal intermediaries: organizations that serve as the administrators for Medicare claims processing by contract with CMS.

Flexner report: an influential report on the quality of medical education. The report resulted in major changes in curriculum and facilities responsible for medical education.

Foreign Medical Graduates Examination in Medical Sciences (FMGEMS): a licensing exam for international medical graduates, taken along with an English proficiency test.

For-profit hospital: operates with the goal of making a profit and distributing it to shareholders.

Foundling asylum: A place for abandoned or unwanted infants.

Fraud: misrepresentation, deceit.

Gross national product (GNP): measures what U.S. residents and corporations produced, regardless of their location in the world, and excludes the productivity of foreign-owned businesses in the United States.

Gross domestic product (GDP): measures only the value of goods and services produced in the United States, whether by U.S.- or foreign-owned businesses.

Group practice: three or more physicians practicing together (two physicians working together is usually referred to as a partnership).

Health center (in Indian Health Service): a facility, physically separated from a hospital, with a full range of ambulatory services including at least primary care physicians, nursing, pharmacy, laboratory, and X-ray, which are available at least forty hours a week for outpatient care.

Health Insurance Portability and Accountability Act of 1996 (HIPAA): A U.S. law designed to provide privacy standards to protect patients' medical records and other health information provided to health plans, doctors, hospitals, and other health care providers.

Health literacy: The ability of an individual to access, understand, and use health-related information and services to make appropriate health decisions.

Health savings account (HSA): money (usually pretax dollars) placed in an account to be used strictly for health care services.

Health station (in Indian Health Service): a facility, physically separated from a hospital and health center, where primary care physician services are available on a regularly scheduled basis but for less than fifty hours a week.

High-deductible health plan (HDHP): catastrophic health insurance which has a very high deductible (may be as much as $5,000). Usually paired with a Health Savings Account, it does not pay for health care until the deductible is met either through out-of-pocket payments or payments from the HSA.

Hill-Burton Act: authorized federal grants to states to plan and assist in construction of hospitals in areas needing facilities. In return for the funding, hospitals had to agree to provide services without discrimination and to serve a fair portion of needy patients.

Health Insurance Portability and Accountability Act of 1996 (HIPAA): 1996 legislation that made wide-range changes to health insurance coverage rules and to the standardization and confidentiality of patient medical records.

Human immunodeficiency virus (HIV): first detected in the United States in the early 1980s among gay men, HIV is now found in males and females, homosexuals and heterosexuals, children and adults. It results in the body's inability to ward off infections.

Homeopathy: treatment and prevention of disease, mainly through the use of "remedies" and involving a focus on the whole person rather than a symptom or disease.

Hospice: a concept of care that provides pain management and other comfort care for those who can no longer benefit from curative care.

Immutable factors: those that cannot be changed.

Indigent: unable to pay.

Indemnity: regarding health insurance, reimbursement for the cost of care.

Infant mortality: death in the first year of life.

Inflation: a general increase in prices.

Institute of Medicine (IOM): an independent, nonprofit organization that provides science-based advice to the nation on biomedical science, medicine, and health. Intensivists: physicians who work in the hospital intensive care unit full-time.

Intermediaries: insurance companies that handle the administrative functions, such as eligibility verification and claims payment, for Medicare.

Intermittent care: care for a few hours a day and not every day of the week.

International medical graduate (IMG): graduates of medical school outside the United States.

Internship: a year of clinical training after medical school is completed; currently referred to as a one-year general residency.

Job lock: the propensity of an employee to stay in a job simply because it offers health insurance.

Leapfrog Group: a group of employers who try to use the way they purchase health care benefits to influence the quality and cost of health care services.

Liaison Committee on Medical Education (LCME): official accrediting body for medical schools.

Licensed practical nurse (LPN): provides nursing care to patients under the direction of a physician, dentist, podiatrist, optometrist, or registered nurse. LPN responsibilities are similar to, but more limited than, those of registered nurses.

Life expectancy: can be expressed in terms of how long someone is expected to live, or in terms of how much longer someone is expected to live at a specific age.

Macro view: looking at the health of a population or community.

Malignant neoplasm: a more formal term for cancer. Malignant neoplasms include a large number of different types of malignancies.

Managed care: a system of health care insurance based on primary care physicians as gatekeepers, referral for specialty care, and cost management through case management.

Medicaid: The federal/state government program of health care for the very poor.

Medically underserved communities (MUCs): areas, often rural, with a shortage of health care providers.

Medicare: The federal government program of health care for the population 65 years of age and over.

Medicare Part A: coverage for primarily inpatient care. Enrollees pay no premiums.

Medicare Part B: primarily covers outpatient services. It is partially funded by the government and partially by recipients through a premium paid by the recipient.

Medicare Part C: basically an option for Medicare recipients to be enrolled in a managed care program rather than Part B and D.

Medicare Part D: Medicare Prescription Drug Improvement and Modernization Act.

Medigap: insurance that covers charges not covered by Medicare. The insurance must be purchased separately in the commercial insurance market and is not a benefit the government pays.

Medline: (Medical Literature Analysis and Retrieval System Online) is the premier bibliographic database of the U.S. National Library of Medicine (NLM) that contains approximately 13 million references to journal articles in life sciences with a concentration on biomedicine.

MedlinePlus: provides answers to health questions, information on drugs, and other health news.

Micro view: looking at the health of the individual patient.

Monopoly: exclusive control by one group of the means of producing or selling a commodity or service.

Moral hazard: the propensity of people who are insured to use more medical services than if they were not insured.

Morbidity: the state of being ill or the prevalence of disease.

Mortality rates: death rates.

Multi-specialty group: physicians of different specialty training in group practice together.

Mutable factors: those that can be changed.

National Board of Medical Examiners: board that developed a national exam for medical licensing.

National Practitioner Data Bank (NPDB): national information system to identify and discipline those who engage in unprofessional behavior; and to restrict the ability of incompetent physicians, dentists, and other health care practitioners to move from state to state without disclosure or discovery of previous medical malpractice payment and adverse action history.

Nonprofit hospital: also known as a voluntary hospital, the mission of nonprofit hospitals is based on turning any profits back into the organization to provide care rather than distributing profits to shareholders. Therefore, nonprofit hospitals have no

shareholders, have voluntary boards of trustees, and provide a portion of care to poor and uninsured individuals.

Nurse practitioner: a nurse trained above the RN level to provide many primary care functions directly to patients.

Nurse-midwife: nurse trained beyond the RN level to provide women's health care, including uncomplicated childbirth.

Ophthalmologist: a medical doctor (MD) with a specialty in medical and surgical treatment of eye diseases.

Optometrist (OD): a person trained to examine, diagnose diseases and vision conditions, and conduct the primary care of the eye.

Orthodontics: The branch of dentistry dealing with treatment of improper bite (often through the use of braces).

Osteopath (DO): a physician whose training includes bone manipulation in addition to other medical training.

Outcomes measurement: a focus of health care quality that reviews how a patient responds to a specific course of treatment.

Palliative care: care focused on relief of pain and other symptoms of serious illness.

Peer Review Organization (PRO): an organization that contracts with CMS to oversee the Medicare program for cost containment and quality of medical care provided to recipients.

Periodontics: The branch of dentistry dealing with treatment of diseases of the gums.

Pharmacist: a professional who dispenses medications and counsels patients on their proper use and any adverse affects that may occur.

Physician Assistant (PA): a person licensed to practice primary care medicine with supervision by a physician.

Physician-hospital organizations (PHO): Physicians and hospitals form their own preferred provider networks to contract with insurance companies or directly with employers to provide care to groups of consumers (patients) at a discounted rate.

Podiatrist: a doctor of medicine who diagnoses and treats diseases of the foot and related or governing structures by medical, surgical, or other means.

Point-of-service insurance plan (POS): somewhat of a hybrid of an HMO and PPO insurance plan.

Preadmission review: review of the patients' records prior to hospital admission to determine the appropriateness of hospital admission.

Preexisting condition: history of an illness and treatment for that illness prior to purchasing insurance.

Preferred provider organization (PPO): a network of health care providers affiliated with a particular health insurance plan that offers patients reduced costs while they are being treated within the network but does not penalize them harshly if the go outside the network. Premiums: the cost of health insurance.

Primary care: prevention services as well as management of disease.

Primary care physician (PCP): the physician, usually specializing in family practice or internal medicine, who is primarily responsible for coordinating care of the patient.

Professional: a person who possesses complex knowledge and is often "licensed" to provide a service or product that cannot be provided by someone unlicensed.

Proprietary: for-profit institutions.

Prospective payment system (PPS): payment for health services determined in advance by patient's treatment and diagnosis rather than by the amount of dollars spent on treatment of the patient. Prosthodontics: The branch of dentistry that deals with the replacement of missing teeth and related mouth or jaw structures by bridges, dentures, or other artificial devices.

Psychiatrists: medical doctors who specialize in the treatment of mental illness including performing medical procedures and prescribing medication.

Psychologists: people with academic doctorates licensed to provide clinical care, counseling, and do research.

Psychotropic drugs: drugs that act primarily upon the central nervous system, where they alter brain function.

PubMed: a database with free access to all users providing citations and abstracts to biomedical and other life science journal literature.

Regional health information organization (RHIO): an organization that works to connect information between various health care providers across a community.

Registered nurse: a trained nurse who has passed the state licensing examination for the designation of RN.

Residency: training in a specialty (and subspecialty) that takes place after medical school; graduate medical education.

Resource-based relative value scale (RBRVS): a payment method for physician services developed by Medicare and based on the value (or work involved) in delivering services.

Retrospective payment: payment to a provider of care for costs of treating a patient after those costs have been incurred.

Safety net hospitals: hospitals that primarily serve those who are poor and uninsured. Although they struggle for funding and resources, they are often tertiary care facilities providing the high-tech trauma care and are centers for medical education.

Senility: loss of cognitive functions related to aging; senility is now redefined as dementia.

Severe acute respiratory syndrome (SARS): a viral respiratory illness caused by a coronavirus, called SARS-associated coronavirus (SARS-CoV). SARS was first reported in Asia in February 2003, and spread to more than two dozen countries in North America, South America, Europe, and Asia before the global outbreak of 2003 was contained.

Single-specialty group: multiple physicians in a group practice, all with the same medical specialty.

Solo practice: one physician working in his own office, treating patients.

Spending down: the practice of paying for medical care (particularly nursing home care) from one's own funds until poor enough to qualify for Medicaid.

Staff privileges: in this context, hospital privileges grant physicians (or other providers) the right to admit and treat patients in hospitals. Privileges are delineated as to what procedures or treatment physicians are allowed to perform.

Swing beds: hospitals may convert acute care beds to nursing home beds and back to acute care beds as needed.

Teaching hospital: a hospital (not necessarily a university hospital) with at least one approved residency program.

Telehealth: uses technology to provide medical care over distances. It is often used in rural health and home health agencies to transmit vital medical information from the patient by nurses, nurse practitioners, or other medical personnel to a hospital, clinic, or specialty physician. Telemedicine is a form of telehealth in which a physician typically transmits information to a specialist or team of specialists for consultative services to determine appropriate treatment.

Telemedicine: a means of connecting provider and patient from a remote area to consultation with specialty care via phone lines or computer networks.

Tertiary care: care delivered by a specialist, oftentimes in a facility with very specialized equipment.

Therapist: a person who works mainly in rehabilitation to help patients develop skills lost through injury or illness.

Third-party payer: insurance, benefit plan, government entity, or other entity paying for the health care services a patient receives.

United States Medical Licensing Examination (USMLE): the exam that is the basis for state licensing and insurance of physicians.

Utilization review: an administrative review, by hospital or insurance company, to verify that medical care was necessary or to verify that patients are receiving appropriate preventive care.

Variation: a variety of approaches to treat the same medical condition.

Voluntary hospitals: Hospitals supported by donations and volunteer workers. They are somewhat of a precursor to nonprofit hospitals.

Women, Infants, and Children (WIC): a special supplemental nutrition program for women, infants, and children up to age 5 who are at nutritional risk; it provides nutritious foods to supplement diets, information on healthy eating, and referrals to health care.

Index